BSAVA Manual of Veterinary Care

Editor:

Sue Dallas VN CertEd

Rodbaston College, Rodbaston,
Penkridge, Staffordshire ST19 5TH

Series Editor for
BSAVA Manuals of
Veterinary Nursing

Gill Simpson BVM&S MRCVS

Rose Cottage, Edgehead,
Midlothian EH37 5RL

Published by:
British Small Animal Veterinary Association
Woodrow House, 1 Telford Way, Waterwells Business Park,
Quedgeley, Gloucester GL2 4AB, United Kingdom

A company limited by guarantee in England.
Registered company no. 2837793.
Registered as a charity.

Copyright © 1999 BSAVA

Figures 2.9–2.15 are copyright Marc Henrie ASC.
Figures 3.3, 3.8–3.12, 3.14, 3.17, 3.20, 3.21 are copyright Alan Robinson.
The following figures were drawn by S.J. Elmhurst BA Hons and are printed
with her permission: 2.20, 2.32–2.34, 4.13–4.29, 4.32, 4.36, 4.38, 6.5, 6.20,
7.1, 7.3, 7.6, 7.7, 7.11.

A catalogue recorded for this book is available from the British Library.

ISBN 0 905412 49 8

The publishers and contributors cannot take responsibility for information
provided on dosages and methods of application of drugs mentioned in
this publication. Details of this kind must be verified by individual users
from the appropriate literature.

Typeset by: Fusion Design, Fordingbridge, Hampshire.

Printed by: Lookers, Upton, Poole, Dorset.

Contents

Contributors

Sally Anne Argyle MVB CertSAC MRCVS
Department of Veterinary Pharmacology, University of Glasgow Veterinary School, Bearsden Road, Bearsden, Glasgow G61 1QH

Sue Badger VN
Department of Veterinary Nursing, University of Bristol, Langford House, Langford, Bristol BS40 5DU

Sue Dallas VN CertEd
Rodbaston College, Rodbaston, Penkridge, Staffordshire ST19 5TH

Sarah Heath BVSc MRCVS
Behavioural Referrals, 11 Cotevbrook Drive, Upton, Chester CH2 1RA

Paula Hotston-Moore VN
Glovers Field, Shipham, Winscombe, North Somerest BS25 1ST

Joy Howell VN DipAVN (Surgical)
2 Blymhill Lawn, Near Shifnal, Shropshire TF11 8LT

Anna Meredith MA VetMB Cert LAS Cert Zoo Med MRCVS
Department of Veterinary Clinical Studies, RDSVS, Hospital for Small Animals, Easter Bush Veterinary Centre, Roslin, Midlothian EH25 9RG

Margaret Moore MA VN CertEd FETC MIScT
Cerberus Training & Consultancy, Yewgate Cottage, Remenham Hill, Henley-on-Thames, Oxfordshire RG9 3ES

George Malynicz BVetMed MRCVS
22 Coolgardie Avenue, Chigwell, Essex IG7 5AY

Judith Philipson PhD
School of Care, Health and the Sciences, Edinburgh's Telford College, Crewe Toll, Edinburgh EH4 2NZ

Sharon Redrobe BSc BVetMed BSc CertLAS MRCVS
Department of Veterinary Clinical Studies, RDSVS, Hospital for Small Animals, Easter Bush Veterinary Centre, Roslin, Midlothian EH25 9RG

Jean Turner VN
Greenway, 1 Eastcote Lane, Northolt, Middlesex UB5 5RE

Trevor Turner BVetMed MRCVS FRSH
Greenway, 1 Eastcote Lane, Northolt, Middlesex UB5 5RE

Kim Willoughby BVMS PhD MRCVS
University of Liverpool Small Animal Hospital, Crown Street, Liverpool L7 7EX

Foreword

This trilogy of veterinary nursing manuals marks another significant landmark in the history of BSAVA Publications. The rise in status of the veterinary nurse within companion animal practice together with the new syllabus under the S/NVQ training scheme has meant that, after three editions spanning 15 years, *Practical Veterinary Nursing* has reached the end of its useful life. However, it was felt that there still was a need for a publication to complement the established textbook *Veterinary Nursing* (formerly Jones's Animal Nursing) published by Butterworth Heinemann on behalf of the BSAVA.

Based on the extremely successful BSAVA Manual formula of a logical, user-friendly approach, this exciting new series of three manuals caters for all levels of staff working with animals, whether it be in veterinary practice or other areas of animal care.

The editors of each of the manuals, Sue Dallas, Margaret Moore and Alasdair Hotston Moore, together with the series editor Gill Simpson, are to be congratulated on bringing together a wide range of talented contributors, both veterinary surgeons and veterinary nurses, to write individual chapters in an impressively easy-to-read format. They have succeeded in the difficult task of maintaining a continuity of style throughout. Each chapter opens with a summary of the information contained therein. The liberal use of tables and illustrations adds to the appeal of the layout, making the information accessible and highly practical in nature.

The *Manual of Veterinary Care* is a perfect introduction to those wishing to pursue a career working with animals. The *Manual of Veterinary Nursing* is written for student veterinary nurses studying for the new vocational qualification. The *Manual of Advanced Veterinary Nursing* has been designed for qualified veterinary nurses who are already working in practice and who either wish to take the Diploma in Advanced Veterinary Nursing (Surgical) or (Medical) or who just wish to expand their knowledge and further their education. There is, at present, no textbook that deals with the advanced course. This book provides both the necessary theoretical background and practical information, all in an easy-to-read style.

This three-volume series is certain to become an essential addition to the libraries of veterinary practices, training colleges and a wide range of animal care establishments.

P. Harvey Locke BVSc MRCVS
BSAVA President 1999–2000

Series preface

The veterinary profession has developed rapidly in recent years and the role of the ancillary staff in the small animal veterinary practice has increased in importance and diversity. Small animal practice in the new millennium will focus on the team approach to total animal care. Within this team should be adequately and appropriately trained personnel.

The aim of the BSAVA Manuals of Veterinary Nursing is to assist in the training and education of staff who are responsible for the care of animals, either within the veterinary practice or in other establishments which have responsibility for the welfare of animals. The series has been produced for the use of animal care personnel through to veterinary nurses studying for Advanced Diploma but the books fundamentally address the requirements for good nursing care.

The first book, the *Manual of Veterinary Care*, acts as an introduction to the care of small animals kept as pets, exploring the opportunities available for employment with animals, then progressing to describe basic animal care techniques. The second volume, the *Manual of Veterinary Nursing*, aims to assist those student veterinary nurses who are training for a formal qualification. It has been compiled with the needs of the Vocational Qualification in Veterinary Nursing in mind. With the development of veterinary nursing as a profession in its own right the remit of the qualified veterinary nurse is expanding. The objective of the *Manual of Advanced Veterinary Nursing* is to aid qualified veterinary nurses in developing their knowledge and skills. The inclusion of more advanced techniques should assist these nurses in fulfilling their essential role in the modern veterinary practice.

Multiple authors, both veterinary surgeons and veterinary nurses, have been involved in writing these books. Indeed, many sections have been co-written by veterinary surgeons and veterinary nurses working together to give a comprehensive approach to subject areas. Where appropriate, authors have contributed to more than one book, which gives continuity of content and style.

Having been associated with the education and training of veterinary nurses for some years, I am delighted to have been involved with these publications. I am grateful to all the authors who have contributed. Many thanks to Marion Jowett from BSAVA for directing the project and to the volume editors who have worked extremely hard to ensure these manuals are succinct and well presented. In particular I should like to thank BSAVA, who have supported the concept and publication of these manuals with the aim not only to improve the education of veterinary nurses but to improve animal care at all levels.

Gill Simpson
August 1999

Preface

There is an increasing need for competence and understanding of basic animal care in the many multidisciplinary areas of animal ownership, both in the home and in the workplace. This book has been specifically written with those needs in mind. It is intended as a basic book, providing knowledge from which the skills of an animal carer can develop.

The *Manual of Veterinary Care* is essential reading for those who wish to work with animals as part of a career. The chapter on 'Living and working with animals' provides insight into the long and varied relationships between people and animals. It also gives information, including entry requirements, qualifications, examining bodies and progression, on a range of careers from the animal care sector to veterinary nursing.

Dogs, cats and other animal species commonly sharing the human household or workplace require care specific to their individual needs. Management of animal housing, animal law and the use of medicines are described here and expanded in the *Manual of Veterinary Nursing*. Both volumes seek to provide a clear guide to animal carers on quality care and the demands of legislation. They link the care of well and sick animals, and give information on effective medication under veterinary supervision.

The chapters on basic first aid for animals and veterinary terminology provide a foundation for the clinical information given in the later volumes in the Series.

The *Manual of Veterinary Care* is written in a clear, easy-to-read format and is well illustrated throughout with photographs and with tables containing essential information.

Thanks go particularly to the authors who by their expertise have provided knowledge required by all who work with and care for animals.

Sue Dallas
August 1999

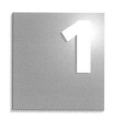

1 Living and working with animals

Sue Badger and Sarah Heath

This chapter is designed to give information on:

- The historical relationship between humans and domestic animals
- The bond with companion animals
- Benefits and responsibilities of pet ownership
- Adequate socialization and habituation
- The 'five freedoms'
- Opportunities and qualifications for working with animals

The historical relationship between humans and animals

Throughout history animals have played an important role in human society, whether as food animals, work animals or purely companions.

In the developing world animals are still kept as part of the agricultural systems that exist there, either directly as food animals or indirectly as working animals acting as beasts of burden or protectors of livestock.

These utilitarian motives for keeping animals are also present in western cultures. Animals still play an important role in food production, but their social role has altered and the keeping of animals purely for companionship is often associated with the western world.

Although pet keeping in the relatively affluent west is certainly on the increase, and the industries that have grown up around pets have now reached phenomenal proportions, this culture of living alongside other species is one that dates back a long way (Figure 1.1) and exists in cultures around the world.

Hunter-gatherers

The domestication of animals by humans almost certainly began in Palaeolithic times. There is evidence that the young of many mammalian species were kept in captivity by the people of that era, at least for short periods. In northern Israel a 12,000-year-old Palaeolithic tomb was uncovered that contained the remains of a human and also those of a dog. The dead person's hand was resting on the dog's shoulder and this has been taken to indicate some form of relationship between the two during their lives.

Evidence from the time of the hunter-gatherer suggests

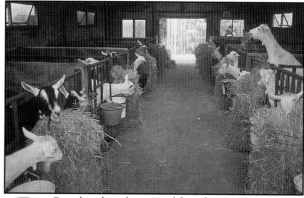

1.1 *Goats have been domesticated for at least 9000 years. Courtesy of I. Thomas.*

that humans had a respect for animals, which extended across a range of species. There have been reports of a variety of species being kept as companions between the 16th and 19th centuries BC and it has been suggested that, by caring for a few members of a species, humans were able to earn respect from the wild animals and so improve their hunting success. This is just one of many theories that have been put forward to explain why hunter-gatherer societies lived so closely with other species, but it is commonly accepted that at this time there was a level of respect and trust between humans and their animal companions.

Agriculture

This relationship appears to have altered around the time that people moved to a more settled agricultural lifestyle about 10,000 years ago. Wild animals were now kept away from human settlements (Figure 1.2) in order to decrease the risk of damage to crops and livestock, and domesticated animals were confined in order to prevent this valuable food

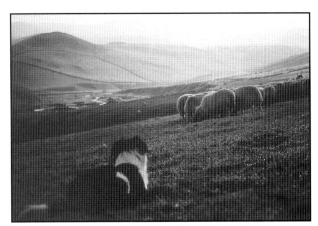

1.2 The Border Collie is an excellent example of a longstanding working relationship between dogs and humans (in this case the shepherd).
Courtesy of Dr S. Crispin.

source from roaming too far from home. Humans began to dominate animals, rather than respect them, and yet at the same time there was a move toward animals being incorporated into religious and cultural activities.

Dogs as pets

Dogs are thought to have been the first companion animal to be domesticated and there is some debate as to when this process began. Until recently it was widely accepted that canine domestication began some 15,000 years ago, but some authors now believe that it may have been even earlier.

Certainly the domestic dog shows the greatest range of size and shape of any of the domesticated species. The ancestor of the domestic dog was the wolf and it is believed that the diversity seen between breeds of dogs occurs in part because different subspecies of wolf were domesticated independently in different parts of the world.

The probability that any animal of a wild species reared by humans will remain tame when it reaches adulthood depends to a large extent on the social behaviour of that species and its compatibility with human social structures. The success of the dog as a companion animal stems from the fact that it fits so well into the human family. After all, both species rely on a hierarchical system and, provided that the two species maintain their respective positions within that hierarchy, the dog can live very successfully as a member of a human pack.

Cats as pets

The cat is classed as a domesticated animal, but it has retained much of its independence: whilst benefiting from the close association with humans, it has never totally given in to the concept of being owned. Juliet Clutton-Brock (see Further reading) describes the cat as 'an exploiting captive' and a 'carnivore that enjoys the company of man'.

There is some debate over the exact timing of feline domestication but it is accepted that it began in Egypt and is likely to have been associated with the development of settled agriculture. Grain stores attract large quantities of vermin and small wild cats are likely to have been attracted closer to the human communities by the easy supply of food. Those cats that were prepared to come closest to people stood the best chance of catching more vermin and so a selection process for bold and confident individuals began.

This process of selection for individuals who tolerated human proximity is thought to have been aided by the practice of confining cats to temples. In Ancient Egypt,

around 5000 years ago, the cat was revered as a deity and it is the divine status of the cat that is thought to have delayed its spread into other parts of the world.

Eventually cats started to move out along the trade routes and domestic cats had reached India by about 200 BC, where they probably hybridized with the local wild cat and then spread to the Far East. It was not until AD 400 that the Romans began to adopt cats as their primary controllers of rats and mice.

In modern times their distribution has become global, but cats are believed to be most popular in Australasia, North America and Western Europe, although there are some cat-loving countries outside these areas – notably Algeria, Israel and Indonesia. The extent to which cats are 'owned' varies considerably from one country to another and in many Mediterranean cities there are large populations of strays, as many tourists can testify.

Fashion

During the process of domestication both the dog and the cat have undergone periods of popularity and revulsion. In the case of the cat its history of tremendous swings in popularity is evident in its ability to invoke extreme feelings of both love and hatred to this day. It has been worshipped as a deity in Ancient Egypt and persecuted as a symbol of the devil in medieval Europe. It is now a highly popular companion animal throughout much of the world (Figure 1.3).

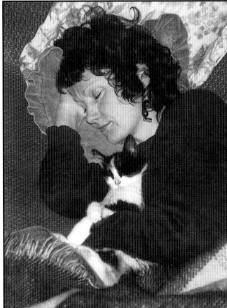

1.3 The cat is fast becoming the most popular species of pet in the UK. *Courtesy of R. Gibb.*

The dog was associated with death in some ancient civilizations and it is reported that bodies of the deceased were put out for the dogs to consume in order that the souls of the dead would be passed through the dog and on into the after life. This rather morbid practice is believed to have evolved into a more positive belief that the dog was able to cure illness and prevent death. Today a far more scientific approach leads us to believe that companion animals are indeed good for human health.

Other pets

Although dogs and cats are undoubtedly the most talked about species in the realm of companion animals, there is a wide range of other species that have an important place in human society. They range from the gerbil and hamster to the horse.

The horse is believed to have started its association with humans too late in history for it to take on any religious significance, but there is no doubt that it rapidly took on a role of great importance. The horse provided power and speed well in excess of that of cattle. As the cow took on a purely utilitarian role in Greek and Roman civilizations, the horse was afforded the respect and prestige that once belonged to cattle.

The companion animal

Pet keeping is often associated with the concept of companionship but it can also have other functions. Pets can be owned primarily for the assistance that they can offer (for example, dogs trained to assist blind, deaf or otherwise disabled owners). Alternatively, they may be kept as an ornament, a status symbol or even as an expression of the owner's own personality. Pet keeping can also be a hobby and the practices of showing pets, such as cats, dogs and rabbits, or keeping collections of ornamental fish or birds are common in western cultures.

Keeping animals purely for companionship involves an understanding and appreciation of the complex relationship that develops between pet and owner. This relationship is often referred to as the human–animal bond and can be compared in many respects to the bond that forms between human companions.

It is commonly assumed, especially by those who are not pet owners, that keeping pets is a symbol of social inadequacy, since they regard the pet as a substitute for a child or human companion. Interestingly pet ownership occurs significantly more often in families with children than in those without and research has suggested that dog ownership is associated with greater family cohesion.

The bond between pet and owner will depend on a number of factors, including the personality of both the human and the animal. It is well established that the way in which an animal is reared will significantly affect the level of attachment that it forms with its human companions. Good levels of socialization and habituation and appropriate experiences of being handled by humans in the early weeks of life will increase the suitability of animals for a role as a companion animal, but other factors need to be considered. Similarity in social structure will make it easier for an animal to 'fit in' with the human way of life. Although ornamental fish are numerically very popular as pets in various cultures throughout the world, most people would agree that they do not provide companionship in the same way as a cat or a dog.

Benefits and responsibilities of pet ownership

Benefits
Owning a companion animal provides many benefits for both pet and owner. Traditionally these benefits have been measured in terms of fulfilling social and emotional needs, but recent research has highlighted the benefits of pet ownership in terms of both physiological and psychological health.

Pets have been found to promote wellbeing in children and elderly people alike. Specific studies (for example, into the use of dogs in therapy for autistic children and the level of morale in elderly women living with or without pets) have shown that the benefits of pet ownership are significant. The role of pets in reducing levels of stress in humans has been an area of great interest and studies have consistently found that pet owners deal more positively with stressful events than non-owners.

All of this information points to the important role of companion animals in society but it must be remembered that keeping pets brings not only benefits but also responsibilities.

Responsibilities
The responsibilities of pet owners can be divided into those involving social, legal and welfare considerations.

Social responsibilities
Social responsibility relates to how the animal fits into society and how the ownership of that animal affects others. These responsibilities are more pronounced in the case of the cat and the dog than they are for more housebound pets such as fish and cage birds, since they have more interaction with people other than their owners. Some of the social responsibilities also have legal implications: there is legislation that controls the effect of pets on society.

Socialization
Domestic pets do not integrate into human society automatically, but need to be taught that living in close association with people is both acceptable and pleasurable. If animals are kept in isolation during their early development they will fail to integrate. As adults they will be social misfits who cannot relate to the people they come into contact with.

Socialization and habituation are often talked about in relation to dogs and cats, but it is important to remember that any species that is to be kept as a companion animal needs to go through this process of learning to relate to other species and to their environment. It is a subject that is often overlooked in relation to the smaller pets for children, such as hamsters and rabbits. As young children want to pick up and cuddle these animals, it is essential that the pets learn to accept handling.

It is not only the degree of socialization and habituation that is important when preparing an animal for its role as a companion, but also the quality. Too much interaction of a boisterous nature can have the opposite effect and make an animal nervous and apprehensive. Socialization needs to be controlled and handling needs to take place in a suitable way.

The most sensitive phase of behavioural development is very early in life, but the process of socialization and habituation needs to continue throughout the first year of life. The responsibility for ensuring that the process takes place in the most beneficial way possible therefore rests with both the breeder and the owner.

Legal and moral responsibilities
Owners need to be aware of their legal position and should be familiar with those pieces of legislation that affect them and their pet (see Chapter 10).

Pet owners also have moral responsibilities, which relate to respecting the rights and feelings of those who do not own animals. The attitudes of others and their requirements for personal space are important and owners need to be aware that not everyone wants to come into contact with their pet. One of the main ways in which owners can show respect in this area is to keep their pets under a suitable level of control.

Keeping animals under control is usually associated with dogs and most people are aware of the need to train dogs to at least a minimum level of obedience.

Cat owners are also aware of a need to keep their pets under some degree of control. Obviously this is limited by the fact that many cats spend long periods away from their owners and the law reflects this fact by placing less responsibility on cat owners.

Although owners of fish, small children's pets and caged birds may not have considered their responsibility to make their pets acceptable members of society, it is important to remember that these pets also need to be kept under control. Recent legal cases relating to damage caused by small rodents who escaped into neighbouring flats highlight this point.

Keeping pets under control is not only necessary in order to comply with the law, but it also promotes the positive image of pets in society and helps to counteract the very vocal anti-pet lobby.

Public health

Cleaning up after pets when they have fouled in public places is a social responsibility as well as a legal one. It is important from the point of view of hygiene, especially in areas where young children play, but it is also an aesthetic consideration. Most people find the presence of animal excreta in public places offensive and cleaning up after pets helps from a public relations point of view to increase the positive image of pet keeping.

Welfare responsibilities

Welfare responsibilities relate to the obvious considerations of caring adequately for animals. Owners can be guided by the five freedoms:

- Freedom from hunger and malnutrition
- Freedom from thermal or physical distress
- Freedom from disease or injury
- Freedom to express most normal behaviour
- Freedom from fear and stress.

The results of failure to provide the first three freedoms are likely to be very obvious and the majority of successful cruelty prosecutions relate to these areas of welfare. However, the final two are equally important and owner education is vital if problems in these areas are to be avoided.

An understanding of the species that is being kept is essential if the owner is to ensure that the animal can express its normal behaviours. For example, the keeping of cats as house pets has increased in recent years, and these animals need facilities within the house environment to express natural behaviours. The increase of keeping exotic pets is an area of education that deserves particular attention.

Freedom from fear is probably the most difficult to assess. Although it is often related to situations of abuse, it is important to remember that an undersocialized or underhabituated individual is likely to experience fear in everyday situations. Prevention of this through adequate socialization and habituation is therefore important from a welfare point of view.

Working with animals

Many people feel an affinity for animals and recognize the importance of their role in society. For the majority that affinity will result in pet ownership and pets have a place in more than half of the homes in the UK.

For a substantial number of people, owning a pet is only part of the picture and the idea of spending more time in the company of animals and working with them appeals to a wide section of individuals. This type of work can be demanding, tiring, dirty and sometimes distressing, but also extremely rewarding. Patience, dedication, a strong stomach, a caring attitude, organizational skills and a capacity for hard work over long hours are just a few of the qualities that are required. Good human interpersonal skills are also valuable, since working with animals very often involves working with people as well.

In today's society animals still fulfil a variety of roles, from companions to sources of food, and there is a wide range of possibilities for people wishing to work with them. The different areas of work are described below under broad headings.

It is not possible to give details of every occupation and training course available in each area, firstly because of limitations of space and secondly because training is constantly changing and evolving. Addresses of relevant organizations from whom further information can be obtained are listed at the end of the chapter.

Veterinary work

Veterinary surgeon

Six universities in the UK offer courses leading to a veterinary degree. Entry requirements are extremely high and this is generally regarded as the most difficult degree course to enter. For the talented few who succeed, opportunities may arise in large or small animal practices, zoos, research, private or government sectors and abroad. The Royal College of Veterinary Surgeons can provide further information.

Veterinary nurse

Currently the training to become a veterinary nurse takes 2 years. It requires applicants to be over 17 and have at least five GCSEs at Grade C or above, including English and either a science and a maths subject or two science subjects. NVQs at levels 2 and 3 were introduced in June 1998 and now form an integral part of the training scheme. Degree courses are also being introduced.

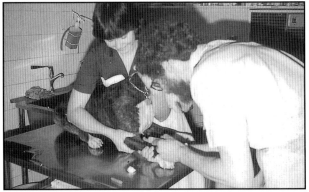

1.4 *A veterinary surgeon and a qualified veterinary nurse anaesthetizing a patient prior to surgery.*

In addition to veterinary practices, veterinary nurses can work in a number of organizations caring for animals. These include laboratories, zoos, universities, colleges, pharmaceutical companies, petfood companies, and breeding and boarding kennels.

Qualified veterinary nurses may go on to take a Diploma in Advanced Veterinary Nursing. This is another 2-year course which is studied for whilst working in practice. The British Veterinary Nursing Association should be contacted for more information on the training involved for both courses.

Animal technician (UK)

There are almost 300 laboratories and breeding establishments in the United Kingdom employing animal technicians, most of whom are members of the Institute of Animal Technology. The Institute organizes examinations at three levels: First Certificate, Membership and Fellowship. In order to take the First Certificate the candidate should be working full-time in the field of animal husbandry.

Charities

Royal Society for the Prevention of Cruelty to Animals (RSPCA)

The RSPCA and the SSPCA (Scottish Society for the Prevention of Cruelty to Animals) run an all-year-round service rescuing animals in danger and treating those that are sick or injured. In 1995 the RSPCA rehomed over 80,000 domestic animals and treated more than 14,000 wild animals at their three wildlife hospitals. The main career it offers is as an inspector.

Inspector

Both the RSPCA and the SSPCA recruit new inspectors by advertising in the national press, usually on an annual basis. The work involves:

- Visiting and inspecting places where animals are kept
- Giving advice about the care of animals and the conditions in which they are kept
- Rescuing animals in danger
- Dealing with cases of cruelty
- Collecting and transporting animals from animal centres, veterinary surgeries and private homes.

There are more than 300 inspectors in the UK providing 24-hour cover for animals in need. Entry requirements include:

- Being physically fit
- Ability to work alone and under pressure
- A good level of general education, with at least GCSE English and a science subject
- Organizational skills
- A driving licence.

If accepted, a challenging 6-month training course has to be completed which covers animal-related topics ranging from animal protection law to handling and rescuing animals safely.

Animal care assistant

An animal care assistant works as part of a team at an RSPCA or SSPCA centre where unwanted or injured animals are taken in and cared for with the ultimate aim of rehoming them or returning them to the wild. The assistant is responsible for:

- Cleaning of living quarters
- Dealing with animals that die from their injuries
- Relocating wild animals
- Rehoming domesticated animals.

The work can be hard and often upsetting but brings its own rewards. Necessary attributes include:

- Common sense
- Physical fitness
- A love of animals
- Good interpersonal skills
- Commitment
- A good standard of education, with passes at GCSE in English and maths.

A useful body to contact is the Animal Care Industry Training Organization, who can provide information on NVQs in animal care, modern apprenticeships and general career advice.

Veterinary surgeon and veterinary nurse

Opportunities for RSPCA veterinary surgeons and veterinary nurses also exist. Vacancies are often advertised in the careers section of the *Guardian* and relevant professional journals.

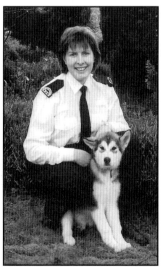

1.5 *An SSPCA inspector with a Husky, a breed that demonstrates some of the physical qualities of the ancestral wolf.*

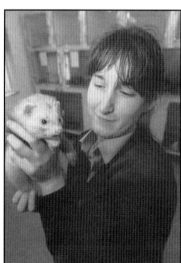

1.6 *Working with animal charities often means dealing with a wide variety of species.*

Blue Cross

The Blue Cross employs over 200 people within its animal rescue centres and head office. It runs three hospitals and a clinic in London and 10 adoption centres, and has an equine welfare department on two sites. Vacancies for positions with The Blue Cross are advertised in either the local or national press, depending on the seniority of the post.

Animal welfare assistant

Animal welfare assistants work in each adoption centre. Their duties include:

- Day-to-day care of the animals
- Feeding
- Cleaning kennels
- Grooming
- Walking dogs
- Administering medical treatment under supervision.

Groom

Grooms are employed at each of the equine welfare sites. Prior experience of working with horses is preferred but not essential. A groom's tasks include:

- Mucking out
- Feeding
- Grooming
- Riding
- General everyday care of the horses, with special attention to any that are sick.

Other staff

There is a small number of other specialist staff, including:

- Ambulance drivers
- Radiographers
- Laboratory technicians
- Night superintendents
- Hospital managers
- Support staff.

    Volunteers are often needed for walking dogs, grooming animals and other general assistance.

Veterinary surgeon

The Blue Cross employs 18 qualified veterinary surgeons, as well as locums when necessary.

Veterinary nurse

All Blue Cross hospitals are approved training centres for veterinary nurses and they usually have a long waiting list. Several qualified veterinary nurses are employed within the organization.

People's Dispensary for Sick Animals (PDSA)

The PDSA was established to provide free veterinary treatment for sick and injured domestic pets whose owners are unable to afford private veterinary fees. The organization does not run boarding kennels or catteries, nor is it involved in large animal practice. It runs 44 veterinary centres in major towns and cities throughout the UK.

Veterinary staff

The PDSA employs around 200 veterinary surgeons and over 250 veterinary centre nursing staff. Vacancies for qualified veterinary staff are advertised in the *Veterinary Record*.

Animal care auxiliaries

Animal care auxiliaries are employed at a limited number of centres. They:

- Care for in-patients
- Clean premises
- Look after security.

Guide Dogs for the Blind Association (GDBA)

The GDBA breeds and trains working dogs to assist visually impaired people in their everyday life. To accomplish this it employs three basic levels of staff.

Kennel staff

Kennel staff need to:

- Be over 18
- Be educated to GCSE standard (Grade D or above)
- Have some experience with animals and people
- Be in good physical health.

    They are responsible for:

- Cleaning kennels
- Feeding
- Grooming
- Assisting in the education of dogs
- Taking care of sick or postoperative dogs or puppies.

Guide dog trainer

Entry requirements are slightly higher than for kennel staff. In addition a trainer must be:

- Confident in dealing with groups of people as well as dogs
- Prepared to walk many miles a day in all weathers.

    The trainer begins to help the young dog adjust to the routine of training. When the dog is ready it is passed on for its advanced training.

Guide dog mobility instructor

An instructor must have five GCSEs, including English, maths and a science subject at Grade C or above, and ideally a social science subject.
    The instructor takes over from the trainer and:

- Leads the dog through the final stages of training
- Matches it with a compatible visually impaired student
- Undertakes a 4-week period of intensive training of the dog with the student, helping them to work as a unit before they return home
- Eases this transition by making after-care visits.

Hearing Dogs for Deaf People

This organization, a much more recent and smaller one than GDBA, trains dogs to react to sounds such as a doorbell or a crying baby and to lead their deaf owner to the source of the sound.

The range of jobs is similar to those with guide dogs. Applicants need to have:

- Experience of dog behaviour and training
- A caring and responsible attitude to both animals and people
- Clear speech and communication skills.

Although a knowledge of sign language would be helpful, training is given at the centre. A good standard of education is expected, though no specific examinations are required.

National Canine Defence League

This charity specializes in caring for stray and abandoned dogs. Kennel staff are appointed by individual kennel managers. A list of kennels is available from the head office.

General work with dogs, cats and small animals

Most colleges of agriculture now include full-time and part-time courses in animal care from BTEC Certificate level to First Diploma, BTEC National Diploma and BTEC Higher National Diploma. Up-to-date information on these should be sought from a local Careers Advice Centre. Many of these courses will be of value in any of the careers mentioned here.

Kennel/cattery work

Vacancies for employment in boarding, breeding and training kennels and in catteries are generally advertised in local newspapers. Working in kennels involves:

- Early starts, on weekdays and at weekends
- Often being outside in all sorts of weather conditions.

Although no formal qualifications are necessary for this type of work, various colleges offer courses in basic animal care (NVQs). There is also the Canine Studies Institute (CSI) Small Animal Care Certificate. One of the best sources of information on local training centres is the nearest Careers Advice Centre.

A list of boarding and breeding catteries may be obtained from Cats Protection. Information about dog kennels can be requested from the Kennel Club and about quarantine kennels from the Ministry of Agriculture, Fisheries and Food.

Dog grooming

There are over 2000 grooming salons in the UK, some of which are part of other pet-related establishments such as pet shops, garden centres and kennels. As with kennel work, positions are generally advertised locally. Obviously a good deal of patience is required as well as a firm but gentle way with animals. The City and Guilds Dog Grooming Certificate 775 is the main qualification but is not mandatory as many people learn 'on the job'. More information can be found by contacting the British Dog Groomers Association.

Dog training

There is a multitude of opportunities for dog training work, from shepherding, work in the police force, drug detection with Customs and Excise, and firearms and explosives work in the Royal Army Veterinary Corps to the training of guide dogs, hearing dogs for the deaf, search and rescue dogs and so on.

The British Institute of Professional Dog Trainers offers a correspondence course and a practical competence course aimed principally at professional dog handlers. There are three certificate levels: bronze, silver and gold. Different levels of membership are open to people working professionally with animals and who fulfil the Institute's criteria.

Pet shops

More than half of Britain's homes have at least one pet. As well as cats and dogs, other animals have become popular over recent years and many people now keep birds, tropical fish, small mammals, reptiles and amphibians. In this country there are more than 3500 pet shops. Pet superstores and garden centres that have pet sections grow in number every year.

A City and Guilds qualification can be studied through a correspondence course run by the Pet Care Trust.

Pet shop workers should demonstrate:

- A wide knowledge of different species
- Knowledge of their nutritional and living requirements
- A high standard of customer care.

Work with horses

The British Horse Society (BHS) is the organization that can give the most information about work with horses. Such work covers a very wide range of activities.

Riding instructor

The BHS oversees examinations at centres throughout the country from the basic Stage 1 through Assistant Instructor, Intermediate Instructor and BHS Instructor to the Fellowship award, which is a recognition of excellence in the field of horsemanship. There are other awards for Driving, Working and Heavy Horses and for teaching riding to disabled people.

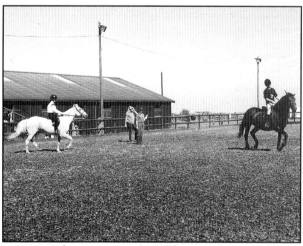

1.7 *Riding instructor working with young riders. Courtesy of S. Dallas.*

Groom

A good groom is a highly regarded person who cares for horses that may be worth many thousands of pounds. Work may be:

- On a stud farm looking after mares and foals
- In a racing stable
- At an international showjumper's yard.

As well as qualifications that may be taken through the BHS, the National Pony Society offers certificates, diplomas and NVQs up to Level 3.

Farriery

Those wishing to be farriers have to register under the Farriers (Registration) Acts following successful completion of an apprenticeship and passing the examination for the Diploma of the Worshipful Company of Farriers. Information can be obtained from the Farriery Training Service.

Racing

Most jockeys begin as apprentices with one of the racing yards in this country. The British Racing School also runs a variety of courses (S/NVQs at Levels 1–3) for the horse industry. There are some opportunities for the talented to become jockeys and certainly most would be expected to 'ride out'. New recruits generally start through one of the racing schools at Newmarket or Doncaster.

Work with farm animals

To make a career of working with farm animals (Figure 1.8) generally means starting by finding employment or work experience on a farm. This can be done in a number of ways, from advertising in the national *Farmers Weekly* to approaching local farmers.

Farms vary enormously, from remote hill farms with beef cattle and sheep to specialist indoor pig and poultry farms. Some young people wanting to take up this type of work might not like or approve of the intensive farming of animals and could be better suited to working in organic or non-intensive farming. In this case it would be useful to contact the British Organic Farmers and also Working Weekends on Organic Farms (WWOOF).

It would be sensible to try working for several weekends on different kinds of farms to get a feel for what one would prefer. On any farm the work will almost certainly involve early morning starts and long and often unsociable hours.

Government-sponsored training schemes for young people may be available through local Training and Enterprise Councils (TECs) and offer training that leads to NVQ Level 2 or 3. Some of the time would be spent in day or block release at college and the remainder would be on a commercial unit under the supervision of a farmer. Trainees receive a training allowance during the programme.

There are various courses at higher levels from National Certificate to Higher National Diploma. Entry requirements vary in accordance with the level at which entry is made. For example, the National Diploma, which is offered by most Colleges of Agriculture, demands four GCSEs at Grade C or above, with at least two of the subjects being sciences. The National Diploma is a 3-year full-time course, with the middle year being spent on an approved farm. Further information can be obtained from ATB-Landbase, which is the industry training organization for agriculture.

Zoos and wildlife parks

Zoos and wildlife parks employ people to look after the animals (Figure 1.9) and to educate and supervise the visiting public. General information may be obtained from the Zoological Society of London and the Association of British Wild Animal Keepers.

Zoo keeper

Zoo keepers need to:

- Be extremely knowledgeable about the animals in their care
- Be prepared to work unsociable hours
- Be prepared to work outside in all weathers, possibly feeding infants at 3-hourly intervals, day and night
- Get on well with the public
- Be capable of answering questions about the animals in their care
- Have stamina and commitment as well as a love of animals.

There are many applicants for posts as keepers and only a few opportunities. Keepers are often recruited for the summer season only, and then the best of these are kept for permanent employment.

1.8 *Working with farm animals involves being outside in all weathers.*
Courtesy of I. Thomas.

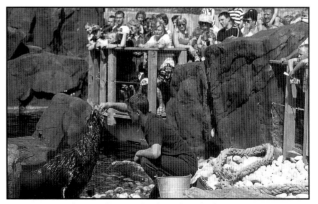

1.9 *Working with animals often also involves contact with the general public.*
Courtesy of Bristol Zoo Gardens.

For its own keepers, the Zoological Society of London provides a training scheme that is part of the career structure at London and Whipsnade Zoos. For those living elsewhere in the UK a correspondence course is run by the National Extension College for the City and Guilds Certificate in Zoo Animal Management, the final part of which is of a practical nature and can only be taken whilst working with captive wild animals.

Conclusion

It has not been possible to cover every aspect of working with animals, but hopefully the reader will have gained a flavour of what is on offer and will be able to follow up areas of personal interest by contacting organizations direct. Since many of these are charities and their finances are tight, it is always appreciated when enquirers enclose a stamped addressed envelope.

The criteria to be met for working with animals in any capacity are very similar. Applicants will be favoured who can demonstrate an interest in animal welfare and behaviour along with some previous experience of animal work, whether voluntary or paid; a commitment to animals without being over-sentimental; a willingness to work long, hard and often unsociable hours; and the ability to relate well to people. The rewards for those who go on to make a career of working with animals, while not necessarily great in financial terms, can be very enriching in many other ways.

Further reading

Appleby P (1994) *How to Work with Dogs*. How to Books, Plymbridge House, Estover Road, Plymouth.

Bartley L, Kingston P, Steadman H *et al.* (1996) *Work with Animals*. Department of Education and Employment, Thames Ditton.

Bradshaw JSW (1992) *The Behaviour of the Domestic Cat*. CAB International, Wallingford, Oxon.

Clutton-Brock J (1987) *A Natural History of Domesticated Animals*. Cambridge University Press/British Museum (Natural History).

Manning A and Serpell J (eds) (1994) *Animals and Human Society: Changing Perspectives*. Routledge, London.

Morgan J (1996) *How to Work with Horses*. How to Books, Plymbridge House, Estover Road, Plymouth.

Robinson I (ed.) (1995) *The Waltham Book of Human Animal Interaction: Benefits and Responsibilities of Pet Ownership*. Pergamon Press, Oxford.

Serpell J (ed.) (1995) *The Domestic Dog – its Evolution, Behaviour and Interactions with People*. Cambridge University Press, Cambridge.

Shepherd A (1997) *Careers Working with Animals*, 8th edn. Kogan Page, London.

UFAW *Careers Information Sheet*. Universities Federation for Animal Welfare, Potters Bar.

Useful addresses

Dogs

British Institue of Professional Dog Trainers
Bowstone Gate, Nr Disley, Cheshire SK12 2AW

Guide Dogs for the Blind Association
Hillfields, Burghfield, Reading, Berkshire RG7 3YG

Hearing Dogs for Deaf People
The Training Centre, London Road (A40), Lewknor, Oxfordshire OX9 5RY

National Canine Defence League
17 Wakley Street, London EC1V 7LT

Horses

The British Horse Society
Stoneleigh Park, Kenilworth, Warwickshire CV8 2LR

The British Racing School
Snailwell Road, Newmarket, Suffolk CB8 7NU

The Farriery Training Service
Sefton House, Adam Court, Newark Road, Peterborough PE1 5PP

The National Pony Society
Willingdon House, 102 High Street, Alton, Hampshire GU34 1EN

Farm Animals

ATB-Landbase
Warwickshire Careers Service, 10 Northgate Street, Warwick CV34 4SR

British Organic Farmers
The Soil Association, 40-56 Victoria Street, Bristol BS1 6BY

Working Weekends on Organic Farms
19 Bradford Road, Lewes, East Sussex BN7 1RB

Zoos and Wildlife Parks

The Association of British Wild Animal Keepers
12 Tackley Road, Eastville, Bristol BS5 6UQ

The National Extension College
18 Brooklands Avenue, Cambridge CB2 2HN

The Zoological Society of London
Regent's Park, London NW1 4RY

General

Blue Cross
Field Centre, Home Close Farm, Shilton Road, Burford, Oxfordshire OX18 4PF

British Veterinary Nursing Association
Level 15, Terminus House, Terminus Street, Harlow, Essex CM20 1AX

People's Dispensary for Sick Animals
Whitechapel Way, Priorslee, Telford, Shropshire TF2 9PQ

Royal College of Veterinary Surgeons
Belgravia House, 62–64 Horseferry Road, London SW1P 2AF

Royal Society for the Prevention of Cruelty to Animals
Causeway, Horsham, West Sussex RH12 1HG

Universities Federation for Animal Welfare (UFAW)
8 Hamilton Close, South Mimms, Potters Bar, Hertfordshire

2 General care and management of the dog

Jean and Trevor Turner

This chapter is designed to give information on:

- The responsibility, cost and commitment involved with dog owning
- Considerations involved in selection of a dog
- The popular dog breeds (an overview)
- Basic principles involved in puppy and dog care, including breeding
- Basic nutrition and feeding
- Normal canine behaviour
- Normal behaviour and development of puppies, particularly in relation to training
- Dog-related activities

Introduction

Rescue organizations are overwhelmed with requests for rehoming unwanted pets. Many lovely puppies, acquired with joy and enthusiasm, end up in a very short time as 'people failures', and new homes are sought for them either through the advertisement columns of local newspapers or via national or local canine rescue organizations. Some of these dogs are in rescue solely as a result of ignorance on the part of owners who simply failed to realize the commitment required when taking a dog into their home.

Charity organizations have done much with their publicity campaigns (e.g. 'A dog is for life, not just for Christmas') but still many of these 'people failures' could be avoided with a little more education.

This chapter explains the advantages and disadvantages of dog owning in general and with respect to particular types of dog. The popular breeds are looked at objectively and the classification of pedigree dogs is explained. Emphasis is placed on the care, training and control required when owning a dog. If the determination to proceed remains after informed consideration of the advantages and disadvantages, owning a dog should give mutual pleasure and satisfaction.

Considerations before acquiring a dog

Before purchasing or even giving a home to a dog, consideration should be given to certain aspects involved when sharing a home with a dog (Figure 2.1). For example:

- What are the reasons for wanting a dog?
- What costs are involved (both for the initial acquisition and for maintenance)?

2.1 Considerations before acquiring a dog

Reasons for wanting a dog

- Companionship
- Protection and guarding
- To grow up with children in the family
- To show, to work in obedience, or other dog-related activities
- Breeding and puppy rearing
- Retired owners benefit from regular exercise required by their pet
- Hypertension – therapeutic effect.

Costs (initial and ongoing) compared with means

- Cost of acquisition
  - Even rescue animals are chargeable
  - Pedigree animals can cost up to several hundred pounds
- Maintenance costs
  - Feeding (increases with size of dog)
  - Veterinary fees
  - General care
  - Health insurance (most insurance policies do not cover maintenance costs such as vaccination and dentistry)
  - Grooming costs (can cost up to £50 every 6 weeks with full-coated dogs)
  - Holiday costs (dog sitters and kennels).

Responsibilities of owning a dog

- Do you have enough time available?
- Would the dog be left alone for long periods?
- Are there facilities for exercising the dog?
- Is family lifestyle sufficiently flexible?

- What are the responsibilities of owning a dog?
- Is the family's lifestyle sufficiently flexible?
- What about the ongoing commitment?

Today we are all part of a consumer-driven society, but dogs (unlike the majority of consumer products) interact with their owners. They will give immediate unstinting and generous love and affection. In return it must be ensured that sufficient time and money are available to care for the pet properly. Owners must make sure that the dog is not the one that does all the giving, receiving little or nothing in return.

It is most important that novice owners, with the commendable desire to own a dog, are aware of the breadth of commitment – which extends beyond feeding, housing and grooming (Figure 2.2). Once the novelty of acquisition has passed, this commitment continues and will be required for the natural life of the dog – probably 10–15 years.

An important factor to bear in mind is that all dogs are pack animals and they do need some company for a fair proportion of the day. A lonely or bored dog cannot be blamed if it resorts to destructive or other antisocial behaviour. A pet is not something that can simply be parked in a corner: as a member of the family a dog is entitled to consideration. Owning a dog is a partnership.

Selecting a dog

Having decided that a dog is a suitable pet, the next decision is which kind of dog to have.

Dogs, like clothes, may reflect their owner's personality but can also be the subject of fashion. This is sometimes rational. After the Second World War new houses and gardens were smaller and Miniature Poodles enjoyed unrivalled popularity. They did not shed their hair, they were biddable and they fitted in with the prevailing conditions. With their increasing popularity certain undesirable traits became apparent: ear problems became rife, and necessary coat attention became a burden for many inexperienced owners. Their popularity waned and today the Cavalier King Charles Spaniel has replaced the Miniature Poodle as the popular pet in the town community. Compared with the Poodle, the demands of this spaniel's coat care are minimal.

The German Shepherd Dog (Alsatian), the Labrador Retriever and the Golden Retriever are still the most popular among those who favour larger pedigree breeds. Mongrels or mixed breeds, with all their variations (often unpredictable), are still by far the most popular pet dogs.

The decision about which kind of dog to own cannot be taken lightly and should only be made after seeking adequate appropriate advice. Although tempting, the acquisition of a puppy from a neighbour's litter may not be ideal. Evaluate the situation and your preferences. Making a short list of breeds or types of dog in which you have an interest and visiting some of the larger dog shows will be time well spent. Selection of a pet needs care and there are many factors to be considered (Figure 2.3).

For example, bigger breeds (e.g. Dalmatian, Labrador Retriever) in general need more exercise, attention and food. Beagles and Bassets (Figure 2.4) may appeal on looks but, bred for generations as hunt pack animals, they need a great deal of attention and control.

Size

Domestic dogs show more variation in size than any other mammal. They range from tiny Chihuahuas, weighing less than a kilogram, to Irish Wolfhounds, St Bernards and Great Danes weighing up to 100 kg. If humans showed as much variation, they could vary from our present height to giants over seven storeys high.

The sizes of home and garden influence the choice of size of dog. There is a move towards owning larger dogs but these are often clumsy in the normal sized house. A Great Dane would clearly be unsuitable in a one-bedroomed flat on the 11th floor of a skyscraper block; an exuberant wag from its tail can easily clear a coffe table.

The larger the dog, the greater is the volume of waste, both urine and faeces. This is a factor to be taken into consideration for those with a tiny garden. The fouling of

2.2 Ongoing time commitments

- Purchasing, preparing and feeding food
- Grooming (especially time consuming with full-coated breeds)
- House cleaning (for removal of shed hair and control of parasites)
- Play and exercise – up to 2 hours a day with some of the more athletic dogs (in bad weather as well as good; the commitment extends beyond pleasant summer days to times when it is cold and raining. Dogs seldom care about the weather, provided that they are about to be taken for that exciting routine walk)
- Looking after sick or ageing dog.

2.3 Considerations in selection of type

- Size – are your preferences practical?
- Life span – the larger the dog, in general, the shorter its potential lifespan
- Coat – length, colour, texture (the shorter the coat, the easier it is to maintain; long coats involve more grooming time)
- Activity levels and temperament of the dog
- Purebred, crossbred or mongrel
- Adult or puppy
- Source – breeder, rescue kennels, response to advertisement
- Bitch or dog
- Veterinary costs (consider insurance).

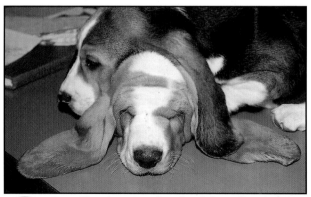

2.4 *Basset Hounds are appealing, though demanding as pets. Photo: Trevor Turner.*

public places can be subject to stringent bylaws and is unpleasant and antisocial. Is the owner prepared to clear up after their Irish Wolfhound or would they prefer to cope with the more manageable volume produced by the Bearded Collie or, better still, the Miniature Pinscher?

It is also worth considering the dog's potential life span. In very broad terms: the larger the dog, the shorter will be its life span.

All these size considerations are the same, whether the intention is to purchase a pedigree puppy or to give a home to a stray from the local rescue centre.

Coat

The Afghan Hound (see Figure 2.9) looks immaculate when presented for exhibition at a show but it is not just 'wash and go'. This beautiful coat is the result of hours of work. Without regular grooming, a full-coated dog will quickly become a matted mess and in pain and discomfort as a result of the knotted coat.

One of the saddest and relatively common sights seen in veterinary practice is an Old English Sheepdog whose coat is so matted that it imprisons the animal as effectively as a suit of armour. The dog has to be heavily sedated or anaesthetized to be clipped out and freed from its own coat (Figure 2.5). This is frequently due to ignorance on the part of the owner.

Short-coated dogs require little time and effort to keep them groomed.

Activity

The ages and activity levels of those members of the family likely to have most contact with the family pet also

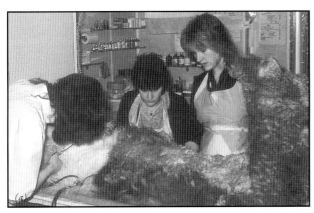

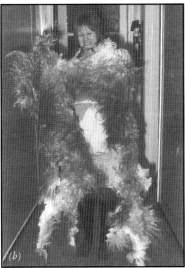

2.5 *(a) Three people working on a badly matted Old English Sheepdog. (b) A mat cut from an Old English Sheepdog undergroomed for 6 months.*

influence choice. Extremely athletic and exuberant animals such as gundogs or hounds are not very suitable for infirm elderly owners, who may have difficulty walking and are living in tiny accommodation. One of the smaller, less active breeds (e.g. King Charles Spaniel or Pekingese) may be more suitable. On the other hand, a lively Labrador could be ideal for a family with teenagers.

Activity is not directly proportional to size. St Bernards, for example, although sharing the title of giant breed with Irish Wolfhounds, are considerably less active. Even among the gundogs activity levels vary: Cocker and Springer Spaniels are active and inquisitive, whereas Sussex and Clumber Spaniels tend to be more sedate.

Purebred, crossbred or mongrel?

Should the dog be pedigree or mongrel? Figure 2.6 outlines the different definitions.

Mongrel

Temperament, coat and size when fully grown can be predicted with reasonable accuracy in a pedigree puppy. This is less certain with a crossbred and virtually impossible with a mongrel. Be warned: charming mongrel puppies of unknown parentage can sometimes provide surprises when they become adult, both in size and in temperament. Always try to acquire as much information as possible about any mixed breed before making a hasty decision.

In the matter of choice, much depends on the owner's life style, budget and individual preferences. Before acquiring the pet, it is always sensible to find out as much as possible about the characteristics of each type of dog of interest – even if the final choice is a mongrel. For example, should the mongrel have mainly terrier characteristics, its potential owner will be at an advantage if they have some knowledge of terriers.

Purebred

If the choice is in favour of a purebred dog, further choices then have to be made. More than 180 different breeds are recognized by the Kennel Club (KC) and this number is increasing all the time. Purebreds are looked at in detail in the section on popular dog breeds later in this chapter.

Anyone wishing to acquire a purebred dog should study the Kennel Club's *Illustrated Breed Standards*. Each breed is illustrated, its basic conformation is described and each standard includes some indication of the behaviour and temperament of the animal.

Crufts Dog Show, the largest annual dog show in the world, has a 'Discover Dogs' section in which the majority of the breeds recognized by the Kennel Club are represented, with knowledgeable breed club members on hand who are willing to advise aspiring owners. 'Discover Dogs' also takes place each year in London in November as a separate event.

2.6 Terminology

- *Purebred* A dog whose parents are both of the same breed
- *Pedigree* A purebred dog whose ancestors are recorded on a pedigree form
- *Crossbred* A dog whose parents are purebred but not of the same breed
- *Mongrel* A dog whose parents are of mixed breed, usually unplanned.

2.7 Advantages and disadvantages of dogs and bitches

Advantages	Disadvantages
Bitches	
More companionable More biddable Less aggressive to other dogs	In oestrus at approximately 6-monthly intervals Attractive to male dogs for approximately 3 weeks Can produce unwanted puppies
Dogs	
Do not have seasons Usually larger and less nervous Can be larger Usually bolder than bitches	Can be more aggressive with other dogs Can roam Urine marking common

Dog or bitch?

The advantages and disadvantages of bitches and dogs are outlined in Figure 2.7. For example, bitches tend to be more home loving and less likely to wander than dogs but they do come into season (heat) about twice a year unless they are neutered (see section on breeding).

Adult or puppy?

Adult dogs

The acquisition of an adult dog sometimes presents advantages. For example, elderly or infirm owners are not presented with the problems of training a young dog with the attendant trauma that sometimes is encountered. Middle-aged and elderly dogs are often in need of a good home due to unforeseen or unfortunate circumstances. These dogs can be the most difficult to rehome yet often make excellent pets for less active people.

There are many genuine reasons why an adult dog has to be rehomed. These include: loss of job or home by the original owners; owners dying, emigrating or changing their home or work; and breeders disposing of adult stock no longer suitable for showing or breeding. The reasons for disposal of a loved family dog may be unexpected, unavoidable and entirely genuine. Ask about the reasons. Sometimes the stress of the situation is very apparent in the dog.

Strays

Adult strays present different problems. They are often of an independent nature with little need or desire for human contact, particularly if they have been fending for themselves for any length of time. Stray male dogs may be oversexed, and searching for a bitch in heat may have been the reason for the original loss of home. The medical history is usually unknown, which means that vaccination is essential. Vigilance must be practised when introducing the adult stray to your home, particularly if young children are involved.

Puppies

Offering a home to an adult dog is commendable and should be encouraged but there are risks attached. Acquiring a puppy is the traditional way of commencing dog ownership and perhaps presents less risk.

When choosing a puppy consider the following:

- Puppies reared well should never show aggression and should be bold and inquisitive
- Always avoid the timid puppy, or the one that cries or appears afraid of being handled, irrespective of its breeding
- If purchasing a pedigree puppy from a breeder, ask to see the bitch. In some cases both parents may be seen. Also ask to see any other adult stock that may be available. Temperament, size and general characteristics can then be assessed.

Selecting the correct pedigree puppy may involve a great deal of effort, time, travel and, perhaps, some inconvenience. That puppy should, with luck, remain part of the family for perhaps a dozen years, a fact that puts a journey of several hundred miles into perspective.

A well bred, well reared pedigree puppy will cost several hundred pounds (depending on the breed). Considering the average life span of the breed, the purchase price is cheap when compared with set-up costs for other hobbies. Paying £400 for a puppy with a life expectancy of, say, 10 years represents a capital investment of only £40 per year – a meagre amount in proportion to the pleasure derived.

Reputable and caring breeders will:

- Spend time ensuring that the prospective buyer and the puppy are suited
- Discuss and provide information about grooming, exercise, feeding, the cost involved in training and its achievement
- Encourage a potential purchaser to see the litter, with their dam, at 4–5 weeks of age. The buyer can then consider the acquisition, discuss any queries and concerns and return when the puppy is 8–9 weeks old. Worming, vaccination and feeding should be discussed at the time of collection.

There should be no attempt to try to persuade the breeder to release the puppy before it is ready to leave the dam. No one will benefit, least of all the puppy and the new owner. Leaving the 'nest' too early can result in a lack of socialization with the littermates and be detrimental to development in the long term.

Source

Answering an advertisement or going direct to a breeder might be the choice of source for a new pedigree pet. However, rescue centres have many pedigree dogs of all ages. Usually these dogs represent 'people failures' – enthusiastic first-time owners who, completely ignorant of the responsibilities and oblivious of the ongoing commitment, have found themselves unable to cope. This emphasizes the need to consider all aspects of the commitment of dog ownership before taking the step.

Cost

Selection may be influenced by cost. Pedigree puppies cost more but there is the advantage of knowing, in broad terms, what their temperament, eventual size, conformation and coat type are going to be.

Ongoing costs

The cost of buying the pet is only the initial consideration. Ongoing costs such as annual vaccinations, regular health checks and worming add to the maintenance expenses. Coat attention in any of the full-coated breeds is also a recurrent cost unless owners are prepared to learn how to do this themselves and buy the necessary equipment – and have the necessary time available.

Although the size of the dog is unlikely to affect the cost of vaccination and routine veterinary maintenance, it is directly related to the costs of feeding and any medication.

Health insurance

Some breeds have inherent disorders that can involve ongoing veterinary costs and drugs. Many of these can be covered by pet health insurance which, depending on the conditions of the policy, may include some hereditary conditions. Always read the policy conditions carefully. Premiums depend on the level of cover selected.

Time commitment

An owner's commitment of time is very important for their dog. Dogs are social animals and they thrive in groups. This does not mean that it is necessary to acquire several dogs. Provided there is sufficient interaction with the family, the dog will consider the pack to include the family members and be perfectly integrated and happy even if it is the only dog on the premises.

For people who live alone, some dogs (e.g. German Shepherd Dog) tend to be very much one-person dogs. Knowledge of such a tendency is a good background when searching for the right dog.

Dominance

It is essential that one member of the family acts as the 'pack leader' as far as the dog is concerned and makes their position of supremacy clear at the outset. This does not mean that the leader has to be aggressive or harsh with the pet in order to establish dominance. However, the natural pack system is hierarchical and all members of the family should play a part in interacting and enforcing the necessary dominance hierarchy.

Local dog training classes will show how to dominate through reward. Training classes are often sponsored by local authorities and are available in most areas. They teach the subtle methods by which dominance is established and maintained. It is useful to have the time to participate in training classes, particularly in the early months after the dog has come to share the family home.

Clear decisions on these issues, established before acquiring the pet, will ensure that yet another dog does not enter the apparently unending stream of 'people failures'.

Popular dog breeds

The Breed Standard issued by the Kennel Club, after close consultation with members of the breed club or society, is a description of how the ideal specimen of any particular breed should look, behave and move. It is a description of perfection and not intended as a guide to breed identification.

Newly imported breeds receive recognition via the Imported Breeds register. Once a breed is accepted and at least 10 dogs of the breed have been registered, an Interim Breed Standard is published by the KC and soon another breed will be recognized.

The Fédération Cynologique Internationale (FCI) is a canine authority which represents almost 50 countries, including Britain (since the KC is affiliated) but not the American Kennel Club. Altogether over 400 breeds are recognized and in consequence FCI has 10 separate groups. Some countries, including many in Europe, depend entirely on the FCI while others have organized their national kennel clubs to follow either the British or the American pattern.

Breed groups

The KC's separate breed standards are divided into Sporting and Non-sporting and are organized into seven groups (Figures 2.8–2.15). From the breed name it is not always easy to decide into which group the dog should be placed. For example:

- The Australian Silky Terrier, the English Toy Terrier and the Yorkshire Terrier are not grouped as terriers but are placed in the Toy group
- The Boston Terrier and Tibetan Terrier are placed in the Utility group.

Popular breeds are drawn from virtually all the groups. For example:

- Bassets and Beagles are members of the Hound group
- English Setters, retrievers and spaniels are in the Gundog group
- Staffordshire Bull Terriers (Staffies) and West Highland White Terriers (Westies) are in the Terrier group
- Poodles (Standard, Miniature and Toy), Schnauzers, Shih Tzus and Shar Peis are all part of the Utility group

2.8 Classification of breeds recognized by the Kennel Club

Group	Characteristics
Sporting	
Hound	Hunting dogs, either by sight (e.g. Greyhound) or by scent (e.g. Foxhound) Not all have 'hound' in the name (e.g. Beagle, Rhodesian Ridgeback)
Gundog	Originally trained to the gun Includes pointers, setters, spaniels and retrievers as well as Viszla, Weimeraner
Terrier	Originally developed in Britain as farm dogs to go to earth after rats. Terriers are to digging as sight hounds are to running and scent hounds to tracking. All have 'Terrier' in their name
Non-sporting	
Working	Contains the guarding dogs (e.g. Dobermann, St Bernard)
Pastoral	Contains all the herding dogs – collies, sheepdogs and Corgi
Toy	Companion (lap or pillow) dogs and mostly small
Utility	All the rest – group has no common factor (in contrast to American Kennel Club non-sporting group). Many of the breeds have working backgrounds (e.g. Schnauzer, Dalmatian) but essentially today they are companion dogs

- German Shepherd Dogs, Great Danes and Boxers are examples of the Working group, which now comprises the guarding breeds
- The Border Collie, Rough Collie and Old English Sheepdog, although working dogs, were split from the Working group in January 1999 to form part of the new Pastoral group, which comprises the herding dogs and is similar to the Herding Group of the American Kennel Club (AKC)
- The Utility group contains all the breeds that will not comfortably fit elsewhere, and broadly conforms with the Non-Sporting group of the AKC
- The Cavalier King Charles Spaniel is not, as perhaps would be expected, a member of the Gundog group (as a spaniel) but is in the Toy group – despite the fact that Cavaliers seen in pet practice often weigh over 20 kg
- Dogs in the Toy group are all considered to be lap or pillow dogs, hence the anomalies with size. Other anomalies are also apparent: the Shih Tzu is placed in the Toy group by the AKC but is in the Utility group in Britain
- Large breeds such as the Irish Wolfhound, Great Dane and St Bernard are often referred to as giant breeds, but there is no 'Giant' group. The Irish Wolfhound is placed in the Hound group; the St Bernard and Great Dane are in the Working group.

The function of the KC's group system is to organize the exhibition of dogs for judging purposes. With the exception of the Utility group, each group has common factors that are fairly obvious. This does not mean that every hound or every member of the Toy group is the same but it does follow that certain generalizations do apply.

2.9 Hounds

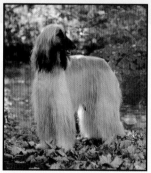
Afghan Hound. © Marc Henrie ASC.

These are hunting dogs. They can hunt by either sight or smell. Dogs have the most efficient sense of smell of all the domestic species. They can detect the scent of a substance at one hundredth of the strength at which it is detectable by humans.

- *Scent hounds* depend on their noses to follow the scent of their quarry. Examples are Bloodhound, Basset, Beagle and Foxhound.
- *Sight, gaze or coursing hounds* depend on their good eyesight and speed to bring down their quarry. Examples are Greyhound, Whippet, Afghan and Saluki.

Traditionally, hunting packs have been drawn from scent hounds; hence there are packs of Foxhounds or Bassets but seldom Greyhounds or Salukis.

Hounds all have the tendency to hunt what they consider 'fair game', i.e. suitable bait. It can be a problem if this happens to be a neighbour's cat or cherished Poodle. Take care when owning that long-awaited Beagle: this tendency is never far below the surface and occurs spontaneously, irrespective of training and close bonding with the family.

The most popular pet hounds today are Beagle, Basset, Afghan and Whippet.

2.10 Gundogs

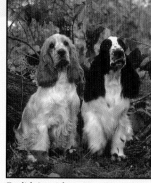
English Spaniels. © Marc Henrie ASC.

All gundogs work in one way or another with the person carrying the gun. They are divided into various subgroups:

- *Pointers and setters* locate and indicate where the game is stationed
- *Retrievers* retrieve the shot game, traditionally without damaging the carcass
- *Spaniels* are really pointing setters and will not only find the game but also put the fowl up for the gun
- ·HPR (hunt, point and retrieve) gundogs are multipurpose. They include Viszla, German Pointer and Weimeraner.

Gundog coats, whether short as in the Weimeraner or long and wavy as in setters and retrievers, tend to be of the low maintenance type, i.e. they do not mat easily and are generally waterproof so that the dog can withstand the worst weather the shooting season can bring.

The American Cocker Spaniel is an exception. Although derived from the English Cocker Spaniel with the typical gundog coat, the coat of the American Cocker Spaniel has been developed so that it is exaggeratedly bushy and would be a disadvantage in working in the rough in Britain. It is certainly not a low-maintenance coat.

The most popular Gundog breeds are Golden Retriever, Labrador, Cocker Spaniel, Springer Spaniel (both English and Welsh) and Weimeraner.

2.11 Terriers

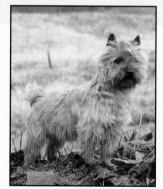
Cairn Terrier. © Marc Henrie ASC.

Terriers were originally bred to kill vermin. They can be thought of as canine pest control officers. Each breed may have a preference for a certain type of prey but they are all quick off the mark.

Terriers have been popular as pets for generations. Today Staffordshire Bull Terriers are probably the most popular. Scottish Terriers, West Highland Whites and Cairns are also very popular.

- Terriers are renowned for longevity
- They do not have large appetites and thus are economical to keep as pets
- They show variation in size from the Airedale Terrier, which is the largest, to the West Highland White Terrier and the Cairn Terrier, which are the smallest.
- The Yorkshire Terrier is a member of the Toy group, and so is not the smallest breed in the Terrier group.

Originally the Utility and the Working breeds formed one group but it became unwieldy as more breeds received recognition. It was therefore subdivided into the Working group and the Utility group. In 1999, for a similar reason, the Working Group was further subdivided into the primarily guarding breeds, which remained within the Working group, and the primarily herding breeds, which became the Pastoral group.

2.12 Working group

This now comprises the guarding dogs.

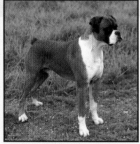
Boxer. © Marc Henrie ASC.

- It contains many popular and well-known breeds; for example, Boxer, Dobermann, Great Dane, Rottweiler and St Bernard
- Perhaps less well known Working breeds are Bernese Mountain Dog, Bullmastiff, Giant Schnauzer and Siberian Husky.
- The German Shepherd Dog is no longer a member of the Working group – it is now in the Pastoral group.

2.13 Pastoral group

This comprises all the herding and shepherding dogs.

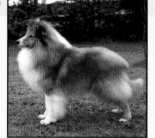
Shetland Sheepdog.
© Marc Henrie ASC.

- Obvious examples are Welsh Sheepdog, the collies, Old English Sheepdog and German Shepherd Dog
- Other examples are Samoyed, Shetland Sheep Dog and Lancashire Heeler.

2.14 Toy group

This contains all the small companion dogs. They are indoor dogs rather than used to living outside. Because of their small size their exercise requirements are not excessive.

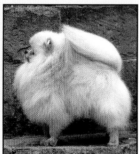
Pomeranian. © Marc Henrie ASC.

- Toy breeds make ideal companions in urban areas. They are easily carried and usually readily accepted on public transport
- Toy breeds are good pets for the infirm, the elderly and those with a sedentary lifestyle
- The current most popular Toy breed is the Cavalier King Charles Spaniel, whose show weight should not exceed 8 kg. With the Pekingese, it is one of the larger members of the group.

Toy group continues ▶

2.14 Toy group *continued*

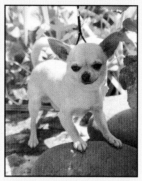
Chihuahua. © Marc Henrie ASC.

- After the King Charles, the next most popular Toy breeds are probably Yorkshire Terrier, Pekingese and Chihuahua
- The Chihuahua is the smallest member of the group, with a preferred show weight of 1–1.8 kg
- Other popular Toy dogs include Papillon, Pomeranian and Pug.

2.15 Utility group

The Utility group is similar to the AKC's Non-Sporting group. Paradoxically it is defined by what it is not: it contains all the breeds that do not fit comfortably into the other groups. Thus it is difficult to find a common theme by which the group can be recognized.

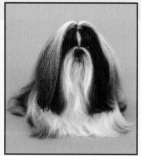
Shih Tzu. © Marc Henrie ASC.

- First and foremost, the Utility breeds are companion dogs, but many originally performed working, herding or sporting functions
- Most are originally foreign imports
- The four popular Tibetan breeds are included: Tibetan Spaniel, Tibetan Terrier, Lhasa Apso and Shih Tzu
- The Schnauzer and Miniature Schnauzer are included, although their temperament is closer to that of terriers
- Spitz breeds and the Chow Chow are in the Utility group
- Many brachycephalic dogs (i.e. those with foreshortened muzzles) are in this group, including British Bulldog, French Bulldog and the American counterpart: Boston Terrier
- The three sizes of Poodle are in the Utility group; Miniature and Toy Poodles are the most popular
- The famous carriage dog, the Dalmatian, is in the Utility group.

Inherited genetic defects

It is recognized that in some breeds there are problems of an inherited nature which have been unwittingly introduced while attempting to breed selectively for other desirable characteristics according to the breed standard. In consequence there are joint British Veterinary Association/ Kennel Club Health Schemes available that endeavour to control the problems.

The most common defects are the following.

- *Hip dysplasia* involves an abnormality of the hip joint leading to pain and crippling lameness at an early age. Under the Scheme, dogs over 1 year old are X-rayed in a standard position and a score is awarded. Breeders are urged to use only animals with a score well below the breed's mean score. There is also a scheme for a similar condition affecting the elbow

- *Eye defects* with different genetic origins affect many breeds. For testing under the Scheme, dogs are referred to a veterinary ophthalmologist appointed to a special BVA eye panel. Due to the varying age of onset (depending on the condition), annual retesting is advised. Irish Setter, collies, Labrador Retriever, Poodles and spaniels are among those affected
- *Conditions affecting the eyelids* can also affect certain breeds and are of a hereditary nature. These include entropion (in-turning) and ectropion (out-turning). Spaniels, bulldogs, Newfoundland and St Bernard are among the breeds affected
- *Merle colouring* (a pattern of coat colour consisting usually of patches of black on a lighter blue or grey background) can be associated with hearing and sight defects. In consequence, merle-coloured dogs (mainly collies) should never be mated together as this is likely to increase the incidence of abnormalities.

Puppy care

Preparation for a new arrival

Adequate preparations should be made for the new puppy (Figure 2.16).

It is imperative that the following are obtained from the breeder:

- Details of worming, vaccination and any medical history together with dates
- A precise diet sheet, including recommended quantities and type of food.

The diet sheet should be taken along on the first visit to the veterinary surgeon. Certain changes may be advised and ways to implement these can be discussed. A puppy is quickly upset by incorrect quantities of strange food fed at irregular times and this can result in chronic diarrhoea.

2.16 Preparation for a new puppy

- Food (only alter diet gradually)
- Suitable bed (consider cardboard box initially)
- Bedding (acrylic or small blankets)
- Supply of newspapers
- Bowls for food and water
- Collar, lead, brush and comb
- Towels and bathing utensils.

Development, behaviour and training of puppies

A 'timetable' of puppy development is outlined in Figure 2.17.

Early weeks

For the first 3 weeks of life the puppies and the bitch should be regarded as a single unit. The needs of the puppies revolve around food, warmth, rest, defecation and urination. There is a simple repertoire of reflex behaviour which dovetails with the instinctive maternal responses of the bitch. These include lying on her side in order to provide access to food supplies, licking ('topping and

tailing') the puppies to stimulate urination and defecation, and clearing up after her offspring. All responsible breeders try to ensure that there is little disruption of the bitch and puppies during these first vital 3 weeks.

Socialization

Socialization period

As the puppies develop sight and hearing, at around 3 weeks old, they start to explore and interact with each other. The period from 3 to 12 weeks is known as the socialization period and experiences acquired during this time can profoundly affect temperament and attitude of the puppy. For example, so-called singletons (single puppies in a litter), deprived of interaction with litter mates, may experience difficulties with other dogs in later life. This can also occur with puppies removed from a litter before they are 6 weeks old. Very dominant or subordinate puppies in the litter may show difficulties with other dogs, or people, when adult.

As the socialization period proceeds, the bitch spends less and less time with her puppies but her presence is advantageous to ensure emotional stability in the offspring. Puppies that are hand reared are often superb in their interaction with people but can exhibit bizarre behaviour with other dogs.

Nervousness

Puppies reared by excessively nervous bitches may show nervousness themselves. Therefore, contrary to the foregoing advice, this would be a good reason for early weaning. Unfortunately it is commonly believed in dog circles that breeding from a nervous bitch will calm her down – clearly little thought is given to the temperament of the puppies.

Puppies and people

It has been shown that puppies reared in a home environment are generally more confident with people than puppies reared in kennels. In order to establish well integrated pets in society, it is advisable for breeders to ensure that puppies are part of the family household from approximately 3 weeks of age. The puppies should be handled by as wide a range of people as possible, including men, women and children, and should be exposed to a wide variety of everyday household sights and sounds.

Puppies tend to be most inquisitive at around 5 weeks of age and therefore exposure to new experiences is most advantageous if arranged as early in the socialization process as possible.

2.17 Puppy development

Age of puppy	Development
0–3 weeks	Puppies and bitch are a single unit which should be disrupted as little as possible
Approx. 3 weeks	Puppies develop sight and hearing
3–12 weeks	Socialization period
18–24 months	Development continues to maturity, often up to 18–24 months

Puppies and other dogs

Although it is medically advantageous to isolate a puppy from other dogs until after vaccination, this is incompatible with socialization, which must be commenced much earlier than the 14 weeks of age at which the vaccinated puppy is considered to be safe.

The older puppy

From about 14 weeks of age the puppy tends to become less spontaneous in its reaction to new sights and sounds. Development, however, continues often up to the age of about 2 years.

Temperament testing

Temperament testing can be valuable in young puppies even while they are still in the primary socialization period (3–12 weeks) but one should recognize the limitations. Puppies should be observed as part of the litter (i.e. with the bitch) for sociability, playfulness and activity levels. Puppies showing signs of overactivity, uncontrollable biting or growling, shyness or nervousness will probably turn out to be unsuitable as family pets. Individual puppies can then be separated and assessed.

Toilet training

The mother instinctively toilet trains the puppy from an early age. As soon as the puppies are able to move about, the dam encourages them to urinate and defecate away from the nest. The new owner should continue this process. A change of surface (e.g. encouraging the puppy to use grass instead of the carpet or vinyl surfaces of the home) will reinforce the behaviour and ensure that early toilet training is established.

Novice owners are often confused regarding training. They are advised that it should start as early as possible, but they then find that training classes will not usually accept dogs until they are 4–6 months old. The confusion arises because these classes are for basic obedience training, which requires more maturity and is very different from early toilet 'programming' and socialization.

Socialization and early training

On leaving the litter the puppy has lost its source of food, warmth, comfort, playmates and companionship. Initially it is very important that there are not too many new experiences for the puppy to absorb all at once.

- Organize the bed and feeds, preferably in a quiet secluded area. A bed made from a cardboard box is a sensible choice initially
- Gradually introduce new noises and all the sounds of the new home. It is possible that the new puppy will never have experienced the sound of a television, telephone or washing machine
- Introduce toys gradually – puppies are great chewers
- Provide the puppy with its *own* toys; there are many commercially available and these are better than providing old shoes. To a puppy, the smell of a worn shoe will be the same whether it is one long since discarded or has only been worn once or twice – a puppy cannot be expected to differentiate.

Training cannot be accomplished quickly. To be successful it must be slow and methodical and is often tedious, but a well trained dog is ample reward.

Young puppies can be taught to sit from an early age but are incapable of exercising self-control. Thus they will sit in return for food reward but cannot be expected to remain sitting. This can only be taught at a later age. Early training can involve sitting on command, walking on a lead, coming when called.

Puppy classes

Veterinary practices can play an important role in providing puppy classes for clients. The primary role of the puppy class is to continue the socialization of the puppy with a variety of other dogs and people while the puppy is still young and receptive. The classes also provide a useful forum for the exchange of ideas and tips, and to demonstrate handling, training and certain products such as recommended foods and training aids.

Successful puppy classes have between four and eight puppies per instructor. Owners should be encouraged to ask about the behaviour and health of their puppies.

Weekly classes are ideal and owners should be encouraged to attend these until the puppies are about 14–16 weeks of age, when they can graduate to adult training classes. Details of adult classes should be available at the practice and can also be obtained from the information services of the local authority.

Play and exercise

Play and exercise should be part of the daily routine, not reserved just for weekends when the family has more time. The sessions are also an opportunity for interaction, which aids the bonding process and prevents unwanted attention-seeking behaviour. The younger the puppy, the more frequently repetitive the play sessions must be in order to be effective.

Owners should be advised that playing with their pets is a fundamental part of the bonding and training process, but certain precautions are necessary (Figure 2.18).

It is important that every member of the family is involved in play sessions and maintains control over the puppy. Children in particular should be encouraged to play with the puppy and to maintain gentle control. They should be taught that control does not mean punishment.

2.18 **Play precautions**

- Ensure that toys are large and sturdy enough to withstand chewing and cannot be swallowed or cause obstruction
- Do *not* give old shoes or discarded clothing – the puppy is unable to differentiate between 'his' shoe or scarf and yours
- Check toys regularly and discard when broken or worn
- Do not allow the puppy to become dominant by demanding a play session
- Examine mouth, ears and eyes as part of 'play' routine
- Give treats forcibly as part of routine to accustom puppy to administration of oral medicines later on.

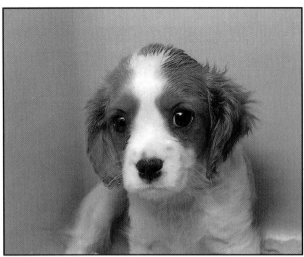

2.19 *A young King Charles Cavalier Spaniel. Photo: Trevor Turner.*

Handling a puppy

Puppies should be taught to accept and enjoy all forms of handling from family members from a very early age. This should involve:

- Lifting and carrying
- Grooming
- Examining every part of the body, particularly feet, ears, eyes and mouth.

The puppy should become used to having its mouth opened (forcible administration of enjoyable treats forms part of this routine) so that later on it will accept pill giving when this becomes necessary. It is important with any oral administration that the owner is taught the correct method so that pain or discomfort is avoided, otherwise the puppy may become mouth-shy. If this does occur it will take a long time before handling of the mouth or face will be tolerated with ease.

- Handling exercises can be structured to include handling of the face, feet, ears, skin and hair coat
- Once this is established the handling can be extended to include tooth brushing, grooming, nail trimming and grasping the muzzle and the nape of the neck
- These activities can then be extended to times when the puppy is eating or playing with a toy. 'Tablet' administration can be phased in at this stage
- If any of the handling results in signs of fear, resistance, threats or aggression, it should be noted so that training can be concentrated in this area – in a manner so mild that no anxiety is elicited
- Rewards in the form of food should very soon increase the puppy's tolerance. The level of interaction can then be increased when the puppy shows no fear
- Start off with very short sessions and increase the length and intensity as the puppy's confidence is gained.

Training is a slow continuous process, which can be tedious but if any attempt is made to rush the process it is unlikely to be successful.

Confinement in a pen or cage

Puppies in the home engage in destructive behaviour, particularly if bored. The simplest form of prevention involves separating the puppy so that the behaviour cannot be expressed.

Owners frequently feel that confinement in a cage is cruel but it is less inhumane than owners sometimes being driven to lose their temper with the puppy on returning home and finding that wholesale expensive destruction has taken place.

Training to a pen or cage is an excellent way to curb many behaviour problems, including house soiling, destructiveness, digging, escaping, chewing of furniture and carpets and raiding dustbins.

Training by using a cage or crate

Folding wire 'puppy pens' are available from all major pet shops and are also widely advertised in the dog press. They are convenient since they can be collapsed for easy storage when not in use and are available in various sizes, up to approximately 1 m x 1 m x 1 m.

For smaller puppies, plastic carrying crates (which are easily cleaned) can be used. The following guidelines apply:

- The crate or cage should not be regarded as a prison for the puppy
- As a training aid it can be used to confine the puppy for periods during the day and can also be used as a sleeping area
- These confinement periods should never exceed 3–4 hours at any one time
- The puppy can be encouraged to use the confined area by placing food there and the prison concept can easily be dispelled by tossing food into the area and getting the puppy to go in to fetch it
- Lavish praise should be used when the puppy enters of its own accord, together with food rewards as appropriate
- Initially confinement periods should be as short as possible but it is important not to allow the pet out if it is barking or whining. Try to distract the puppy's attention with a sharp noise or even a food reward. When it is quiet, even if only for a few seconds, open the cage.

Toilet training with a cage

The cage is a great aid to toilet training since it can be used as a substitute for the nest. From 3 to 4 weeks of age puppies attempt to avoid soiling their nest. The puppy must be taken out of the cage frequently in order that toilet training can progress, but avoid removing the puppy when it is whining or demanding to be released. Only a few seconds of quietness are necessary in order to establish that the owner rather than the puppy is in control. Food rewards and voice act as deterrents to the puppy's demands to be released. Once the puppy is quiet, release it immediately. When it is voiding appropriately, use a command word which will become associated with the act.

Collars and leads

A puppy should be trained to accept a collar and lead from 6 weeks of age onwards. A light puppy collar and lead and a game around the living room are all that is required initially. Later on, when attending obedience classes, a check collar or head collar might be advised (Figure 2.20).

2.20 Collars and leads

- Collar should be adjusted loosely enough to be comfortable but not loose enough to be pulled over the head
- Traditionally of leather but modern collars often of nylon material, which is strong, durable and hygienic
- Collar should be broad rather than narrow.

Check collars and chains can be useful in training but must be used with caution since they can cause injury if used harshly.

Slip leads: collar and lead are continuous. Similar to check collar. The collar (or loop if continuous) must be applied correctly so that the collar or 'noose' around the neck slackens as soon as neck pressure is reduced.

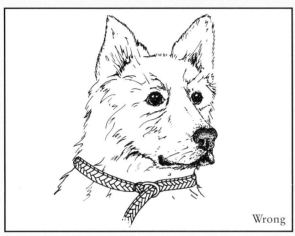

Wrong

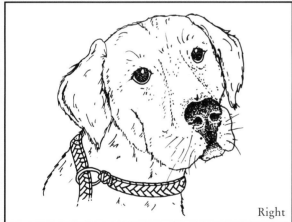

Right

Check collar.

General care of the dog

Regular exercise, feeding, grooming and veterinary check-ups are just as essential for the adult dog as for the puppy.

Veterinary care

Contact with a veterinary surgeon should be established as soon as possible and is usually made at inoculation. The puppy can be immunized against several diseases (Figure 2.21) including infectious bronchitis. All these diseases require regular boosting of immunity and the veterinary surgeon will give advice regarding frequency.

Regular medical check-ups are also required and

2.21 Vaccination

Routine vaccination is normally provided against:

- Distemper (canine distemper virus)
- Infectious canine hepatitis (canine adenovirus 1)
- Canine enteritis (parvovirus)
- Kennel cough (canine adenovirus 2, canine parainfluenza virus)
- Leptospirosis (*Leptospira icterohaemorrhagiae, Leptospira canicola*)

for most adult dogs this is usually twice a year. Teeth, eyes, ears, heart and lungs are checked, advice is given on routine worming and appropriate medication is prescribed. Any concerns regarding behaviour, feeding, weight problems, exercise, etc. should be discussed at this time.

Grooming

Grooming is necessary for all dogs, irrespective of coat length. With heavy-coated breeds (e.g. Old English Sheepdog) it can be very time-consuming.

- Grooming is not only concerned with the coat – it involves attention to skin, feet, ears and eyes as well
- As a result of grooming, the dog looks and feels better and there is good skin health
- Regular and careful grooming plays a role in the human/ pet bond, for which body contact is a vital part
- Grooming also gently asserts owner dominance
- The regular routine of grooming alerts the owner to any problems so that veterinary advice can be sought at an early stage.

More details on grooming are given in Chapter 6. There is a wide range of grooming equipment available (Figure 2.22) but seek veterinary or breed specialist advice before selection.

- Short-coated dogs probably only need grooming a couple of times a week with a slicker and brush
- Heavy-coated breeds need daily grooming to prevent hair matting, which is unpleasant for the dog. More specialized grooming equipment is required (see Figure 2.22)
- Many terriers need stripping, since clipping softens the coat and will not help any potential show career. If exhibition is intended advice should be sought from an expert at an early stage
- Provided grooming is carried out regularly, most dogs enjoy it. Start the puppy off at an early age and make it a game.

Bathing

Too frequent bathing removes natural oils from the coat but specially formulated shampoos and conditioners are available (see Chapter 6). Anti-parasitic shampoos, widely used for flea control, have the disadvantage of lack of residual effect to prevent reinfestation. Flea control with sprays or spot-on preparations should be considered.

2.22 Basic grooming equipment

Equipment	Uses and comments	Short coats[1]	Long coats
Bristle brush	Unlikely to damage coat Useful for cleaning short-haired dogs and putting finish on longer coats Flexible bristles cannot penetrate thick coats	✓	✓
Pin brush	Useful for longer coats Used gently, will penetrate better than bristles because less flexible and will not damage hair		✓
Slicker brush	Hooks assist in pulling out dead hair Useful for undercoat but care is necessary	✓	
Hound glove	Useful for removing dead undercoat in short-coated breeds	✓	
Rubber-toothed brush	Gentle and well tolerated Useful for general grooming	✓	
Combs	Handled combs generally easier to use, particularly for long periods		✓
Rake comb	Useful for dematting Care necessary Can cause pain and injury to skin		✓
Dematting comb	Used to cut through dense mats Instruction in use essential		✓
Stripping comb	Used principally for trimming terriers	✓	✓

1 – Wash leather or piece of silk for final gloss.
For detailed descriptions of grooming equipment, see Chapter 6.

Ears

Ears should be inspected regularly when grooming. If irritation or an accumulation of wax or hair is apparent, a veterinary surgeon should be consulted. Ear disease often starts with mild scratching or head shaking, followed by smell or discharge.

Eyes

Dogs with very prominent eyes suffer from tear overflow and staining. If neglected, this can lead to infection and eczema. Veterinary advice should be sought if necessary.

Mouth and teeth

The mouth and teeth should be checked when grooming. Some breeds (e.g. spaniels) often have deep skinfolds around the lower lip and these can become infected. If the problem is extensive, seek veterinary advice.

Convenience foods, with the concomitant lack of gnawing and chewing, may encourage a build-up of dental calculus (tartar). Without regular inspection of the mouth, halitosis is often the first sign. Special 'chews' and foods are available that help to alleviate the problem (see section on dry diets in this chapter).

Anogenital hygiene

Part of the grooming routine should include checking anal and genital areas. Most dogs take care of their own intimate hygiene but soiling is not uncommon in heavy-coated dogs. Diarrhoea, urinary infections, genital diseases and senility all exacerbate the problem.

Some dogs (e.g. Yorkshire Terrier) can be prone to faecal mats across the anus, preventing further defecation. This is unpleasant for dog and owner. Daily inspection, and cleaning if necessary, is recommended, especially with elderly dogs.

Beds

Beds and bedding suitable for all types of adult dogs are compared in Figure 2.23.

2.23 Beds and bedding

Type	Advantages and disadvantages
Beds	
Wicker basket	Traditional Difficult to clean and deflea Easily destroyed
Plastic moulded beds	Modern version of traditional basket Hygienic and available in wide range of sizes and colours Recommended
Soft beds	Traditionally shaped and made from foam and plastic Liked by owners and dogs Suitable for smaller or elderly dogs Easily chewed Can be washed
Metal-framed beds	Popular with medium-sized and larger dogs Difficult for some dogs to get into
Bedding	
Acrylic fur fabric	Hard-wearing and hygienic Recommended
Fabric-covered foam pads	Give good support Washable Chewable
Bean bags	Liked by elderly animals Easily destroyed Can be 'arranged' by dog Waterproof covers are available
Blankets	Traditional Warm and cosy Chewable Difficult to launder

Signs of illness

Signs of illness include lassitude, skin irritation and scratching, inappetence, polyuria (frequent urination) and diarrhoea.

Lassitude

Dogs vary in their activity level according to breed and disposition. Many normal dogs sleep for up to 16 hours a day; puppies and older dogs may sleep even longer.

Excessive scratching

Healthy dogs will scratch occasionally but excessive licking, scratching and nibbling may be a sign of disease.

Inappetence

Lack of appetite may be a sign of illness. Most dogs have a good appetite but bitches in whelp or in a phantom pregnancy will often eat less.

Urination

Bitches urinate less frequently than dogs, except when in oestrus (heat). Male dogs usually urinate (empty the bladder, in contrast to depositing small quantities of urine to mark territory) at least three times a day. More frequent urination, particularly with straining, may be a sign of ill health.

Defecation

From once to four times a day can be normal, depending on age, breed and diet. A greater frequency, even without a change in consistency, can be a sign of illness.

Diarrhoea

This is an increase in frequency and volume with an unformed stool. The term is often used incorrectly to describe a loose stool, which may be due to environmental factors such as stress and temperature coupled with the dog's innate habit of devouring scarcely edible food.

Respiration and temperature

Temperature and the rate and rhythm of respiration give indications of health. Normal rates are shown in Figure 2.24. An excited dog can have a temperature of 40°C and a heart rate of 80–100 beats per minute.

Rectal temperature should be taken with a lubricated thermometer inserted for the appropriate time. A suitable thermometer (either mercury or electronic) should be part of the pet's own first aid kit (Figure 2.25).

Other signs

Warm dry nose

A warm dry nose should not be considered a sign of ill health – dogs frequently have warm dry noses in centrally heated homes.

Doggy odours

A 'doggy' smell may indicate that a problem is present. There are many causes for this odour – ear or skin disease, bad teeth, anal or genital problems and severe systemic disease. If the odour persists after bathing and grooming, a trip to the veterinary surgery is indicated.

Obesity

Healthy dogs, irrespective of their breed, should not be obese (Figure 2.26). The skin should be supple and move freely over well defined muscles. If the dog is getting fat, seek professional advice. There are many specialized diets available.

2.24 Normal values in the dog

Temperature:	38.3–38.7°C
Heart rate:	60–140 beats per minute
Respiratory rate:	10–30 breaths per minute

2.25 First aid box

It is always worth having a pet's first aid box separate from the family's first aid kit. In this way everything is readily to hand in an emergency. Essential contents should include:

- Thermometer
- Scissors
- Tweezers (for grass seeds)
- Assorted bandages and dressings
- Adhesive tape for fixing dressings
- Cotton wool
- Cotton buds
- Suitable antiseptic
- Muzzle (bandage can be used)
- Pen torch
- Hand magnifying glass.

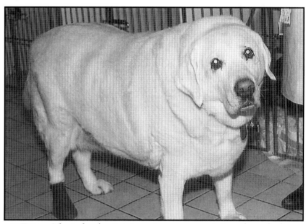

2.26 *The Labrador Retriever is a common victim of overfeeding.*

Breeding

Having acquired a dog and enjoyed the experience, owners often think of breeding. This should be considered very carefully. Rescue centres are full of mongrel, crossbred and purebred dogs that are no longer wanted. Is it right to bring more dogs into the world when faced with so many unwanted animals? This is a particular problem in respect of mongrel or crossbred litters.

A litter of puppies can be fun and is instructive, and many families will breed just one litter in order to share the experience, particularly if there are children involved. Before deciding on such a course discuss the matter with the professionals – dog breeders, veterinary surgeons and other experienced dog owners. The lovable family of little puppies will soon grow up and it is essential that good homes are guaranteed, otherwise some may become rescue dogs.

Two misconceptions concerning breeding are:

- A nervous bitch will become more stable following a litter
- Mating a highly sexed male dog will reduce sex urge.

Both statements are untrue.

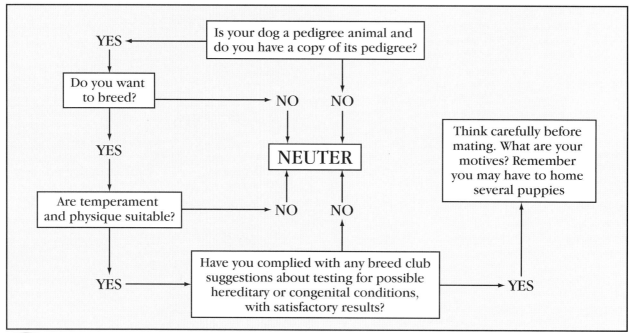

In the UK, professional breeders are controlled under the Breeding of Dogs Act. This requires premises to be licensed when more than two bitches are kept for the purposes of breeding for sale (Chapter 10).

Many owners elect to keep a bitch in preference to a dog because they are more companionable, more biddable, less likely to roam and are generally less aggressive towards other dogs. The disadvantage is the 6-monthly oestrus or heat period, which lasts for approximately 3 weeks. This is when the bitch is attractive to male dogs and will allow mating. Most bitches come into season for the first time when they are approximately 6–7 months of age (range, 4–24 months). For the majority of bitches oestrus recurs every 6 months but some large breeds may only cycle every 12–18 months, whereas some toy breeds cycle every 3–4 months.

Neutering

If it is decided not to breed, sterilization should be considered (Figure 2.27).

With pet dogs, many veterinary surgeons do advise neutering, especially for pets kept in an essentially urban or suburban environment. Neutering reduces wanderlust in male dogs, reduces aggressive behaviour and makes the animal more companionable and biddable. In bitches it eliminates the inconvenience of oestrus (heat).

Neutering is advocated by the majority of rescue organizations in order to reduce the number of unwanted puppies. It is routinely practised by most organizations with service dogs, such as Guide Dogs for the Blind, Hearing Dogs for Deaf People and Dogs for the Disabled.

Sterilization can be by chemical means, using synthetic hormones, or by irreversible surgery.

Mismating

Despite every care some bitches will be accidentally mismated when in heat. Should this occur, do not delay. Veterinary treatment is available that will avert unwanted pregnancy but the need for treatment is urgent. Depending on the factors involved, termination and

neutering may be possible. The veterinary surgeon will advise.

Whelping

- Pregnancy lasts approximately 63 days (range 57–70)
- Immediately prior to whelping the bitch may be restless and off her food, and may start bedmaking. This is the first stage
- Once the bitch starts to strain forcefully (second stage) a puppy should be born within one hour. If it is not, veterinary advice should be sought
- Anterior and posterior presentation (puppy delivered forwards or backwards) are normal in the dog
- Often the placenta (afterbirth) is not expelled after each puppy but two or three may be expelled together. Bitches instinctively eat the placenta
- Fetal fluids in the bitch are often green or brown
- It is worth consulting a veterinary surgeon within 24 hours of whelping.

Care of the elderly dog

Life expectancy in the dog ranges from 7–10 years in bulldogs and some giant breeds to practically double that in some spaniels and small terriers. Like people, dogs are generally living longer, due to modern developments in health care and nutrition.

Signs of senility

With the onset of senility dogs have a capacity for deep and prolonged sleep. Care should be taken when they are in this state: if disturbed they may wake with a start and snap at the nearest object.

There are many ways of making life more comfortable for the elderly dog (summarized in Figure 2.28):

- Rapid and extreme *temperature changes* should be avoided. An old dog spending all day in a warm living room should not be shut in a cold outhouse at night

2.28 Care of the elderly dog

- Boost inoculations regularly, according to manufacturer's instructions
- Avoid rapid temperature changes
- Avoid stress of boarding if possible
- Avoid obesity
- Check for pressure sores
- Do not allow to stray at exercise
- Groom regularly and check nails, ears and teeth
- Do not over exercise
- Check water intake frequently.

- Avoid *boarding* if possible. This may precipitate terminal illness due to stress
- Regular reinforcement of protection against the preventable diseases, according to manufacturer's instructions, is well worthwhile
- Take advice regarding *diet* from your veterinary surgeon. As joints stiffen and exercise becomes more difficult, ensure that the dog does not become obese. Obesity is often a problem due to reduced exercise because of stiffness
- Check for *bed sores* over bony prominences in contact with ground when resting. They are often difficult to heal
- Ensure that the old dog does not *stray* too far when at exercise. It can easily become disorientated due to deteriorating sight, smell and hearing. Fetch the dog rather than call when out at exercise
- Check *teeth and gums* regularly for signs of disease and infection
- Check and trim overgrown *nails* regularly. Frequent attention will make walking more comfortable
- With the onset of senility, dogs often become *apprehensive*, craving owner's company. Disorientation and restlessness often also occur. If concerned, seek veterinary advice: medication is available that can help.
- *Hearing* acuity is lost with age. Often the old dog becomes more vocal, or fails to come when called
- Ensure the dog is not *overexercised*. Most old dogs, eager to start the walk, do not have the stamina to finish. Reduce the length and duration of the exercise
- Monitor *water intake* and seek veterinary advice if an increase noted
- Offer *food* in smaller more frequent meals.
- Old dogs often have *arthritis*: a shallower feeding dish sometimes helps in the case of a stiff neck, as does raising the dish off the floor for a taller dog.

Feeding dogs

Dogs, like all living animals, require food on a regular basis in order to stay alive. The food also has to provide a correct diet for the animal to remain healthy.

If there are any doubts regarding the quality of nutrition supplied to a dog, the type of food that should be fed or the water intake, a veterinary surgeon should be consulted. Advice is freely available in this highly specialized area.

 Any changes made to a dog's diet must be introduced gradually, in a slow and controlled fashion. In this way, bowel upsets are more likely to be avoided.

Nutrients

Food contains a complex collection of raw materials called nutrients. A nutrient is any food constituent that helps to support life. This is commonly interpreted as providing energy and consequently nutrients are usually thought of as fats, carbohydrates or proteins. However, supplying energy is only one function of a nutrient. They are essential for all body functions, including the formation and repair of structural components such as muscles and bones, and also the cells lining the bowel, all of which require constant renewal.

In addition, nutrients play a part in the transportation of substances into, around and out of the body.

Nutrients are divided into six basic classes:

- Water
- Carbohydrates
- Proteins
- Fats
- Minerals
- Vitamins.

Some nutrients are involved in all body functions except the production of energy. Water and some of the minerals are examples.

Others, including vitamins, minerals and (most importantly) water, provide the necessary substances to initiate and effect repair of tissues and aid the complex processes involved in maintaining the structure and function of the body.

Vitamins are essential for most of the metabolic (chemical) reactions that take place within the body.

Some nutrients are not capable of being manufactured within the body and are therefore 'essential', i.e. they must be provided in the food the dog eats. Others are 'non-essential', in that the body will manufacture them from other nutrients supplied in the food.

- The science of *nutrition* is the understanding of these complex processes.
- *Digestion* is the name given to the chemical process whereby food that has been eaten is broken down in the gut into simple compounds which can be absorbed and used by the body for any of the processes described. Unlike cud-chewing animals such as the cow, the dog has a relatively simple digestive tract. It can deal with most foodstuffs but, unlike the ruminant, it cannot break down complex plant materials such as cellulose.
- *Absorption* is the transport of the products of digestion across the wall of the gut and into the body. Both the circulatory and the lymphatic systems play a part.

Minerals

Some nutrients are only required in very minute quantities. These include minerals. Essential minerals can be divided into two groups, depending on their concentration in the diet:

- The major or macrominerals include calcium, phosphorus, sodium, potassium and magnesium and are usually required in milligram quantities
- The so-called trace elements, or microminerals, are only required in microgram quantities; they include iron, copper, zinc, manganese and iodine, all of which are essential for the body to function but need only be present in minute quantities.

Calcium

The balance of minerals in the diet is just as important as the range and absolute quantity available. For example, if puppies of the larger breeds are oversupplemented with calcium, the calcium/phosphorus ratio (Ca/P ratio) becomes disturbed. Since these two elements are closely linked, both nutritionally and metabolically, problems can arise resulting in serious deformities affecting the growing bones, most commonly those of the limbs.

For generations dogs were traditionally fed the scraps from the table and these usually consisted of a random collection of nutrients which could result in nutritional imbalances. Dogs depicted in some of the portraits painted in the 17th and 18th centuries show bizarre limb angulations.

Traditionally, well fed dogs were given raw meat. Today it is known that raw meat is seriously lacking in calcium. If raw meat is fed to a puppy without any supplementation it is likely to result in serious and irreversible bone deformities – which could well be the reason for the odd postures of some of the dogs depicted in the paintings.

Food processing

Some nutrients are destroyed by processing, particularly if high temperatures are involved.

- Proteins (essential building blocks for growth and repair of muscle and tissues) can be denatured or destroyed if overheated
- Some vitamins are thermolabile and will be destroyed by cooking. This applies to vitamin A and some of the vitamins of the B complex.

On the other hand, certain foods are improved by cooking. Starch, for example, is relatively indigestible for the dog but if it is cooked it is partially converted into sugars which are a useful form of energy that the dog can utilize.

Raw fish such as herrings are oily and a good source of energy but contain an enzyme called thiaminase, which destroys thiamine (vitamin B_1). This is a necessary dietary nutrient in the dog and helps to provide a metabolic pathway making available some of the energy from the food that is digested. Cooking the fish destroys the thiaminase. Overprocessing during canning can also destroy this important vitamin.

Eggs, perhaps one of the best sources of protein available, should always be fed cooked since raw egg white contains the enzyme avidin, which destroys the B vitamin biotin. Cooking destroys this enzyme.

Types of pet food

There are two major types of food fed to dogs:

- Home-prepared
- Commercially produced.

Home-prepared fresh foods and commercially prepared foods all have advantages and disadvantages, summarized in Figure 2.29.

Homemade foods

Dogs can be fed nutritious and highly palatable homemade diets if the owner is willing to spend the necessary time, money and care in selecting and preparing the food. It is frequently difficult to produce a balanced diet, because the owner's criteria may not be based on sound nutritional guidelines. For example:

- Fresh foods are often highly palatable because they are prepared from ingredients that the owner perceives the animal likes best
- In some cases, the owner chooses ingredients that are the least expensive.

In the long run homemade foods often prove to be more expensive and sometimes, despite every effort, remain seriously unbalanced.

Commercial dog foods

Recent surveys have shown that over 90% of dog owners in this country feed commercially prepared foods as at least the main part of the diet.

2.29 Advantages and disadvantages of various types of dog food

Type	Advantages	Disadvantages
Fresh	Highly palatable	Difficult to balance Labour intensive to prepare
Frozen prepared	Highly palatable Well balanced Usually complete, only need thawing	Takes up freezer space
Canned	No refrigeration Durable container Vermin proof Highly palatable Highly digestible	Expensive means of preservation Heavy to handle Opened cans need refrigeration
Semi-moist	No refrigeration Palatable Easy to handle	Need refrigeration once opened Humectants can cause diarrhoea
Dry	No refrigeration Long shelf life even when opened Energy dense, contain only 10% water	May have low fat content May not be palatable to some dogs, especially small breeds Some vitamins may be destroyed in processing Digestibility lower

These are generally available as:

- Dry (moisture content 5–12%)
- Semi-moist (moisture content 15–50%)
- Canned (moisture content 72–85%)
- Frozen (moisture content 60–80%).

Whatever their form, commercially prepared pet foods may be formulated and sold as either the whole or part of the diet.

- *Complete foods* are formulated to provide all the necessary nutrients with the exception of water
- *Complementary foods* are sufficient for all the animal's nutritional needs only if used in combination with other foods, which are often stated on the label.

Thus complementary foods may be rich in some nutrients but lacking in others. Usually complementary foods are intended to provide a relatively cheap source of energy (e.g. dog biscuits). As such, they can be used to complement the low-energy/high-protein content of most canned dog meats.

Frozen foods

- Frozen foods are similar to fresh foods in that they are usually highly palatable
- They are usually well balanced and are often complete foods
- They have the advantage of needing little preparation other than thawing
- Their major disadvantage is that they need specialized storage and take up valuable freezer space.

Canned foods

- Canned foods require no refrigeration
- They have a durable container that is not easily penetrated by rodents (as can occur with some dry and semi-moist foods when stored in outhouses or garages)
- Their ingredients are usually highly palatable and more digestible than most dry foods
- They are an expensive form of preservation of food
- Each can contains on average 75% water
- They are heavy and difficult to handle
- The contents of any opened cans will quickly spoil if not kept in a refrigerator.

Semi-moist foods

- Semi-moist foods require no refrigeration
- They are almost as palatable as canned food but contain only about 25% water
- Packaging allows easy handling
- The contents deteriorate quickly once the package is opened if not refrigerated
- They contain humectants (moisture retainers) which can cause digestive upsets in some dogs.

Dry foods

- Dry foods are rapidly becoming the most popular form of commercial dog food, particularly for the larger breeds
- Their packaging allows easy handling

- They require no refrigeration
- They have reasonably long shelf lives
- They do not spoil once the package is opened
- They have more nutrients and energy in relation to weight than any other commercial dog food
- On average they contain only approximately 10% moisture and are therefore more economical than foods with a higher moisture content
- If fed dry they have been shown to reduce dental calculus significantly. Development of this property has led to the production of special dry formulations specifically designed to aid oral heath; these products can be obtained both in dry pelleted forms and as food treats, and are safer than bones, which have customarily been used for this purpose
- Without protectants, the fat in dry food will become rancid
- Some dry foods may be too low in fat, which is the natural energy source for the dog. All the major dog food manufacturers are actively addressing this area but it is always important to check the label with any commercial food, dry or otherwise
- The processing and dehydration of dry foods may destroy some of the vitamins
- Palatability of dry foods is often lower than that of other forms of commercial food, particularly for smaller dogs
- Dry foods are easily contaminated by insects and other vermin
- If stored in damp situations they soon become unusable.

Frequency of feeding

- When suckling, puppies feed almost continuously for the first 7–10 days of life. As they develop, the bitch will leave them for increasingly longer periods
- When the puppies are ready to leave the bitch at 6 weeks of age, they should be receiving 4–6 meals a day
- As the puppy grows, the quantity of food should be increased and the frequency decreased so that at 6 months three meals are being fed each day
- This is reduced to two meals a day at approximately 9 months of age
- By the time the dog is mature (which can be from 1 to 2 years of age, depending on breed or type) it can be given one main meal a day.

The above timetable can only be a guide and will depend on many factors:

- Breed or type of dog and associated activity levels (temperament is important – very active or excitable animals burn up energy more quickly and this needs replenishing more frequently, particularly in the young animal)
- Age of dog
- Type and quality of food
- Method of feeding
  - Free choice or ad lib feeding, with food and water always available, is suitable only for a minority of adult dogs that do not overeat
  - Portion-control feeding offered at set times once or twice a day is the most usual method of feeding the pet dog
- Health of the dog (certain conditions, e.g. convalescence, are helped with frequent small meals).

Water

Water is required in greater quantities than all the other nutrients – about two to three times the total dry matter requirements. It is found everywhere in the body and comprises approximately 70% of the total body weight of the dog. It is involved in all the important body functions.

Dogs require approximately 50 ml water/kg body weight per day and it is obtained from several sources:

- 'Metabolic' water – produced when carbohydrates, fats and proteins are broken down by the body
- In the food – fresh and canned food contains approximately 75% water, but dry food only about 10%
- Fluid drunk.

Dehydration is more serious than starvation. It is essential that a plentiful supply of clean drinking water is always available.

If fed a dry complete diet, a dog will appear to be drinking excessively compared with dogs fed fresh or canned food.

Food and water bowls

There are may different types of food and water containers, ranging from disposable to virtually indestructible stainless steel. The ideal container should be:

- Resistant to tipping and chewing by the dog
- Sturdy and unbreakable
- Sufficiently heavy to prevent sliding when the dog is eating
- Relatively silent on the floor surface if it does move
- Resistant to chipping and scratching and to normal disinfectants, boiling water, etc.
- Easy to clean and capable of thorough disinfection, including boiling if required.

Stainless steel is probably the most suitable material at present but it does have the disadvantage of being noisy when the bowl is pushed around on the floor. Large and giant breeds, dogs with arthritic and other conditions may benefit from having bowls raised off the floor. Appropriate stands are commercially available.

Normal canine behaviour

Dogs are social animals and this has contributed to their success in domestication. Pack animals will often form attachments within the pack and these are communicated by signals involving touching, looking and vocalization – similar to those used by people, which makes ownership of a dog very rewarding.

Because dogs are so close to us we tend to anthropomorphize, that is, we endow dogs with our own feelings. There are differences in communication pathways between people and dogs and these can lead to misunderstanding.

Dominance hierarchy

Dominance plays a large part in relationships between pack animals. As dogs reach adulthood (usually at about 2 years of age) many of them attempt to assert their dominance within the pack. Should they be family pets and the 'pack' in this case involves other members of the family, serious problems can arise.

The dominance hierarchy reduces physical conflict between pack members; there are consistent pack rules concerning sharing of resources, especially food. Without the hierarchy, there would be conflict and loss of the pack infrastructure.

Signs of dominance

With some dogs, dominant signals are obvious for even the most naive owner – for example, growling when any member of the family approaches the dog's resting or feeding areas. Other signals are more subtle. For example, the dog that continually craves attention and is continuously petted, fed or let out will assume that the family is subordinate. If there is then what the dog perceives as attempted dominance, such as serious grooming or putting the dog on a lead, problems can arise.

Some dogs may never show any aggression but still consider themselves to be the dominant member of the family pack. Excessive barking is an example. Other dogs may never be aggressive towards any member of the family but become excessively protective: strangers such as the postman, invading what is considered to be pack (family) territory, can be the subject of uncharacteristic barking and aggression.

Unacceptable dominance

Dogs that are dominant in these ways are also often very hard to control. Some breeds, particularly those of the pastoral group such as sheepdogs, collies and German Shepherd Dogs kept as pets, and also guarding dogs such as Boxers, Dobermanns and Rottweilers, can become unacceptably dominant even at a young age. Puppies that show signs of aggression at 8–12 weeks when presented for vaccination can be particularly difficult if owners are inexperienced in reading the subtle signs. Young puppies that growl when being picked up or groomed are showing abnormal signs but many owners think this is amusing behaviour.

It is essential to ensure that the family, not the dog, is always dominant.

Instinct

Many facets of canine behaviour are traditionally considered instinctive. Instinct is a spontaneous act or automatic response without thought and prior learning. A puppy instinctively finds the nipple. A neonate (newly born puppy), if separated from dam and litter mates, will crawl slowly in a circle to make contact with the nipple, dam or other puppies. This is an instinctive response, although behaviourists refer to it as a behaviour pattern, part of which may be inherent, i.e. instinctive, and part acquired as a result of learning.

Reflexes

Reflexes are responses that always result from the same stimulus. They can be simple and basic – scratching in response to an itch. This can occur without the dog even knowing it is happening (dogs will scratch while asleep). With other reflexes the brain has to be involved: a dog will eat when it is hungry but it cannot eat while asleep. Behaviour patterns can be complex mixtures of different reflexes.

Behaviour patterns

Normal canine behaviour is extremely complex. Think of normal canine actions – wagging tails, rising hackles, lapping tongues, scratching the ground with the hind feet after elimination, turning round several times before lying down to rest, etc. Frequently owners will ask, 'Why does my dog do that?' These are common behaviour patterns, whether instinctive or acquired, and are present in all dogs.

Inherent behaviour in breeds

Some breeds have stronger inherent behaviours than others. Thus terriers and hounds are likely to chase rabbits but bulldogs or a Pug are less likely to do so. Inherited behaviour patterns are usually simple and vary from breed to breed. Consider eating, drinking, guarding and herding as examples:

- Dachshunds and Labradors are notoriously greedy eaters
- Sheepdogs are great herders
- Setters are not usually greedy and are not very concerned with herding.

Some complex behaviour patterns are inherited and can be developed with training. Thus sheepdogs become even better herding dogs with training, but any amount of training would be unlikely to make a Pug a good farm dog. Similarly, Greyhounds inherently chase hares but only careful and intensive training results in a winning dog. German Shepherd Dogs and Dobermanns have extremely strong guarding instincts which they combine with aggressiveness if their territory is invaded; this instinct is enhanced with training and becomes a behaviour pattern.

Physical attributes

Normal canine behaviour also partially depends on physical attributes. Bull Terriers have immensely strong jaws: when fighting they grab, hold and attempt to crush. Greyhounds, with lighter jaws, dash in and out when fighting, slashing and tearing as they run.

Intelligence

Intelligence may be an inheritable trait. American Pit Bull Terriers, Welsh Sheepdogs and German Shepherd Dogs have reputations for outstanding trainability (Figure 2.30) and are considered to be more intelligent than other dogs. However, studies have indicated that there is little or no difference in the intelligence of the various breeds.

Predatory behaviour

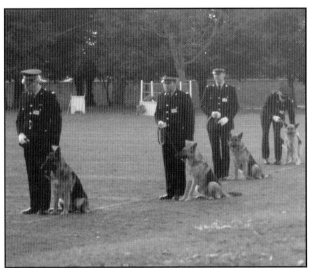

2.30 *German Shepherd Dogs with their police handlers. Courtesy of S. Dallas.*

Family dogs, although basically predators, will integrate with family animals such as cats or rabbits but there are exceptions. For example, some dogs do not like cats: they may tolerate the family cat but any other cat on their territory will be unwelcome. Some dogs are perfectly reliable with the pet rabbit when the family is present but may well try to kill it when unsupervised.

Eating and drinking behaviour

Dogs are naturally sporadic eaters. Killing prey is a pack effort. After eating the prey, dogs will rest until hungry again, when once more they will hunt as a pack.

For predators, unlike grazing animals, food is not freely available and therefore the majority of dogs will overeat given the opportunity. It is therefore not surprising that pet dogs suffer problems of obesity and that ad lib feeding is satisfactory for only a few.

In the pack situation the dominant dog, the pack leader, will eat his fill first. Pet dogs must be trained to be always subordinate during family meals. A sign of dominance by the dog is growling during eating if approached by other family members.

Defecation and normal elimination behaviour

Behaviour patterns accompanying defecation and urination are linked with both sexual behaviour and communication. Male dogs mark their territory by urinating and defecating. Information about other dogs is received by investigating elimination odours such as those of in-season bitches in the proximity.

This organized communication system does not allow for random elimination of faeces and urine. Both sexes follow well set routines which, once established, can be difficult to alter even with intensive training. If the lounge carpet becomes established as the place for elimination, it will be difficult to break the pet of the habit and the residual scent may attract other visiting dogs.

Leg cocking

When urinating, it is normal for male dogs to stand with one leg lifted (cocked). Urination is usually against a vertical surface and the urine is deposited at approximately nose level. Male sex hormones influence this activity and it is also learned from other dogs.

Some male dogs do not learn to cock their legs until fully mature, at 18–24 months of age, and a few normal males never adopt the habit. On the other hand, castration of a leg-cocking male may not result in loss of the habit. In some dogs the behaviour is so strong that even if they lose a hindleg they will still attempt to cock the other leg, balancing on their forelegs if necessary.

Urine marking is also used to indicate possession. This explains the behaviour of the dog that soils its owner's possessions or clothing. Also male dogs will often urinate over the urine of another dog, presumably to mask the smell.

Uncontrolled elimination

Faeces also carry distinctive scents – including that from the anal sacs, which may be emptied in fright. Startled dogs of both sexes will often urinate and defecate involuntarily. This is part of the body's 'fight and flight' reflex, ensuring that the animal is as light as possible, which makes it easier to fight or run.

When dogs show extreme submissive behaviour they

often dribble urine, simultaneously rolling over and raising one leg, exposing the inguinal region. Scolding exacerbates the situation.

Some dogs will lose control and urinate when excited, particularly if immature. Under stress, basic house training can be lost; urination and sometimes defecation in inappropriate places can result.

Elimination behaviour in puppies

Newborn puppies cannot control their basic functions. Defecation and urination are controlled by the bitch, who stimulates them by licking ('topping and tailing'). The bitch then clears up the faeces and urine produced by the puppies, thus reducing the scent for opportunist predators and keeping the nest clean. When the puppies are approximately 3–4 weeks old they move away from the nest to eliminate but the bitch continues to clean up after them to reduce the scent. Sometimes this instinct becomes abnormal and dogs will clear urine and faeces of other dogs; this may be one of the reasons for coprophagia.

Normal sexual behaviour

Sexual behaviour can occur as early as 5 weeks of age in some puppies and they will mount litter mates. This could be an early sign of dominance within the pack or it may have an underlying sexual motive. If it is sexually motivated, this shows that the sex hormones are not the entire reason for sexual behaviour as they have not yet become significant. Although they may initiate and establish certain behaviour patterns, these will often continue long after the hormones have disappeared – for example, the mounting behaviour often observed in neutered animals.

Sexual maturity

The normal age for sexual maturity varies according to breed. Generally pack breeds such as Beagle, Foxhound and the smaller toy breeds mature earlier than the larger breeds. Most dogs are capable of fertile mating between 6 and 10 months of age, but with the slower maturing breeds (e.g. Dobermann, German Shepherd Dog, Wolfhound) breeding is not advised until they are aged 18–24 months.

Bitches usually show signs of first oestrus (heat) between 5 and 15 months of age, with the pack and smaller breeds attaining sexual maturity earlier. Wolfhound bitches will frequently be 18–24 months old before their first oestrus. Greyhounds, Chow Chows and Salukis are also slow to attain sexual maturity.

Sexual behaviour influences other aspects of dog behaviour, e.g. eliminating, marking, communication and pack order.

- In wild packs, female pheromones (marker scents) alert ranging males of imminent oestrus; the bitches responsible will receive increasing attention until they are receptive and allow mating
- Lifelong pairing can occur with wolves and pack dogs in the wild but not with domestic dogs
- Copulation can take up to half an hour, since the dog and the bitch 'tie': the bulbus glandis of the dog is gripped by the vulva of the bitch, preventing withdrawal of the penis until ejaculation has occurred
- Homosexual behaviour is common with dogs of both sexes and may result in very close relationships

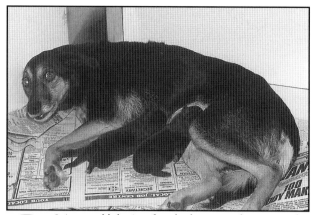

2.31 *It is normal behaviour for a bitch to protect her puppies after whelping.*

- Environment can play a part in successful mating – males appear to be very sensitive to their environment and it is for this reason that bitches are brought to the dog's territory to be mated.

Maternal behaviour

In the wild, pregnant bitches continue to behave normally and run with the pack until 2–3 days before whelping. The bitch then seeks a quiet place in which to make a nest.

A pet bitch needs to be introduced to the area where whelping should take place some weeks before the event, otherwise she is likely to be upset and to carry her offspring around looking for the place of her choice (see Chapter 10 in *BSAVA Manual of Veterinary Nursing*).

It is normal behaviour for the bitch to protect her puppies after whelping (Figure 2.31). Bitches that are well integrated with the family pack will permit other members close contact but strangers may be regarded as a threat.

It is important that the bitch and puppies are left quietly by themselves as much as possible. Constant interference can result in the bitch killing and even eating the puppies. This is instinctive behaviour to ensure that the pack is not threatened by ever constant predators. For similar reasons the bitch may also kill any deformed or weak puppies.

In the nest bitches exhibit very strong maternal behaviour, feeding, licking and cleaning their puppies and ensuring they do not move away from the nest. In the wild, bad mothering instincts are eliminated since natural predators kill offspring from such bitches. Domestication has halted the process in some breeds where handrearing is commonplace because bitches of that particular breed are considered to be 'notoriously bad mothers'.

Puppies' eyes open and their ears become functional at around 2–3 weeks of age. Then the bitch will interact to a far greater degree with the litter, sometimes sharing her food and playing with the puppies. At this time it is normal behaviour for the bitch to vomit the partially digested contents of her stomach for the puppies to eat.

False or phantom pregnancy

Pack bitches tend to coordinate their cycles. After oestrus, some bitches will develop all the signs of pregnancy (including milk production) without having conceived. This may have a part to play in communal puppy rearing. Such phantom pregnancy is very common in pet bitches.

Sounds, signs and signals of normal behaviour

We consider that dogs are fairly easy to 'read'. Facial expressions, tail position and movements, sounds and elimination behaviour are all familiar but in fact much of this expressive language is not understood. Most owners are aware of changes in the behaviour of their pet and veterinary professionals should always take note of an owner's comments when an animal is presented for clinical examination.

Body language, vocalization and scent marking are the essentials of canine expression.

Body language

Signs such as growling, tail movements and facial expressions will indicate intentions. For example:

- The ears are erect or pricked when alert or listening intently but also when preparing to attack
- Eyes are narrowed or half closed when greeting with pleasure or in submission but the eye will be fully open prior to an attack
- Eye contact is an essential part of control by the pack leader and is used when training
  - Staring at a dog, as would the pack leader, may result in submission, in which case the dog will lower its head and turn away
  - If the stare is returned, take care – this can be followed by attack
- The mouth is also used for expression:
  - Some breeds (e.g. Labrador, Dalmatian) will partially draw back their lips in greeting; this is similar to a human grin
  - Drawing the lips back further, showing the pigmentation of the lip edge and more of the teeth, results in the snarl of aggression (Figure 2.32)
- Other signs include raising the hackles (hair erection) around the neck and on the back so that, before attack, the dog looks as large as possible (Figure 2.32)
- Tail wagging and the angle at which the tail is carried are important in communication but are breed dependent. Some dogs have no tail, commonly because of human intervention but occasionally due to nature:
  - The tail is carried at approximately 45° or more from the horizontal when the dog is alert and interested or aggressive – or during play, when instead of standing erect the dog will be crouching on the forelegs in the so-called play bow (Figure 2.33)
  - The tail clamped low over the anus and genitals indicates a fear posture (but Whippets and Italian Greyhounds naturally carry their tails in this position) (Figure 2.34).

Vocalization

- Puppies cry in a variety of tones from the moment of birth:
  - When contented, they make soft whimpering noises
  - When hungry, there is a harsh strident sound often called 'seagulling' since the sound is similar to that made by seagulls
- Puppies start to bark at about 6 weeks of age and will bark with surprise, for defence and as a challenge to other dogs

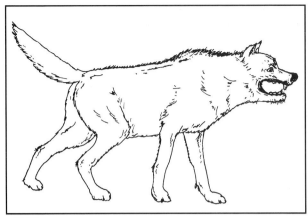

2.32 *Posture of aggression.*

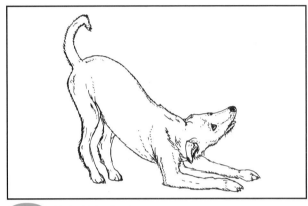

2.33 *Typical 'play-bow' stance.*

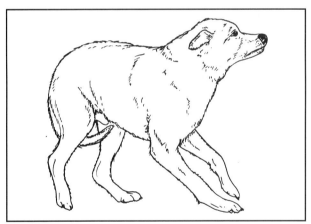

2.34 *Posture of fear.*

- In play, the bark will become softer and is a yap
- In distress, the bark becomes a whine to attract attention
- The howl carries over long distances and is used as a means of communication
- The growl is probably the vocalization that people most misinterpret. It can indicate:
  - Threat
  - Dominant challenge
  - Mock dominance in play
  - A way of 'talking' to their owner, when some dogs use a special low type of growl of varying pitch
- The whimper is a sound made by dogs in submission when they are attempting to appease.

Chemical expression

The sense of smell is particularly well developed in dogs. It is considered to be 40–100 times more sensitive than in humans and is one of the reasons why dogs will linger, sniffing and licking people and other dogs. They are fact-finding regarding contact with other dogs, people and food.

Chemical smells used in normal dog behaviour include those of urine (information about sex, advent of oestrus, etc.), faeces, anal sacs and saliva. There are also numerous sebaceous glands over the body and between the foot pads which act as marker or scent glands.

Activities with dogs

Apart from the more obvious activities that have already been mentioned, there are boundless opportunities (given the inclination) to engage in all manner of dog-related pursuits, both energetic and sedentary (Figure 2.35).

Further information may be obtained from the local veterinary practice, local authority or one of the organizations listed below.

2.35 Activities with dogs

- Participation in normal exercise, from the sedate with toy breeds to the energetic with large breeds
- Dog shows (there are also classes for mongrels)
- Obedience competitions (breed is no barrier)
- Working trials for larger guarding breeds
- Agility competitions, open to all breeds (including mongrels)
- Field trials for gundogs
- Dog racing for Greyhounds, Salukis, Afghans, Whippets
- Drag hunting, mainly for scent hounds – it does not involve chasing or killing other animals but concerns scent recognition
- Sponsored walks, for all adult dogs
- Charity work, for all breeds
- Participation in Pets As Therapy (PAT) scheme sponsored by the PRO-Dogs Charity – involves visiting schools, the elderly and the sick, reinforcing the role played by the companionship of animals. Dogs of any size or type can take part provided they have a reliable temperament with strangers.

Other dog-related activities:

- Breed rescue support (counselling, transport, fostering)
- Helping behind the scenes with exhibitions and competitions (administration, catering, stewarding)
- Puppy walking and socialization schemes:
  - Guide Dogs for the Blind
  - Hearing Dogs for Deaf People
  - Dogs for the Disabled.

Further reading

Geary M (1998) *Purnell Pictorial Encyclopaedia of Dogs*. Purnell, Bristol

Gorman NT (ed.) (1998) *Canine Medicine and Therapeutics*, 4th edn. Blackwell, Oxford

Kennel Club (1998) *Kennel Club's Illustrated Breed Standards*. Ebury Press, London

Lane D and Cooper B (1999) *Veterinary Nursing*, 2nd edn. Butterworth-Heinemann, Oxford

Turner T (1990) *Veterinary Notes for Dog Owners*. Popular Dogs

Journals

Our Dogs, published weekly by Our Dogs Centenary Ltd, Manchester

Dog World, published weekly by Dog World Ltd, Ashford, Kent

Dogs Monthly, published monthly by Our Dogs Centenary Ltd, Manchester

Dogs Today, available from Pankhurst Farm, West End, Woking, Surrey

Useful addresses

Kennel Club
1–5 Clarges Street, London W1Y 8AB
Telephone 020 7493 6651

Assistance Dogs UK
(provides information on all charities involved in training dogs for assistance purposes, including those listed below)
c/o Hearing Dogs for Deaf People (see below)

Dogs for the Disabled
The Old Vicarage, London Road, Ryton-on-Dunsmore, Coventry CV8 2ER
Telephone 01203 302050

From 2000, Frances Hay Centre, Blacklock Hill, Banbury, Oxfordshire OX17 2BS
Telephone 01295 252600

Guide Dogs for the Blind
Hillfields, Burghfield, Reading, Berkshire RG7 3YG
Telephone 01189 835555

Hearing Dogs for Deaf People
London Road, Lewknor, Oxon OX9 5RY
Telephone 0184 435 3898

PAT Dogs
PRO-Dogs National Charity
Rocky Bank, 4 New Road, Ditton, Maidstone, Kent ME20 7RD
Telephone 01732 848499

Support Dogs
2 Little Matlock Way, Stannington, Sheffield, South Yorks S6 6FX
Telephone 01742 320026

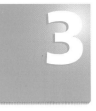

General care and management of the cat

Kim Willoughby

This chapter is designed to give information on:

- Recognition of different breeds of domestic cat
- Basic understanding of genetics and of coat colours and patterns
- General care and everyday management
- Routine veterinary care
- Basic nutrition
- Basic understanding of the normal behavioural characteristics

Introduction

The cat has recently become Britain's most popular pet: more than 7 million cats share our homes, compared with about 6.5 million dogs. It is almost certainly due to changes in society as a whole that cats have overtaken dogs in popularity, as they seem to be able to cope better than dogs in families where they may be alone for the working day (or have the company of other animals). Despite their reputation for solitude, cats are usually very affectionate companions. The vast majority of pet cats in this country are non-pedigree domestic shorthairs, but pedigree cats are gaining favour and many different breeds are commonly encountered in the veterinary practice.

This chapter gives a general introduction to the choice and care of this deservedly popular pet, from kitten through to adulthood, and covers selection of a cat, breed descriptions, introduction to feline genetics, basic breeding advice, general veterinary care and normal behaviour.

Considerations before purchasing a cat

Before acquiring a cat, the practicalities of keeping a pet that may live for 15–20 years must be considered. As with any animal, buying a kitten should not be entered into lightly. All the factors below must be considered before deciding that a cat is a suitable animal for that person or family to keep as a pet.

Cost of keeping a cat (financial and time)

- Feeding: cost of food and time spent
- Equipment: minimal cost in most cases
- Veterinary care: even routine visits can be expensive
- General attention: playing, grooming, etc. (consider two cats if there is little company during the day)
- Arrangements for holidays: convenience balanced against quality and cost.

Outdoor or indoor cat?

- Indoors/outdoors?
- Does a catflap need to be fitted? (This may pose a security risk)
- Is the road outside busy? (Risk of road accident)
- Will the cat have free range in the house? (Some cats may be destructive; also toilet arrangements – provision of a litter tray – need to be made)
- Alternatives (constructing an outdoor run area for the cat, restriction to part of the house only).

Other family members

Consider other occupants of the house too:

- Does everyone want a cat?
- Does anyone have allergies that may be made worse by having a cat in the house?

Many cats end up in rescue centres because a child or other member of the family has asthma or eczema.

Selection of a cat

What kind of cat?

Cats come in many shapes and sizes. Long hair, short hair, curly hair, no hair, highly bred pedigree or local domestic shorthair – all need similar types of care, though some need more than others. For example, longhaired cats need daily grooming while a shorthaired cat may need little more than stroking to keep the coat in good condition.

Unlike the situation with pet dogs, where pedigree animals are popular, for a pet cat many people will choose a non-pedigree domestic shorthair cat. The popularity of pedigree cats is growing, however, and these days they are regularly encountered as pets, not just as breeding or show animals.

Prospective owners who plan to show or breed cats will almost certainly want a pedigree cat. In that case they also have to think about how to avoid the production of half-bred kittens, and of the costs associated with breeding and showing.

The advantages of buying a pedigree cat are that some kind of prediction can often be made about its temperament, and what it will look like as it grows. With a non-pedigree kitten, such things are less predictable.

What age of cat?

Most people, when they decide they want a cat, will opt for a kitten. Kittens are fun, often very energetic and occasionally destructive. If an owner feels they may not be able cope with the needs of a growing kitten, and a 'mad half-hour' every night when the curtains are conquered or pot plants tipped over, then perhaps an adult cat will make a better choice. Rescue catteries, such as those run by Cats Protection, always have much more trouble rehoming unwanted adolescent and adult cats than the adorable cute and cuddly kittens. Giving a home to such a cat can be saving it from a long wait in a cat shelter, or even euthanasia.

Which sex?

Should it be a male (tom) or a female (queen) cat? In a pet household both would usually be neutered, and both make good pets. The cost of neutering can be a consideration for owners, and it should be borne in mind that males are usually cheaper to have neutered than females. While neutered cats are more likely to put on weight than entire cats, obesity is relatively uncommon.

Real differences between the sexes show themselves in entire cats (Figures 3.1 and 3.2).

3.1 Tom cat characteristics

- Toms become 'butch' as the secondary sex characteristics develop, getting large and often stocky, with a broad neck
- Behaviour usually considered inappropriate for pets may develop, such as spraying urine around the house or staying out all night, fighting with the other local bruisers while seeking out the ladies
- Entire males maintain larger territories than neuters, which can put them more at risk from road accidents and infectious diseases.

3.2 Queen cat characteristics

- Entire queens are capable of producing litters of kittens at regular intervals, and it can be hard to tell, especially with a non-pedigree cat, when she is in season, or even when she is pregnant, until it is too late
- Rescue centres have many pregnant cats and kittens as a result of unwanted pregnancies, where the owners cannot find homes for the kittens and no longer want the cat now that she has become a 'problem'
- Even breeders of pedigree cats sometimes have difficulty selling kittens, and so breeding kittens intentionally should not be entered into lightly.

Where to get a cat?

It is preferable to get a kitten from either a private house, a breeder (Figure 3.3) or a cat rescue society (Figure 3.4). In this way, the new owner can learn a bit about the home background of the cat and can often, in the case of a kitten, see the mother. It can be established whether the kitten is used to children or dogs, and the temperament of individual kittens can be assessed in a home environment. With a pedigree cat it may be possible to see the father as well, but

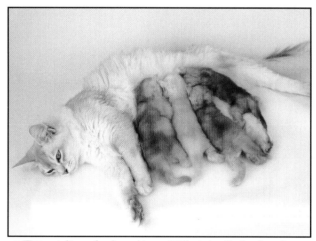

3.3 *A litter of pedigree kittens (Tiffanies) will often have homes arranged even before their birth.*
© *Alan Robinson.*

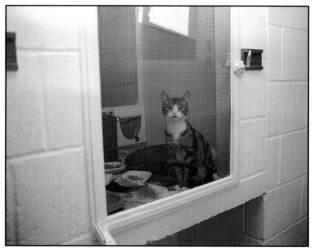

3.4 *An adolescent cat waits at a rescue centre for a home.*

it should be remembered that many breeders do not keep their own stud cat and the queen may have travelled a long way to be mated.

Considerations on choosing an individual cat

How should owners choose 'their' cat? They may have decided that they prefer a male or female kitten, or one of a particular colour, but much of the time they will choose a non-pedigree cat or kitten by instinct, because that ginger one looks nicest, or the little black and white one has a sweet expression.

Pet quality

With a pedigree cat, the breeder will know which cats are 'pet quality' and which are suitable for showing or breeding. This does not imply that pet quality kittens are inferior in any way, other than in terms of the defined breed description in the official 'standard of points' against which cats are judged at shows.

Cat clubs

Where the owner is looking for a cat to show or to breed from, cat clubs and magazines can be a valuable resource in locating a particular breed sought. Most areas have mixed-breed local clubs, and there are nationwide breed clubs. These can be contacted via the registering bodies (Governing Council of the Cat Fancy or the Cat Association of Britain – see 'Useful Addresses' at the end of this chapter), or by purchasing one of the cat magazines widely available in newsagents.

It is also a good idea for the prospective owner to visit a local cat show to meet breeders and see the cats at first hand. Lists are available from the registering bodies.

Home visits

Be prepared for the vendor, especially a pedigree breeder or rescue cattery, to want to 'vet' prospective owners before they let them have a cat. Many rescue societies will want to perform home visits to ensure that their animals are going to good homes, and breeders will usually want to meet owners at least once to decide on their suitability before selling them a pedigree kitten.

Selecting a kitten

Unless the potential owner is knowledgeable about cats it is advisable that someone who is more experienced should go with them to look at or collect a kitten. They should expect to be able to see the whole litter, and the queen, in most circumstances.

It is likely that they will not meet the kittens until they are around 6–8 weeks old, when kittens should be bright and active, curious about strangers and playing with each other and the queen. Kittens that have been reared in the house with human company usually make better pets than those reared in catteries, and are familiar with ordinary household objects like vacuum cleaners.

A simple health check is suggested in Figure 3.5.

While non-pedigree kittens often leave their mothers at around 8 weeks of age, pedigree kittens are usually at least 12 weeks old. All kittens should be fully weaned and (mostly) litter trained before they move to a new home – the queen usually trains the kittens (see 'Kitten development and behaviour' below).

3.5 Basic health check for a kitten

General condition

- **Bright, alert and responsive**. Kittens should be curious and should respond to being stroked by purring, rubbing or pushing against your hand
- **Weight**. Pick the kitten up. It should feel plump and not bony or clammy. The whole litter should be of a similar size. The kitten should not feel limp or floppy; there should be good muscle tone. Kittens should not be pot-bellied
- **Movement**. The kitten should move easily, with no signs of loss of balance or difficulty walking or jumping.

Examination for problems

- Eyes and nose should be clean and free of any discharge. The third eyelid (haws) should not be visible in the corner of the eyes. The kitten should not sneeze or cough. All these can be signs of infectious respiratory disease (Figure 3.6) which may be problematic to treat
- Ears should not be waxy or irritated. This can be a sign of ear mites (watch the kitten for shaking the head or scratching)
- Teeth should be white and clean; gums should not be excessively red or inflamed. The front teeth should meet, though this is not always the case, especially with longhaired cats of Persian type
- The coat should be clean and show no signs of hair loss, sore patches, scaliness, or irritation. Check for parasites such as fleas
- The area under the tail should be clean with no sign of faecal staining on the surrounding hair. Sometimes worms may be seen around the anus. The cat should not have diarrhoea. Always check the sex of the kitten or cat (Figure 3.7)
- The kitten should have no obvious deformities. Check for hernias at the umbilicus (navel), for kinks in the tail, that the ribcage feels normal and not flattened, and that the back and limbs feel normal
- Take the cat or kitten to a veterinarian for a full checkover within a few days to ensure all is well.

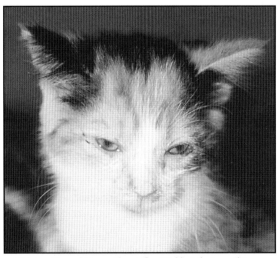

3.6 *Young kitten with cat 'flu. Highly infectious, this disease can be difficult to treat successfully and can leave cats with long-term symptoms.*

Sexing kittens

It can be difficult for the inexperienced to sex kittens accurately. While most breeders can sex kittens as newborns, this takes some practice and experience. At 6 weeks or so, sexing is relatively straightforward.

- With the kitten facing away from you, lift the tail
- Identify the anus, and look below
- A female kitten has the vulva very close to the anus, in a tear shape or slit
- A male kitten has a rounded swelling (within which is the penis) further from the anus and below the larger scrotal swelling.

In the vast majority of male kittens testes will be present in the scrotum by 6 weeks of age, but they are very small.

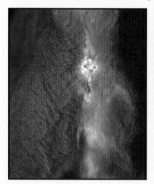 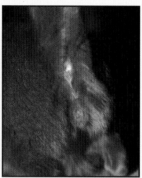

Female adult cat. Note the relationship of the anus and vulva.

Male neutered cat. Note the presence of the scrotum, but absence of testes. The distance from the anus to the penis is much greater in the male than that of the anus to the vulva in the female.

Paperwork

Pedigree kittens should also be vaccinated before sale against at least cat 'flu and enteritis (see below), and a written pedigree, registration transfer certificate and record of vaccination should be supplied at the time of purchase. Many pedigree cat breeders also supply kitten insurance as a kitten 'cover note', valid for 6 weeks or so after purchase.

Popular cat breeds

The majority of the pedigree cat world in the UK is regulated by the Governing Council of the Cat Fancy (GCCF, founded in 1910) in much the same way as the Kennel Club regulates dog breeders. It recognizes new breeds, maintains registers of pedigree cats, runs shows (see 'Activities with cats', below) and sets out the rules by which breeders affiliated to it should behave. The GCCF produces various publications, including the breed descriptions against which cats are judged at cat shows, known as the 'standard of points'. It also organizes the Supreme Show (the 'Crufts' of the cat fancy).

The Cat Association of Britain is a much smaller group affiliated to the Fédération Internationale Féline (FIF), which organizes shows and recognizes breeds in a similar way.

'Breed recognition' means that the particular governing body will accept kitten registrations for that breed, and will allow them to be exhibited at shows. For a new breed to be recognized, a group of breeders must demonstrate their commitment to the breed, that there is sufficient interest in

it, and that it is sufficiently different from other breeds. The new breed can then progress through a process which involves registering a minimum number of cats and kittens and demonstrating their merits at shows before 'full recognition' is granted.

Cat breeds are subdivided into breed sections, in much the same way that dogs are divided into working, toy, etc. The breed sections into which the recognized cat breeds are divided are:

- Longhair
- Semi-longhair
- British
- Foreign
- Burmese
- Oriental
- Siamese

In addition, some other breeds are present but not recognized.

Longhair section

One of the oldest established breeds, the Persian cat is recorded as appearing at cat shows since records began more than 100 years ago. The modern Persian cat probably has its origins in cats imported from Central and Eastern Europe in the latter part of the nineteenth century. However, opinions vary, as longhaired cats have been known in Western Europe for at least 300 years.

Persian

Persian cats occur in almost every colour and pattern, including silver in both silver (black) and golden (brown) forms. The length of the hair allows the differentiation of tipping in ticked tabbies and silvers into *shell* (only extreme tips of hair coloured), *shaded* (intermediate tipping) and *smoke* (most tipping colour). Where black tipping is involved, the shell type is known as *chinchilla*.

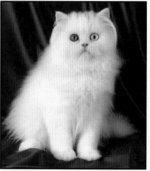

Odd-eyed white Persian.
© Alan Robinson.

The long hair is due to the recessive gene, *l*, but the overall look (or 'type') of the Persian is due to the influence of many genes.

The basic cat has a large body, a round head with small ears, a short nose and very large eyes. The coat should be long and 'double', with soft woolly undercoat and coarser guard hairs, and requires a lot of grooming (i.e. daily) to keep it in good condition. There has been concern that, if the head type is too extreme, cats may suffer from the same problems as brachycephalic (literally, short-nosed) dogs, such as Pekinese and Bulldogs, where the anatomy of the nose and throat can begin to interfere with normal breathing.

Exotic Shorthair

The Exotic Shorthair is originally derived from breeding Persian to British Shorthair, producing a cat of intermediate build with short hair. These cats often have Persian-type faces, but are rarely as extreme as their longhaired relatives. All colours and patterns are acceptable.

Though still longhaired, the coat of the semi-longhaired cats is finer than the Persian, and less liable to matting, so grooming is usually easier. In addition, the very short nose and large eyes of the Persian type is not a feature of the semi-longhairs, so brachycephalic syndrome should not be a problem.

Birman

The Birman cat is a very attractive, colour-pointed cat with distinctive white feet, often known as gloves or gauntlets. The basic cat is of medium build, the head

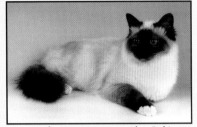

Seal point Birman. © Alan Robinson.

shape is fairly round, and the nose is of medium length. The eyes are blue (Siamese colour restriction) and these cats are recognized in many colours, including the dilute, tabby and tortie forms of all major colours.

Turkish

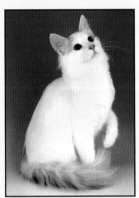

Auburn Turkish Van. © Alan Robinson.

Also called the Turkish Van, this semi-longhaired cat is mostly white, with patches of colour on both ears and tail. Originally only recognized in auburn (orange), other colours are now also bred. The eyes are almost always amber, but can be blue; odd-eyed cats are occasionally seen, and according to some sources can be deaf. A fairly large and muscular cat, the head shape again is not extreme, though somewhat wider and shorter than the Birman. Turkish cats are said to like water and swimming, and are sometimes known as the Turkish swimming cat.

Ragdoll

In looks, Ragdolls are semi-longhair, colour-pointed cats, and can be confused with Birmans, particularly the 'mitted' Ragdoll which has white feet. The other coat patterns are straight colour-point, and bicolour (where the white patches are more extensive than in the mitted form). Ragdolls were quite recently recognized by the GCCF and are becoming popular.

Somali

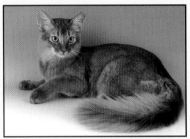

Sorrel Somali. © Alan Robinson.

Another attractive cat, the Somali is the longhaired version of the Abyssinian (see later) and is essentially the same cat of basic 'Foreign type' with long hair. The distinctive ticked tabby pattern of the Abyssinian is well demonstrated in the Somali, where many bands of colour can be seen on each hair. Somalis are recognized in a range of colours similar to those in the Abyssinians.

Maine Coon

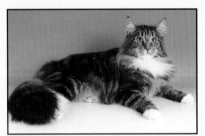

Brown tabby and white Maine Coon. © Alan Robinson.

The Maine Coon is one of the oldest established breeds in the United States. Maine Coons can be very large cats, and males can be in excess of 7 kg in weight. They have long coats, which also tend to be thicker than those of the other semi-longhairs, with the exception of the Norwegian Forest cat. They have large heads in keeping with their body size, and tend to have ear tufts and almost shaggy neck ruffs. There is no restriction on the colours of Maine Coons and they are bred in all colours and patterns, except pointed.

Norwegian Forest

The Norwegian Forest cat is very similar in looks to the Maine Coon, and it takes experience to tell them apart. The coat of this cat is double, with a fluffy undercoat. These cats are large, like the Maine Coon, but are slightly different in type, having the hindlegs slightly longer than the front, and a different 'look' to the face. Again, these cats are available in all the main colours.

This group is derived from the British domestic cat population.

British Shorthair

A stocky cat, with a large, round head, deep chest, cobby body and strong legs, this cat can be very heavy and powerful. Bred in all colours, including colour-point and silver, the solid colours, especially blue, remain in demand, though the other colours are gaining popularity. Though shorthaired, the coat is dense and these cats can withstand cold weather. They are generally good tempered and more 'easygoing' than some other breeds, such as the Foreigns.

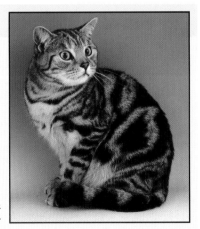

Silver tabby British Shorthair. © Alan Robinson.

British Section continues ▶

Manx

Manx cats are basically British in type but have no tail. This is due to a dominant lethal gene, designated *M*. As the gene is lethal in the homozygote (all *MM* kittens die *in utero*), all Manx cats are heterozygotes (*Mm*). This means that in litters of cats bred Manx to Manx (i.e. *Mm* x *Mm*) there will often be at least one kitten that has a tail (*mm*), inheriting the normal gene from each parent.

As well as lack of a tail, the Manx gene can cause other spinal problems, including spina bifida and fusing of vertebrae. The lack of a tail can take various forms, from cats with no perceptible tail ('rumpies') to those where an obvious stump is present ('rumpie risers' or 'stumpies'). Only the 'rumpie' type is allowed to be shown. Otherwise, Manx cats are similar to British Shorthairs, though they may have slightly longer hindlegs.

This breed has been recognized for many years. If a breed with such a gene mutation were developed today, it is unlikely it would be recognized.

There is also a longhaired version of the Manx, known as Cymric, though this is rarely seen.

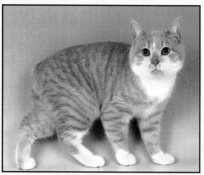

Cream and white Manx.
© Alan Robinson.

Many breeds are represented in the Foreign section – not all of them foreign. 'Foreign' refers rather to the type of cat, not extreme in head shape or size. Though the majority of cats in this section are shorthaired, some have long or even curly hair. These cats usually have a somewhat more demanding temperament than longhairs or British Shorthairs, being similar to Siamese in terms of vocalization and attention-seeking. They are usually very sociable and want to be where the owner is (preferably between them and what they are doing).

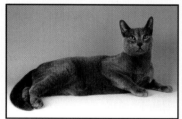

© Alan Robinson.

Russian Blue

The Russian Blue has a slender body type but is muscular, with strong limbs and tail. The head is a medium wedge shape, with prominent whisker pads, and the ears are set high. The coat is double, and mid blue, with silver-tipped guard hairs giving a sheen to the colour. Though white and black variants have been bred, these are rarely encountered.

Korat

The Korat (see Figures 3.26 and 3.27) is another shorthaired blue cat, of rather different type to the Russian: it has a heart-shaped head, large ears and prominent large green eyes. The coat should be heavily tipped with silver, and the body semi-cobby, with strong limbs. The Korat is claimed to be one of the oldest cat breeds, described in the fourteenth century Thai *Cat Book Poems*, but remains rather uncommon. Recently, lilac and pointed variants have been described in the UK.

Abyssinian

The Abyssinian (see Figure 3.17a) has a striking ticked tabby coat, giving it an appearance like rabbit fur, due to the banding of light and dark colour in each individual hair. In type, Abyssinians are moderate, the body is well proportioned and legs slender. The ears are rather large and often have ear tufts. Originally only a few colours were recognized, but recently all the main colours have been produced, and silvers are also now being seen. The Abyssinian is a breed where unusual colour names may be used (e.g. 'usual' for the black tipped tabby) and the light brown gene is present in this breed, producing the sorrel.

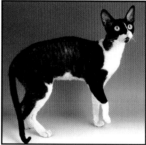

Black and white Cornish Rex.
© Alan Robinson.

Cornish Rex

The Cornish Rex is of basic Foreign type, with a strong head and body, long legs and tail. The distinctive feature of Rex cats is the curly coat. The Cornish Rex usually has a good covering of hair, which is short and wavy. This mutation occurred in Cornwall in the 1950s, and these cats have been bred in a variety of colours, including all the main colours, bicolours and Siamese pointed (so called Si-Rex).

Devon Rex

The Devon Rex, due to a different gene than the Cornish, originated a few years afterwards in neighbouring Devon. The 'rexing' of the hair takes the form of a very short wavy coat, which can be rather sparse in places, especially on the neck and trunk. More extreme in type than the Cornish, the Devon has very large ears and a wider face, and is often likened affectionately to a 'gremlin' or described as pixie-like.

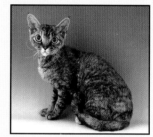

Tortie-tabby Devon Rex.
© Alan Robinson.

Singapura

The Singapura is a breed recently introduced into the UK, with a short close-lying coat, ticked with brown on a delicately coloured background. A small but stocky cat, with rather large eyes and ears, it was originally bred from just four cats in Singapore.

Foreign Section continues ▶

Asian and Burmilla

The Asian and Burmilla have arisen from cross-breeding Burmese with longhair Chinchilla (silver/black tipped Persian), producing cats of basically Burmese type but of

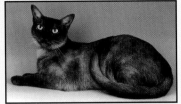

Brown smoke Asian.
© Alan Robinson.

colour, pattern or coat length not found in the Burmese. A great variety of colours are available, and Burmese coloration can re-emerge from Asian x Asian matings, though these cats are not recognized as Burmese.

There are five subgroups of Asians:

- *Burmilla* Colour is shaded (from spine to belly, decreasing in intensity), with pale undercoat. May be silver or non-silver (standard)
- *Smoke* A non-agouti cat, not shaded, any colour combination with silver
- *Tabby* Ticked tabby is most common, but others are produced. All colours
- *Asian Self* Solid colours. The black is known as Bombay
- *Tiffanie* (see Figure 3.3) Semi-longhaired version in all colours and patterns above.

Ocicat

The Ocicat is a spotted cat under development from a Siamese and Abyssinian background. Thought by the original breeders to look like an ocelot, these cats were named Ocicats after their striking boldly spotted coats. Though popular in the United States, these rather large cats are not common in the UK.

Tonkinese

Not a true breed, Tonkinese are produced as a hybrid of Siamese x Burmese, and have features of both. They have one Siamese and one Burmese colour restriction gene (i.e. C^sC^b), and have an intermediate colour and body shape and blue-green eyes. These cats cannot breed true; two Tonkinese bred together produce on average 50% Tonkinese, 25% Siamese and 25% Burmese colouring in their offspring, which are still of intermediate type.

Bengal

Another dramatically spotted cat, the Bengal has resulted from cross-breeding with the wild Asian leopard cat. Temperament may have been questionable in

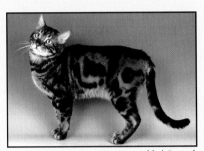

Brown marbled Bengal.
© Alan Robinson.

some of the early generations, but cats now bred are similar to other domesticated cats in temperament. These large, strong cats, in a number of tabby patterns and a variety of colours, have become very popular – more than 1000 were registered in 1998. The type is not extreme, and the coat is plush with a soft undercoat.

3.12 Burmese section

Burmese cats are a breed with a long history. Like the Siamese and Korat, these cats are recorded from the fourteenth century. However, the modern cat derives from a Burmese and Siamese background in the United States in the 1930s and 1940s. The first Burmese recognized was the brown – a rich, dark brown all over due to the effect of Burmese colour restriction on a genetically black cat. Originally only the brown was recognized, then blue, chocolate and lilac, with reds, creams and the tortoiseshell following on. Other colours have been introduced to produce the Asian group (see above), but only 'true' Burmese are included in the Burmese section.

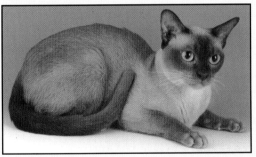

Burmese

The Burmese type is not extreme. The cat has a wedge-shaped head, not as narrow as the Siamese and not as broad as the British. The eyes should be almond shaped, and 'chartreuse' in colour (yellow-green); the ears are medium sized and widely set, with rounded tips. The body is solidly built, and Burmese cats often seem heavier to lift than would be expected for their size. These cats make good pets and are often very affectionate and 'talkative' to their owners.

Chocolate Burmese. © Alan Robinson.

3.13 Oriental section

Oriental Shorthair

The Oriental shorthair is basically a self-coloured cat of Siamese type. It is recognized in many colours and patterns, including all tabby patterns and silver. These cats are named by their colour (e.g. Oriental Black (Figure 3.21a), Oriental Caramel ticked tabby, Oriental Blue (Figure 3.17c)), with two exceptions: the brown cat of Oriental type is called a Havana, and the white is called a Foreign White.

Siamese

The Siamese (see Figure 3.21c) is a very old breed in its native Thailand, being one of the breeds (with the Burmese and Korat) to have its history recorded in the fourteenth century *Cat Book Poems*. First introduced into the UK in the late 1800s, Siamese cats have been exhibited at cat shows since 1871 and have become very popular. The modern Siamese is a medium sized cat, with a long body, limbs and tail, frequently described as svelte. The head is wedge shaped, with a long nose, large ears and medium sized slanted strikingly blue eyes. The development of colour is restricted by the Siamese pattern gene (genotypes C^sC^s) to the 'points' – that is, the mask (muzzle and ears) and extremities of the limbs and tail; the remainder of the coat should be white or a pale creamy colour. As Siamese get older, the points tend to darken and colouration of other areas can develop. The development of colour is also influenced by skin temperature: when cold, the colour is darker. If a Siamese cat is clipped for surgery, for example, the hair may grow in darker. Conversely, a Siamese sleeping on a heated pad can lose colour in the points. Siamese are bred in many colours, including tabby and tortoiseshell patterns.

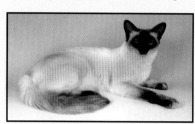

Balinese

The Balinese is a longhaired Siamese, accepted in all Siamese colours. Though longhaired, there is no undercoat, so the coat is long and silky. Sometimes these cats have a tuft or 'beard' on their chins.

Chocolate Balinese. © Alan Robinson.

Recent figures of kittens registered (1997, supplied by GCCF) demonstrate that the most popular are the well established breeds: Persian (8443), Siamese (4873), British Shorthair (4287), Burmese (3327) and Birman (2216). However, some of the more recently recognized breeds are becoming popular, notably the Maine Coon (1296) and Bengal (1222).

Other breeds

Other breeds are very uncommon, but include a long-haired version of the Manx known as the Cymric, and a long-haired rex known as the Selkirk Rex. There is also a hairless cat called the Sphynx and a cat with folded-over ears – the Scottish Fold. In other countries, notably North America, other breeds are also seen, including a cat known as the 'Munchkin', which has short, dachshund-like limbs.

Coat colours and patterns

The majority of pedigree cats are described by a combination of their colour (e.g. blue, seal point, silver tabby) and their 'type' or breed (e.g. Oriental, Persian, Burmese). Thus a full description of a cat might be, for example, 'silver tabby British Shorthair' (see Figure 3.17b), 'blue point Siamese' (see Figure 3.21c), or 'brown tabby and white Maine Coon' (see Figure 3.9), though some breeds can be only one specific colour (e.g. Korat, see Figure 3.26).

It is useful to be able to recognize the more common breeds and to be able to have at least an educated guess at their colour, though some of them are definitely not easy for the amateur (even breeders get it wrong sometimes and have to re-register kittens). A very good way to pick up the different colours and breeds is to visit a local show or, even better, to help with 'vetting-in' at a show early in the morning, when all the cats are examined before going into the show hall. Show managers are usually delighted to be offered extra help at 7.30 a.m.

Basic genetics

Genetic material (genes) is arranged in structures called chromosomes, which are present in the nucleus of every body cell of the cat. These chromosomes are present in pairs: there are two copies of every gene in every cell.

There are two exceptions to this general rule:

- The sex chromosomes – males have one X and one Y chromosome and females have two X chromosomes
- The reproductive cells (eggs and sperm) – only one 'set' of genes is present, so that when these fuse to become a fertilized egg (and eventually a new kitten), two copies are present: one set inherited from the father, and one from the mother.

Individual genes may be described as 'dominant' or 'recessive'. Where a gene is dominant, a single copy on either of the two chromosomes ensures its expression, whereas if a gene is recessive, both copies must be of the recessive gene for it to be expressed. (In a genetic context, 'expressed' means that that character will be produced.)

By convention, the symbols used for gene names are written in italics. Symbols for dominant genes are written in capital letters; symbols for recessive ones are in lower-case letters. The following example (Figure 3.15) demonstrates this principle.

3.15 **Genetics example 1**

Genetic makeup	Basic colour	Genes that can be passed to offspring
BB	Black	*B* (black) only
Bb	Black	*B* (black) or *b* (brown)
bb	Brown	*b* (brown) only

Black (B) is dominant to brown (b).

Gene (symbol)	Effect	Gene (symbol)	Effect
Agouti (A)	Tabby expression	Non-agouti (a)	Self-colour
Mackerel (T^m)	Striped (or spotted) tabby	Abyssinian (T^a)	Abyssinian tabby
		Blotched (t^b)	Blotched (classic) tabby
Black (B)	Black	Brown (b)	Dark brown (chocolate)
		Light brown (b^l)	Medium brown (cinnamon)
Not orange (o)	Normal colour	Orange (O)* (red, ginger)	All pigment altered to orange
Dense (D)	Dense colour	Dilute (d)	Dilutes colour (e.g. black to blue; brown to lilac)
Full-colour (C)	Colour over whole cat	Burmese (c^b)	Burmese colour restriction
		Siamese (c^s)	Siamese colour restriction, blue eyes
		Albino (c)	White, pink eyes
Normal pigment (i)	Full pigment development	Inhibitor (I)	Pigment suppression of some parts of hair shaft; also known as silver gene
Normal colour (w)	Allows expression of all other colour genes	Dominant White (W)	White coat; eyes blue, orange or odd-eyes. Associated with deafness
Normal colour (s)	No white spots	White spotting (S)	White patches or spots¶

Dominant genes are shown in upper case, recessive in lower.   * *Sex-linked gene*   ¶ *Expression variable*

Where both copies of a gene are the same (e.g. *BB* or *bb*), the genetic makeup is known as 'homozygous', and the cat can pass on only that gene to any kittens. Where the cat has one of each (e.g. *Bb*), it is called 'heterozygous', and the cat can pass on either gene; the cat might be described as a black cat 'carrying' brown, for example. Where a dominant gene is present, it is usual to write this as '*B-*', rather than writing *BB* or *Bb*, and this will be done in this section.

The genetics of coat colours are the same for every cat, be it domestic pet or pedigree. The fundamental genes, colours and patterns are listed in Figure 3.16, and are briefly described below. For more detail, consult the 'Further reading' section.

Coat patterns: tabby and self-coloured

The 'tabby' pattern of a cat is controlled by two genes. All cats have tabby (*T*) genes, but whether or not they are expressed is dependent on the agouti (*A*) gene, which determines the banding of pigment on the hair shaft. *Agouti* (*A*) allows banding, and is dominant to non-agouti (*a*). All tabby cats are therefore *A-* (remember, that means *AA* or *Aa*), and all non-tabby (i.e. 'self-coloured') cats are *aa*.

There are three tabby patterns:

- Abyssinian: no stripes as such but a broad ticking of the coat, like rabbit's fur (Figure 3.17a)
- Blotched: the so-called classic tabby with wide stripes (Figure 3.17b)
- Mackerel: the tiger stripe, where the stripes are narrower and tend to break into spots (Figure 3.17c).

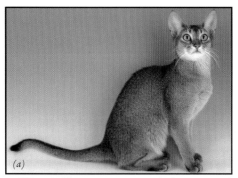 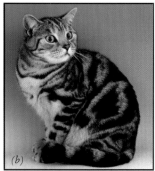 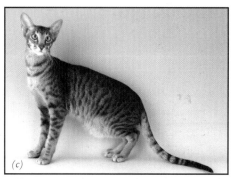

3.17 *Tabby patterns. (a) Usual Abyssinian (ticked) tabby pattern. (b) Blotched (classic) tabby pattern in a silver tabby British Shorthair. (c) Mackerel (spotted) tabby pattern in an Oriental Blue spotted tabby. The stripes tend to break into spots – this feature is sought after in pedigree cats. © Alan Robinson.*

The tabby genes form a 'gene series' in which mackerel is dominant to abyssinian, which is itself dominant to blotched. An example of the influence of these genes is shown in Figure 3.18.

3.18 Genetics example 2

Genetic makeup	Coat pattern and colour
A- T^m- B-	Mackerel tabby, black stripes
aa T^m- B-	Black self
A- T^aT^b bb	Ticked tabby, brown tips to hairs
aa T^aT^b bb	Brown self

Basic coat colours

The basic coat colour genes are:

- black (B)
- brown (b) (also sometimes called chocolate)
- orange (O)
- dominant white (W).

A further light brown gene (b^l) is also seen which is uncommon even in pedigree cats. The black and brown genes behave as expected (see Figure 3.15), provided that neither the orange nor white gene is present.

Orange

The orange gene (Figure 3.19) is a special case because it is on the X chromosome.

3.19 Genetics example 3

Genetic makeup	Coat pattern and colour
A- T^mT- B- X^oY	Ginger mackerel tabby male
aa T^m- B- X^oX	Tortoiseshell (ginger and black) female
A- T^bT^b bb X^oX^o	Ginger classic tabby female
aa T^aT^b bb X^oX	Chocolate tortoiseshell female

A male cat has only one X chromosome. If this carries the orange gene he will be orange (ginger), regardless of the other basic colour genes present, because orange prevents the expression of the basic colours.

A female cat has two X chromosomes. If the combination is X^oX^o she will be ginger, but a combination of X^oX- (i.e., one X chromosome has orange, one does not) leads to 'tortoiseshell', which is a mixture of ginger and black (for example, Figure 3.20). That is why almost all tortoiseshell cats are female. Very occasionally, male 'torties' are seen, but most are sterile, as they must have a chromosomal abnormality.

A further effect of the orange gene is that, very often, tabby markings are produced on a ginger cat (or ginger patches on a tortoiseshell one), whether or not the agouti (A) gene is present. Tortoiseshell cats can also be tabby, known as 'tortie-tabby', where the black is also tabby (see Figure 3.11).

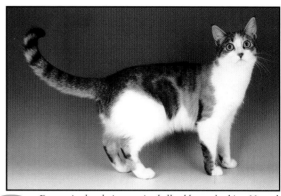

3.20
Domestic shorthair, tortoiseshell tabby and white. Note the tabby markings on the black areas in addition to the ginger. © Alan Robinson.

White

Dominant white (W) is a very special gene, which prevents expression of all other colours (including orange) and produces an all-white cat, with eyes of blue or amber, or even one of each (see Figure 3.8). This gene is also associated in many cats with deafness, due to a deformity in the cochlea in the inner ear.

Modifying genes

The basic colours of black, brown and orange (in their self-coloured, tabby or tortoiseshell forms) can be modified by a number of further genes, the most important of which are the dense (D) and dilute (d) gene pair, and the colour series gene (C), which controls the Siamese and Burmese colour restrictions.

Dilute and dense genes

The dilute gene is a recessive one that dilutes the main colour. The various permutations of the basic colour with the dilute gene produce the three dilute colours: blue (B-dd), lilac ($bbdd$) and cream (X^oX^odd), as well as the blue–cream tortoiseshell pattern (X^oX-B-dd).

Colour series gene

The colour series gene (Figure 3.21) produces:

- Full colour (C): colour develops over the entire cat
- Burmese restriction (c^b): colour is lightened over the body, and though darker on the 'points' (face, ears, feet and tail) it is not as dark as the genetic colour
- Siamese restriction (c^s): the body is very pale with darker points, and the eyes are blue
- Albino (c) – the most recessive gene in the series, pink-eyed albino, not to be confused with dominant white (although both cats are white, the albino has pink eyes and is not associated with deafness).

Other genes

White spotting gene

The white spotting gene is a common one that controls white patches. It has variable expression, from only a small white bib, or perhaps just one toe, through a cat with quite a lot of white (see Figure 3.20), to the cat that has only very small amounts of normal colour, often restricted to the ears and tail – for example, in a cat such as the Turkish Van (see Figure 3.9).

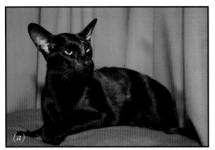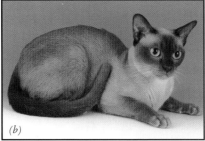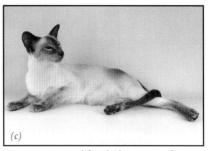

3.21 *The colour series gene. (a) Oriental Black. (b) Chocolate Burmese. The influence of the Burmese gene modifies the brown gene from all-over brown to brown only at the points. (c) Blue point Siamese. The influence of the Siamese gene modifies the colour genes so that they are only developed at the points.* © *Alan Robinson.*

Inhibitor or silver gene

The only other colour gene that might be encountered is the inhibitor (*I*) or silver gene, which suppresses colour on parts of the hair shaft. This gene is dominant, but has some variable expression. Cats with the silver gene can be described as silver (see Figure 3.17b), shaded, smoke, shell or tipped, or given other names depending upon the breed being described, and the basic cat colour. For example, a silver tipped British Shorthair is a genetically black cat with the silver gene. The cat looks white, with a small amount of black tipping to the hair. Though this gene is quite rare in the domestic shorthair population, smoke non-pedigree cats are seen now and again.

Preparation for a new arrival

While in some cases a stray quite literally walks in off the street, in most cases people make a conscious decision to have a cat and some preparations need to be made for the new arrival. The basic equipment required includes:

- Cat carrier
- Bed and bedding
- Food and water bowls
- Litter box
- Scratching post
- Toys

Cat carrier

A suitable box in which to transport the kitten or cat is essential (Figure 3.22). A cardboard box picked up from the local supermarket checkout is not acceptable as a carrying box. Some more substantial corrugated cardboard carriers are available from pet shops, veterinary surgeries, etc. which are satisfactory for relatively short-term use, but they are not secure if left unattended, and cannot be cleaned adequately. Similarly designed plastic versions are available, which are a little better. More substantial carriers are more durable and range from traditional wicker baskets (also difficult to clean) to more sophisticated designs made from covered wire, plastic or fibreglass.

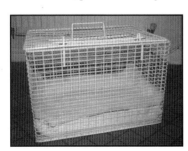

3.22 *Cat carrier.*

Points to bear in mind concerning the design of the carrier include the following:

- It is easier to get a cat in and out of a top-opening container than a side-opening one
- Good visibility is usually desirable for both owner and cat, but some cats prefer being able to hide in a solid-sided carrier
- The carrier should be easy to clean (some have removable trays to make cleaning of in-transit 'accidents' easier).

Beds and bedding

A cardboard box can make a very suitable bed: it has the advantages of low cost, ready availability, ease of re-design (holes can be cut out at appropriate places) and hygienic disposal. A more permanent basket of wicker, plastic or fibreglass may be more aesthetically pleasing, and the plastic versions are easy to clean. Polystyrene bead 'bean bags' are warm and comfortable, but can be a bit too much like a litter box for some cats.

Whatever the basic bed, warm bedding such as a towel, blanket or purpose-designed pad will be much appreciated – cats spend a lot of time sleeping, and a comfortable bed may help to reduce the time they spend sleeping on chairs or their owner's bed.

Feeding equipment

Ceramic, plastic or metal feed bowls are perfectly suitable for home use. Disposable bowls are available but are really needed only in catteries. As cats often have food left out for *ad lib* feeding and often prefer wide, shallow bowls, it is wise to have a feeding mat or tray under the bowl to minimize mess.

Plastic caps are useful to seal catfood cans after use until the next meal. For general hygiene reasons, cat bowls should be washed separately from (or at least after) the general washing up. A fork or spoon for use with catfood should be kept separate from the family cutlery.

Litter box

A litter box is necessary even where a cat has access to outdoors, unless that access is permanent. Litter boxes are almost always made from plastic, and are easy to clean and disinfect. Some designs are covered, or incorporate air-fresheners.

Lining litter trays with purpose-designed liners or even newspaper can help to make cleaning easier. Soiled litter should be removed at least twice daily, using a scoop.

Cat litter is available in many forms:

- Mineral-based types in both 'clumping' (i.e. clumps when wet) and 'non-clumping' varieties;
- Those based on sawdust or newspaper pellets;
- Sand or peat
- 'Reusable' litters.

'Reusable' litters are based on plastic pellets or other inert material that can be cleaned after use; these usually require a special type of tray through which urine can drain into a lower chamber.

 Pregnant women should avoid cleaning litter trays or should use gloves, due to a risk of *Toxoplasma* infection, which may be harmful to the unborn child.

Scratching post

It is a good idea to give a cat or kitten somewhere to scratch, in an effort to dissuade it from scratching the furniture. Scratching posts can be bought from pet stores, or pieces of bark or carpet may be mounted on a wall or other vertical surface. Usually cats are very happy to use these items when they know where they are, though sometimes the addition of catnip may be encouraging.

Toys

A wide variety of toys is available, and most of them involve some kind of chasing/hunting activity – balls, mice, furry toys, toys dangling on the end of a 'fishing line' and so on. Some toys are very popular with individual cats, while others are never played with. A cardboard box with cut-out holes can provide a lot of fun for a cat (or, even better, for two cats) to hide in and jump out of.

Some cats enjoy a lot of attention and will play with their owners for hours, even retrieving objects such as balls of silver paper; others ignore all toys and refuse to play with humans. Pedigree cats, especially the Foreign, Siamese and Burmese types, are often very playful and need time set aside for play.

General cat care

Compared with dogs, cats need less 'maintenance' in terms of walks, grooming, etc. However, they do still need time, effort and money spent on them. The costs of feeding are generally lower than for a dog, but costs of boarding (for holidays), veterinary visits, etc. are not so different.

Grooming

Coat

Most cats groom themselves quite adequately, and do not need their owner to groom them other than regular stroking to make sure there are no grass seeds, etc. stuck to their fur, and keeping them free from parasites. However, longhaired or semi-longhaired cats need regular (daily) grooming to keep their coats in good condition. Without this, unmanageable and uncomfortable mats of hair will result. Longhaired kittens should be groomed with a wide-toothed comb from as young an age as possible.

It is important to groom all over, and not just where the cat will allow it. The problem areas are usually along the back of the thighs, under the tail and under the axillae and chin. If mats develop, they may need to be cut or clipped out, which may have to be done under sedation or general anaesthesia and should not be attempted by the inexperienced.

Even in a shorthaired kitten, weekly use of a flea comb is wise – to give an early warning of parasites – and may be beneficial at times of moulting to help to prevent the development of hairball (an accumulation of hair in the stomach). Hairball causes retching and occasionally more serious illness, and can require veterinary treatment ranging from the use of mild laxatives to surgery in severe cases. A soft bristle brush or rubber brush is used by many people to groom shorthaired pedigree cats, giving them a final shine with a silk handkerchief to keep them looking their best.

Eyes and ears

Apart from the coat, the grooming routine should include inspection of the eyes and ears for evidence of any discharge or other problems. In certain cats, especially where the skin is pale, the eyes may naturally look pinkish, but if there is any concern a veterinary opinion should be sought. Where a cat has deepset eyes (e.g. a Siamese), it is not uncommon for a drop of mucus ('sleepdust') to form at the corner of the eye.

Any breed with a short nose (e.g. Persian, Exotic) may suffer from tear overflow and subsequent staining of the face. This should be bathed and dried carefully, or inflammation may result. A little petroleum jelly may help to prevent tear staining.

Claws

A cat's claws may need attention. The claw grows from the inside, and older layers are removed by scratching to reveal the sharp new claw underneath. A scratching post should be provided so that a cat can exercise the claws, but it may be necessary to clip them occasionally to prevent the worst of scratching on furniture or to stop the claws getting caught on soft blankets, etc. Some older cats have joint problems which prevent them from keeping their own claws in order, leading to overgrowth.

It is not hard to clip a cat's claws, but most cats will object at first, so help may be needed. Gently squeezing the toe will extrude the claw, and the sharp point can be safely cut off (Figure 3.23) using claw clippers.

3.23 Clipping a cat's claws

- It is often easier to sit with the cat on your knee
- The claw can be extruded by gentle pressure on the toe
- The point can be simply cut with sharp nail clippers
- Do not cut above the point, as the tender quick will be damaged
- In older cats, or cats without the opportunity to scratch and exercise their claws, the claws may be quite layered in appearance.

Playing

Most cats like to play and interact with their owners in some way. The sort of toys that are available have been described above, and some time should be set aside to play with the cat every day. Probably the best toy is another cat, but an attentive owner willing to throw a mouse or ball, or dangle something just out of reach, is usually appreciated. Many cats like to retrieve, play hide and seek, or to be chased in fun.

Outdoor access

Most cats will need outdoor access (Figure 3.24). Going outside gives them exercise, the ability to hunt and the opportunity to eat grass, which most cats will do. It also allows them to interact with other cats on common ground, and to establish a territory of their own which they can mark as they feel fit.

Outdoor access can be controlled by the owner opening a door or window, or can be via a catflap.

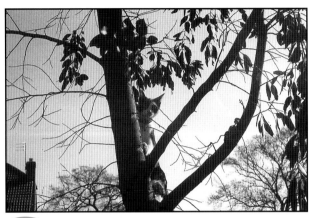

3.24 *Cats enjoy outdoor access.*

Catflaps

Catflaps can have some disadvantages, the most significant of which is that other cats may be able to get in, depending upon how sophisticated the flap is, and that this may be a threat to the resident cat. Most of the time, however, catflaps are very satisfactory. They can be locked at night; they can allow one-way traffic only; and some are electronically operated by a magnet on the cat's collar to prevent unwanted visitors.

Whether a cat has a flap or whether the owner controls outside access, a litter box should still be available for emergencies.

Risks

There are three main hazards with outdoor access:

- Risk of being hit by a car
- Risk of injury by another cat
- Risk of unwanted pregnancy.

Many cats have been injured or killed on the road before their first birthday, and this can be hard to prevent. In some cases, injured cats are never reunited with their owners if they are not easily identifiable, so a cat with outdoor access should either wear a collar or have other identification, such as a microchip implanted.

The risk of injury from other cats arises because cats fight each other to maintain their territories. Cat bites suffered during fights frequently become painful abscesses needing antibacterial therapy.

As for the risk of unwanted pregnancy, pet cats are usually neutered to prevent this, and pedigree cats intended for breeding are not usually allowed unrestricted outdoor access.

Provision for holidays

It is important to stress to an owner that holiday arrangements must be made for a cat.

Pet-sitting

Often, these arrangements will involve simply making sure that a friend or neighbour has a key and is willing to come into the house to feed the cat and clean the litter tray, preferably twice daily, and also, if possible, to play with the cat and provide some social interaction. This system has the advantage of cheapness, and that the cat is not removed from its home environment. An added extra is the security for the holidaying owner of having someone in the house every day. Where a neighbour is not available, there are commercial companies that provide pet or house-sitting services.

Boarding catteries

An alternative for holidays is to put the cat into a boarding cattery. Catteries can be found by looking in the Yellow Pages of the telephone directory or by asking friends, local veterinary surgeons or cat rescue groups for recommendations. All boarding catteries have to be inspected by the local council, but some are better than others. The Feline Advisory Bureau has a system of inspection that is very stringent and they publish a list of approved catteries (see 'Useful addresses'). It should always be possible for an owner to inspect a cattery before booking a place for their cat.

There is wide variety in cattery design, from entirely indoor cages to chalets with outdoor runs, and a broad range in between. Basically, catteries should have individual housing for each cat or household, with sufficient space for sleep and exercise, availability of food, water and a litter box, and heat in the winter. Premises should be clean, and cattery managers should insist that cats boarded with them should have current vaccination certificates against feline enteritis and cat 'flu (see below). Chapter 5 describes cattery construction and management in more detail.

Veterinary attention

Routine veterinary attention includes:

- Vaccination
- Control of internal and external parasites
- Neutering
- Pet identification (tattooing, microchip implantation)
- Consideration of purchase of pet insurance to cover veterinary fees for illness or accident.

Vaccination

There are various vaccines available for cats in the UK (Figure 3.25). These diseases are either common, serious, or both, and some form of vaccination is considered necessary for all cats. Vaccination is discussed in greater detail in the *BSAVA Manual of Veterinary Nursing*, and only a brief summary is presented here.

Cat vaccine components

Available in the UK:
- Feline infectious enteritis (FIE, feline panleucopenia, feline parvovirus)
- Feline herpesvirus (FHV-1, feline viral rhinotracheitis, FVR)
- Feline calicivirus (FCV)
- *Chlamydia psittaci*, var. *felis*
- Feline leukaemia virus (FeLV).

Available elsewhere in Europe, or in the USA:
- Feline coronavirus (FeCoV, feline infectious peritonitis, FIP)
- *Bordetella bronchiseptica*
- Rabies.

Feline infectious enteritis

Feline infectious enteritis is a viral disease, causing depletion of white blood cells (panleucopenia) and thus suppression of the immune system, and also causing severe damage to the lining of the intestine. This disease is often fatal, and affected cats may die within 24 hours or less of becoming ill, though not all affected cats will die. If a pregnant queen is infected (or if she is vaccinated with a live vaccine while pregnant) the virus may damage the kittens within the womb, causing brain damage – specifically, cerebellar hypoplasia. Kittens with cerebellar hypoplasia cannot walk properly, and may have fits or visual problems.

Cat 'flu

So-called cat 'flu is caused by two respiratory viruses: feline herpesvirus and feline calicivirus. Both viruses cause a raised temperature and nasal discharge, but cats often have slightly different clinical signs depending on which virus is involved.

Feline herpesvirus causes quite a severe illness, usually featuring conjunctivitis and rhinitis with discharge from the nose and eyes. More severe cases may have pharyngitis and tracheitis, causing drooling of saliva.

Feline calicivirus usually has milder effects. It does not commonly cause the severe conjunctivitis associated with feline herpesvirus, but is usually associated with mouth ulcers. Occasionally feline calicivirus can cause a lameness syndrome, with a high temperature and shifting lameness, most common in young kittens.

Both viruses produce carrier cats after primary infection, so that recovered cats may transmit the disease to other cats, despite appearing healthy. In addition, some cats never recover fully from cat 'flu and have chronic ocular or nasal discharges for life. It is rarely fatal in healthy adult cats, but young kittens and cats with immunodeficiency (e.g. infected with feline leukaemia virus or feline immunodeficiency virus, or on anti-cancer treatment) may die.

Chlamydiosis

Chlamydia organisms primarily cause conjunctivitis in cats. Chlamydiosis (feline pneumonitis) can be difficult to resolve and may cause problems in breeding catteries, with young kittens being affected most often and most severely.

Feline leukaemia virus (FeLV)

Feline leukaemia is a fatal disease of cats that attacks the white blood cells, causing tumours and other diseases associated with derangement of the immune system. Usually young cats are affected, and an infected queen will transmit the virus to all of her kittens through the placenta, while they are still in the uterus. A blood test is available for FeLV which may be used to diagnose the disease, to eliminate the infection from catteries and to screen cats before vaccination or at rescue catteries before rehoming.

Combined routine vaccinations

Combined feline enteritis and cat 'flu vaccines are the most commonly advised, but more owners are now choosing to have cats vaccinated against feline leukaemia virus and *Chlamydia*. Some manufacturers produce these in a form that allows them to be combined with the more routine vaccinations. Vaccination is usually carried out at 9 and 12 weeks of age, though this regimen may be altered in some circumstances. Booster vaccinations are recommended annually by all manufacturers. For further information on these diseases and vaccination regimens see the *BSAVA Manual of Veterinary Nursing*.

Worming

Cats can play host to a variety of internal parasites, including roundworms, tapeworms and lungworms. Parasites are discussed more fully in the *BSAVA Manual of Veterinary Nursing*, but a brief résumé is given here.

Roundworms

Roundworms can cause problems in young kittens, and routine worming, using a product suitable and safe for kittens, is usually advised. Unlike puppies, kittens are not born with roundworms, but they can be infected by the queen early in life.

Tapeworms

Tapeworms can be transmitted by fleas or by consumption of infected prey. Cats can become reinfested regularly, and may need repeated treatment by either tablet or injectable drugs.

Lungworms

Lungworms are quite common, but rarely cause major disease, though they may be responsible for some cases of mild coughing. Only drugs available from a veterinary surgeon will be suitable to control lungworm infestation.

Fleas

Fleas are very common in cats, and it is an unusual cat who does not pick up some fleas at some stage. Fleas commonly cause skin disease, which can be severe and may need veterinary treatment. There is a peak in flea numbers in the summer, but fleas can be a problem all year round with centrally heated houses. It is usually necessary to treat a cat for fleas at least through the summer months.

There are various control measures. The simple application of insecticide preparations to the coat is common, and these are available as sprays or spot-on style products. An oral preparation which breaks the flea's life cycle is also popular; it can be given in food or by injection.

Where a flea problem is present, it may be necessary to use a spray in the house to kill larvae in the carpet and prevent reinfestation. The control of parasites is also discussed in the *BSAVA Manual of Veterinary Nursing*.

Neutering

It is usual to neuter cats not intended for breeding. This has the advantage of preventing the birth of unwanted kittens, and also of altering the less socially acceptable habits of the entire cat:

- Queens that are not neutered will come into call around every 3 weeks, and can have unpredictable behaviour, including aggression and spraying of urine around the house
- Entire males can be aggressive, and will often spray in the house after sexual maturity.

Spraying is a form of territory marking and can be difficult to stop once the behaviour has become established, as the cat will return to the marked area to reinforce the signal.

Neutering is usually carried out from around 5 months of age, though some advocate earlier neutering. For both sexes general anaesthesia is required.

- Male cats are castrated, having both testes removed via the scrotum
- Female cats have a complete ovariohysterectomy (i.e. the ovaries, oviducts, uterus and cervix are removed) in a procedure usually termed 'spaying'.

Spaying can be carried out by a flank incision or midline (midline is often suggested for Siamese cats as the coat tends to re-grow darker in a shaved patch).

There are many local names for neutering, so do not be surprised if an owner asks for advice on the best age to 'dress' a cat, or when male cats should be 'doctored'. Routine surgical procedures are covered in the *BSAVA Manual of Veterinary Nursing*.

Feeding cats

It is important to recognize that cats have very specific nutritional needs, different from those of dogs, humans and other omnivores. This is because cats are true carnivores and must have a high proportion of meat or other animal tissues in their diet. It is therefore necessary to consider carefully what to feed a cat, and to recognize that table scraps are unlikely to be adequate.

Macronutrients

The macronutrients are protein, fat and carbohydrate.

Protein

Protein requirement, in both quantity and quality, is one of the most important nutritional differences between cats and dogs. Proteins are made up of chains of amino acids, some of which are essential (i.e. have to be consumed in their final form) and some of which are non-essential (i.e. can be synthesized by the cat).

Being strict carnivores, cats have an absolute requirement for meat in their diet. The cat is unable to synthesize certain amino acids (taurine and arginine) found only in animal protein sources and cannot meet these needs from protein of non-animal sources. If these amino-acids are not available in sufficient quantity, deficiency diseases will occur. Taurine deficiency causes serious eye and heart problems; arginine deficiency causes grave metabolic disease.

The cat's reliance on protein does not stop with the supply of essential amino acids. Though protein is usually regarded as a 'body-building' food, most important in growth, pregnancy and lactation, cats also rely on protein to meet part of their energy needs. The protein part of a feline diet should therefore comprise at least 30–40% of the dry matter of a complete food for a healthy cat, which is twice as much as a dog needs. Cats cannot get enough protein from dogfood, and their special amino acid needs mean that they cannot tolerate a vegetarian diet either.

Fat

Fat is another important factor in the feline diet, accounting for about 10% of intake. Fat is important not only as a concentrated energy source, but also as a source of essential fatty acids, and is another reflection of the cat's status as a carnivore. Omnivores can synthesize arachidonic acid from its precursor, linoleic acid, but the cat cannot and it needs animal fat in the diet.

Fat is also a valuable source of the fat-soluble vitamins A, D and E, and the cat requires animal-sourced vitamin A, being unable to produce it from carotene (the vegetable source) as omnivores can. Furthermore, fat makes a diet palatable to cats, and is often used in this way by petfood manufacturers.

Carbohydrate

The remainder of the cat's diet will often come from carbohydrate, a useful source of energy and bulk, and which may also include micronutrients, depending on the source (e.g. B vitamins from wholegrain wheat). As carnivores, cats can survive relying largely on protein and fat for energy sources, but carbohydrates can be useful at times of nutritional stress, and are usually present in commercially prepared foods. Starch sources (cereals, etc.) must be pre-cooked before being fed to cats.

Micronutrients

The micronutrients are vitamins and minerals.

Vitamins

Cats require an animal source of vitamin A, found in fat, but it is important that they do not receive too much vitamin A, as this can lead to skeletal disease. Excessive vitamin A consumption usually occurs in cats with a high consumption of liver, and so feeding liver should be restricted to (at the most) a once-a-week treat, if it is fed at all.

Vitamin E can also cause problems for cats, as it can be destroyed in contact with some fish oils, leading to the painful deficiency disease of pansteatitis (yellow fat disease), where the body fat of the cat becomes inflamed. Feeding cats on a diet with a high proportion of oily fish is therefore to be discouraged, and this includes excessive use of some commercially available products sold as 'complementary' foods.

A further problem with fish is that it can contain an enzyme that destroys the vitamin thiamine (vitamin B_1), causing thiamine deficiency and leading to neuromuscular disease. High levels of some preservatives in brawn-type foods can also break down thiamine and cause thiamine deficiency.

Another vitamin compromised in cats is pyridoxine (vitamin B_6), for which cats have a high requirement. The other vitamins will usually present no cause for concern in a varied diet.

Minerals

The most important minerals are calcium and phosphorus, which must be present in the diet in the correct proportions to allow for healthy bone growth and maintenance. A cat hunting for itself in the wild and consuming the small bones of rodents or birds naturally provides itself with a balanced source. It is important to remember that lean meat will not provide this balance, and supplementation will often be needed if a homemade diet is fed.

Over-supplementation is as dangerous as under-supplementation, and the amounts of any extra calcium and phosphorus given must be calculated properly. Other minerals will usually be present in sufficient quantities in a varied diet.

Water

Water is a basic requirement, essential for all body processes. Cats can concentrate their urine a great deal if required, but water must always be available. The use of dried foods increases the cat's need for water; this will be discussed below.

Milk

Most cats like milk, and it is a valuable source of calcium, protein, fat and vitamins.

Some cats, as they reach adulthood, are unable to digest milk properly. They lack an enzyme in the intestine which breaks down lactose (the milk sugar) and this can lead to diarrhoea. Special cat milks are available which may help to prevent this problem.

For kittens at weaning, a queen's milk replacement is usually preferable to cow's milk. Some cat breeders suggest the use of goat's milk, though this may not be readily available.

Basic nutritional requirements

Nutrition for various stages of the cat's life, including for some disease states, is described in more detail in Chapter 6.

- In general terms, an active adult cat has a calorie (energy) requirement of approximately 85 kilocalories (kcal) per kilogram bodyweight, falling to around 70 kcal/kg for a cat that is less active
- Growing kittens and pregnant queens have higher calorie requirements than this: approximately 100 kcal/kg
- Lactating queens have the highest requirements of all: up to 250 kcal/kg at peak milk production (around 2–4 weeks after kittening).

Although these daily feeding requirements are expressed as energy, it should be remembered that protein is an important source of energy for cats, and that these requirements must be met with a diet balanced for macro- and micronutrients. The higher energy requirements for kittens and pregnant or lactating queens are most easily met by increasing the quantity of fat in the diet, as it is a more concentrated form of energy. Inspection of most prepared foods intended for this group of cats will usually show an increased fat content to help to meet the energy requirements without adding extra bulk, as might be the case if carbohydrate sources are used.

Feeding habits

Cats do not tend to have 'meals' in the same way as dogs or humans do, and are more likely to return to their bowl for a snack at a number of stages during the day. Fed in this way (*ad lib*), cats rarely become overweight. In the occasional case of an overweight or even obese cat, some form of calorie restriction has to be practised.

Types of diets available

The choice is basically between commercially available foods and homemade diets. Although the choice of fresh feeding is uncommon, it is preferred by some breeders.

Fresh (homemade) diet

With a homemade diet it is very important to ensure that no deficiencies or excesses are produced. It can be difficult to achieve a balanced diet, though the cat will often supplement the supplied diet by hunting if outdoor access is allowed.

It is beyond the scope of this chapter to formulate homemade diets but, in general terms:

- Three parts of an animal-derived protein food (meat, fish, eggs, cheese) to one part of carbohydrate (cooked rice, bread, potatoes) will be adequate if combined with a vitamin/mineral mix
- It is usually necessary to give full-cream milk to cats on home-made diets in order to help to meet their calcium needs, though a calcium supplement can also be used
- It is important to remember the general advice about avoiding excesses of liver and fish, to prevent nutritionally related diseases.

Commercially manufactured diet

There is a wide variety of commercial catfoods. They may be presented as canned, semi-moist or dry, and may be either complete (designed to be fed as the entire diet) or complementary (designed to be used as part of a balanced diet). It is common for cats to be fed a mixture of different foods, with perhaps the canned food being given as meals, and dry or semi-moist food left out during the day.

Canned foods

Canned foods remain the most popular in the UK. Similar in nutritional terms to the canned foods are the premium 'tray' foods – individual portions, cooked in a foil tray.

- Most complete canned foods are around 75–80% water, with a balanced mix of protein (around 8%), fat (around 5%) and carbohydrate, and a certified quantity of vitamins and minerals
- An average adult cat (around 4 kg bodyweight) requires approximately one can (400 g) per day
- It is usually necessary to supply a fresh serving at least twice daily when using canned food, as it tends to dry out, lose palatability and become at risk of spoiling
- A food designed for adult cats will usually be sufficient for the needs of pregnant and lactating queens, though of course larger quantities will be required
- Also available in cans are kitten diets, which are higher in fat, protein and vitamins, and which are also eminently suitable for use with pregnant or lactating queens, having a higher calorie content in a smaller volume
- After weaning, kittens should still be fed at least three times a day until around 5–6 months, and should have access to milk or milk-substitute.

Dried foods

Dried foods are the next most commonly used foods. They are usually designed as complete diets.

- The major difference in nutritional terms is the percentage of water, which is less than half the water content of a canned food. A cat on a dried food diet must drink extra water (or milk) to make up the difference
- While canned foods usually rely on animal protein sources alone, some dried foods contain vegetable protein in addition
- Around 100 g of complete dried food, along with about 200 ml of water, is sufficient for an adult cat weighing 4 kg
- Dry food has the advantage that it does not appreciably spoil through the day, though the highly palatable fat on the surface does diminish with time
- Dry food is better for the cat's teeth and gums, and will help to reduce tartar build-up
- Dry food should be introduced gradually into a cat's diet, and may be soaked with water, milk or gravy at first. Changing abruptly to dry food before the cat has had a chance to adapt to increased drinking habits may result in the formation of crystals in the urine, which can be life threatening
- Kitten dry food formulations are also available, as are some 'senior' diets with lower energy concentrations to help to prevent obesity in the less active older cat, and with lower protein, which may assist in lessening the effects of renal failure, a common problem in older cats.

Semi-moist foods

Semi-moist foods have never really gained much popularity in the UK. With a dough-like texture, they are similar to true dry foods in their advantage of convenience and in the requirement for additional water consumption.

These foods can contain a preservative, propylene glycol, which may cause anaemia by reducing the life span of feline red blood cells. Although this is not common, problems may be seen where there is underlying disease.

Complementary foods

All the foods above have been described from the point of view that they are complete, as are most of the catfoods generally available. There are also some complementary foods available, which are designed to be fed as part of a balanced diet, or as part of a homemade diet. As long as they are used as they are intended, there is unlikely to be any problem in feeding complementary foods, but some owners do not realize that these food are not intended as complete diets and this can cause problems.

Perhaps the best known of these are the high-fish canned foods, which can cause pansteatitis due to lack of vitamin E (see above). It is important that owners examine the label of catfood and use the contents as directed.

Another type of complementary food, rarely fed except by cat breeders, is 'brawn', a high-meat product usually produced in a plastic sausage-like skin. Most of these foods are not complete, and may contain high levels of sulphur dioxide as a preservative, which can destroy thiamine and cause thiamine deficiency.

Breeding

It is not usually advisable to breed intentionally from non-pedigree cats; there are so many cats crowding cat shelters that producing more kittens will generally be discouraged by veterinary surgeons or rescue societies.

Reproduction is covered in more detail in the *BSAVA Manual of Veterinary Nursing* but is summarized briefly here.

Signs of oestrus

The queen cat is seasonally polyoestrous (i.e. comes into heat, or on call, many times during a breeding season). When 'on call' she will usually rub against items of furniture, especially marking with the side of her face. If she can find a low chair or table, she will often rub her back along that.

The cardinal sign of calling is lordosis, where the back is flexed downward to push the vulva upward, and she may attempt to entice other cats to mount her, regardless of their sex or ability. This performance is usually accompanied by a loud and persistent yowling call, and she may lie writhing on the ground on her side or back, crying in a most alarming manner. It is not unusual for owners to fail to recognize the signs of calling, and to ring the veterinary surgeon for advice, believing the cat to be in pain.

Breeding season

The breeding season for cats in the UK is from around March to September, though there is individual variation within this and some queens will call all year round, especially pedigree cats of Foreign or Oriental type.

Puberty

The queen will usually reach puberty at between 6 and 15 months, though this depends on breed, date of birth and weight. Cats of the Foreign, Oriental or Siamese type are more precocious; British and Persian cats tend to reach puberty later. Kittens born early in the year may come into call that summer or autumn, while they are little more than kittens themselves.

Males are generally fertile by 5–6 months, but there is similar breed variation on the development of appropriate sexual behaviour.

Mating

Where an owner intends to breed from a cat, it is generally advised that the animal should be at least 12 months old and at most 4 years old at mating. The novice breeder can get a lot of help and advice (at times contradictory) from other cat breeders. It is often a good idea to contact the original breeder for advice on selection of stud, etc., but local or national cat clubs are also valuable sources of information about the location of suitable males.

It is usual for a queen to be taken to the stud cat within the first few days of her starting to call, and for her to remain with him for a week or more. The stud owner will usually observe mating.

It is important that queens are mated frequently, as the stimulation of mating is required to induce ovulation. If a cat is not mated, she will call for around 10 days. After successful mating(s) and ovulation, she will usually come off call within 2–3 days. The gestation period is around 63 days.

Obviously an entire queen, whether pedigree or not, who gets out while on call makes her own arrangements on selection of a male and frequency of mating. There will often be a number of entire males queuing up outside the owner's house awaiting an escape by a calling queen.

Kitten development and behaviour

As kittens usually spend the first few months of their lives with the queen, a great deal of the behavioural influence comes from her and from her owners.

Neonates

At birth, a kitten is blind, mostly deaf (eyes and ears open around 10–14 days) and unable to regulate its own body temperature. It can crawl along the queen's abdomen, seeking a nipple, treading to assist in milk 'let down' and often purring, surprisingly loudly. An individual kitten often has a preference for a particular nipple, and those nearest the back are most favoured. Happy, feeding kittens are quiet; cold or hungry kittens vocalize to let the dam know their distress.

For the first month after parturition the kittens are largely immobile, remaining in the nest feeding (Figure 3.26). The queen stimulates them to urinate and defecate by licking the perineal area, and either consumes the waste or removes it from the nest for disposal elsewhere. Should the queen feel threatened, she will carry the kittens to another nest, by the scruff of the neck – a reflex relaxation of the kitten makes this safe for both queen and kitten and this is a useful method of restraint in later life.

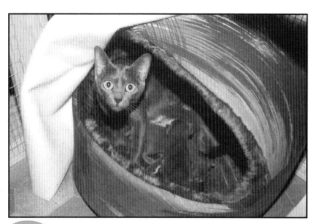

3.26 *Three-week-old Korat kittens in the nest with the queen.*

Contact with the mother during the first month is very important for normal behavioural development of kittens. If the mother dies a foster mother is best, but if this is not possible, quality human contact and handling for at least 20 minutes a day will help to reduce potential problems. More detail on the care of neonatal kittens is given in the *BSAVA Manual of Veterinary Nursing*.

Weaning

As kittens become more mobile at around the end of the first month, they start to leave the nest and the queen starts to become slightly more resistant to their demands for feeding. She presents them with solid food, and teaches them how to bury their faeces and urine.

From this age the normal social contact between kittens matures rapidly as recognition and play behaviour patterns develop. The kitten can already discriminate between the calls of the queen and other kittens, and those of a potential threat, such as growls or sudden unexpected sounds. The senses of vision and smell are also well developed, and weaning on to solid food can start (Figure 3.27). In free-ranging cats, the mother will start to bring in prey at this stage, and though it will be many weeks before the kitten is a competent predator itself, it will learn through observation and play.

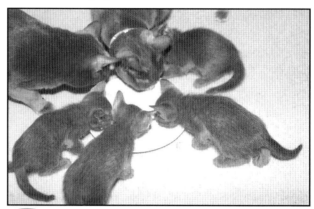

3.27 *Six-week-old Korat kittens at weaning.*

Play behaviour

Play behaviour is a prominent feature of kittens, presumably linked to refining their social and predatory skills, but some patterns seem to have no special function and might perhaps be assumed to be fun. The types of play seen in kittens and cats are often segregated by behaviouralists into social play, object play, locomotor play and self-directed play.

Social play

The patterns used in social play alter as the kittens grow older and more experienced. This form of play starts in the nest and peaks at between 9 and 14 weeks. Kittens will dance sideways, 'bat' at each other with forepaws, lie on their backs, raise themselves on to their haunches, and chase and pounce on each other in a highly ritualized way, all the while with a variety of facial expressions, yowls and growls.

Kittens seem to be able to separate this play from true aggression, and while one or other may be dominant at some times, this position may be rapidly reversed, even in the same encounter. Young kittens will often interact in this way as a 'gang' of three or more, but as they get older often only two kittens are involved in more direct stand-offs. At around 18–20 weeks, actual aggression becomes more common, as does sexual behaviour from the males.

Object play

Object play incorporates some of the features of social play, even though the interaction is with an inanimate object or prey. Kittens will investigate unknown objects intensively (thus the saying, 'Curiosity killed the cat') by observation, sniffing and gentle touching, perhaps from a 'safe' distance and retreating quickly afterwards, and will eventually, especially if the object is small, culminate with batting, chasing and pouncing on it. Kittens will frequently pick up suitably sized objects using one or both paws, for biting or mouthing, and will toss them into the air for further pursuit.

Object play may be better developed in a single kitten, or in hand-reared kittens, where the opportunities for social play with other kittens are unavailable.

This facet of play becomes more important than social play at around 16 weeks, and may be driven by the weaning process. Its persistence seems to depend upon the individual temperament of the cat: some cats will happily play with objects all their lives; others will ignore them after they have grown out of kittenhood. This play is usually considered desirable by owners and can be encouraged by a variety of cat toys available.

Cats are slightly unusual in also using a scoop behaviour to capture an object from a confined space (a box, or from under a chair) by reaching the paw in as far as possible in order to retrieve it. Several toys are designed to exploit this behaviour pattern.

Locomotor play

Locomotor play includes what many owners think of as a kitten's 'mad half-hour' of running about, wild eyed, over many unsuitable objects. A large scratching post may help to divert a kitten from the rival attractions of the curtains or the top of the bookshelves, but even adult cats will indulge in this and send cups or lamps flying, apparently for no good reason. This behaviour is thought to be self-rewarding, i.e. it is just fun.

Self-directed play

Self-directed play is typified by the kitten that chases its tail, or bites its feet. Again, this seems to be purely motivated by fun, rather that having any great purpose. Most cats seem to grow out of these behaviours.

Isolated kittens

A kitten weaned early and reared in isolation (for example, as part of a programme to reduce the level of an infectious disease in a cattery) can suffer as a result of the failure of normal socialization with other adult cats and people. Such kittens need careful handling to ensure that they grow up well balanced.

Activities with cats

Unlike dogs, cats are not usually taken for walks in the country or on the beach, nor do they attend training classes or similar. Cat-orientated activities revolve around playing with owners or suitable toys and, for a few cats, going to cat shows.

Games

It is quite easy to train a tractable cat in some simple activities that can be fun for both owner and cat. Many cats will retrieve objects and will respond to commands similar to those given to dogs ('Sit!', 'Paw!', etc.) in return for an edible reward. Cats will play hide and seek, or other chasing games, with people. Most will 'help' their owners around the house – by lending a paw with tasks such as brushing the floor, or getting between their owner and the computer screen. Some cats like to watch television and there are even videos available for cats to watch.

Cat shows and clubs

Going to cat shows is not solely the domain of the pedigree cat, as there are classes for non-pedigree ('household pet')

cats too. Unlike dogs, neutered cats can also be shown, and have their own classes.

Cat shows are mostly run by local cat clubs, and lists of shows may be obtained from the GCCF or Cat Association of Britain offices (see 'Useful addresses'). As well as running shows, most cat clubs organize social events, which can be a good way for owners to meet others with similar interests.

The rules for showing are quite strict, and the novice is well advised to attend at least one show before considering showing their own cat. All cats are checked on entry to the show hall by a veterinary surgeon, who screens for infectious diseases and veterinary defects. The cats are then 'penned' in cages in which only very specific objects (plain white feed bowl, water bowl, litter tray, blanket) are allowed. The cat is identified only by a number, to ensure impartiality of judging.

Usually, a cat or kitten may be entered in an 'open' class, where it competes against others of the same breed, and then may enter further classes for mixed breeds (e.g. 'Any variety Foreign kitten').

- When a pedigree cat is adult (and entire), it competes for a Challenge Certificate (CC) in the open class. If it wins three of these, the cat becomes a champion
- Champions may compete for a Grand Challenge Certificate (GCC) in a mixed breed open class for champions of their breed group; in a similar way, a cat with three GCCs is a grand champion
- Many clubs also run a best-in-show competition.

The major show in the British cat world is the GCCF Supreme Show, where cats compete for top honours. Here, in addition to the normal classes, there is a special class for grand champions to compete for UK Grand Challenge Certificates. As this show only takes place once a year, just two UKGCCs are needed to become a UK grand champion.

The system outlined for entire cats is exactly mirrored by one for neuters, in which the competition is for premier, grand premier, etc.

Although the GCCF is the major registering body in the UK, there are others and these may have different procedures. They may recognize further breeds, or variants of established breeds (in terms of colour or pattern), and have different show rules and awards. For example, the Cat Association of Britain allows Sphynx to be shown, permits decoration of pens and has different judging procedures.

Further reading

A number of cat magazines are available from newsagents, with articles for those interested in cats. These can be very useful and informative for both clients and professionals, and a good source of information on pedigree cat breeders in specific geographical areas.

Bradbury JWS (1992) *The Behaviour of the Domestic Cat*. CAB International, Wallingford, Oxon.
Pedersen NC (1991) *Feline Husbandry*. American Veterinary Publications Inc., Goleta, California.
Robinson R (1991) *Genetics for Cat Breeders* (3rd edn). Butterworth Heinemann, Oxford.
Taylor D (1989) *The Ultimate Cat Book*. Dorling Kindersley, London.

Turner T and Turner J (1994) *Veterinary Notes for Cat Owners*. Stanley Paul, London.

Walter S (1980) *The Book of the Cat*. Pan Books, London.

Wills JM and Simpson KW (1994) *The Waltham Book of Clinical Nutrition of the Dog and Cat*. Butterworth Heinemann, Oxford.

Useful addresses

Pedigree cat organizations

Pedigree cat clubs may be local or national. These associations maintain lists of affiliated clubs. Many breed clubs operate a rescue scheme for pedigree cats.

Governing Council of the Cat Fancy
4–6 Penel Orlieu, Bridgwater, Somerset TA6 3PG
01278 427575
http://ourworld.compuserve.com/homepages/GCCF_CATS/

Cat Association of Britain
Mill House, Letcombe Regis, Oxon OX12 9JD
01235 766543

Fédération Internationale Féline
General Secretary: Ms Penelope Bydlinski, Little Dene, Lenham Heath, Maidstone, Kent ME17 2BS
01622 850913
http://www2.dk-online.dk/users/kriste_m/fife/fifemain.htm

Other organizations

Feline Advisory Bureau
Headquarters: 'Teaselbury', High Street, Tisbury, Wiltshire SP3 6LD
01747 871872
http://web.ukonline.co.uk/fab/fab.html

The FAB is a charity that supports a number of veterinary surgeons working in the field of feline medicine at a number of the veterinary schools in the UK. It publishes a quarterly journal with articles of general and veterinary interest, and organizes meetings for breeders and veterinary surgeons. It also runs a boarding cattery inspection service, and publishes a guide to catteries.

Association of Pet Behavioural Counsellors
PO Box 46, Worcester, WR8 9YS
01386 751151
http://www.apbc.org.uk

The APBC is a network of behavioural counsellors who, on referral from a veterinary surgeon, can give advice on the management of pet animals exhibiting inappropriate behaviour.

Cat shelters

Two major groups run cat shelters in the UK; numerous small organizations are also involved. Look in the Yellow Pages of the telephone directory for local shelters. Veterinary surgeons often have lists of local groups.

Cats Protection
Headquarters: 17 Kings Road, Horsham, West Sussex RH13 5PN
01403 221900
http://www.cats.org.uk

A charity basically for cat rescue, CP can also sometimes provide support to owners in financial difficulty over neutering of their cats. It publishes leaflets about cat care and infectious diseases.

Royal Society for the Prevention of Cruelty to Animals
Headquarters: Causeway, Horsham, West Sussex RH12 1HG
01403 223284
http://www.rspca.org.uk

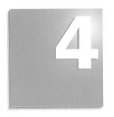

4 General care and management of other pets and wildlife

Anna Meredith and Sharon Redrobe

This chapter is designed to give information on:

- The species of animals kept as exotic pets, and their advantages and disadvantages as pets
- Basic biology, anatomy and husbandry requirements of exotic pets
- How to handle and determine the sex of exotic pets and wildlife safely and humanely
- How to recognize the signs of pain and disease in exotic pets and wildlife
- How to administer basic medication to exotic pets and wildlife

Introduction

Pets other than cats and dogs are extremely popular, and their numbers are on the increase. The rabbit is now the third most popular mammalian pet in the United Kingdom. In addition to small mammals, many people keep birds, reptiles, amphibians, fish and invertebrates as pets. In many veterinary practices, these so-called exotic pets make up a significant proportion of the patient caseload, and some practices now offer specialist expertise in exotic pets.

The expectations of the owners for the level of knowledge and care that these animals should receive is also increasing, and the aim of this chapter is to provide guidance as to the suitability of the various species as pets, and to give a broad introduction to their general husbandry and care.

Abandoned, injured and sick wild animals are also commonly presented for veterinary attention. The requirements and behaviour of wildlife are extremely varied and often differ very significantly from those of domestic animals. This chapter will describe the techniques for caring for wildlife patients, including emergency first aid for the wildlife casualty.

Exotic pets: considerations before purchasing

The main types of pets that are generally available are listed in Figure 4.1.

Unfortunately a lot of pets are purchased on impulse and without any prior thought or planning. This can lead to welfare and disease problems and unwanted animals, as owners

4.1 Types of exotic pets available

Mammals	Rabbit, guinea-pig, chinchilla, hamster, gerbil, rat, mouse, ferret
Birds	Parrot, budgerigar, canary, finch, pigeon
Reptiles	Snake, lizard, tortoise, turtle, terrapin
Amphibians	Frog, toad, salamander, axolotl
Fish	Goldfish, tropical fish
Invertebrates	Stick insect, spider, snail

are not aware of their special requirements. Research and advice from knowledgeable sources should always be sought before acquiring a new pet. Veterinary nurses are often approached for advice on this subject. Points that should be considered are given below.

- The reason for wanting a pet – companionship, special interest, children's pet, education. A reptile would not be suitable for someone wanting a close companion with a lot of interaction
- Facilities and space available – a garden is desirable for rabbits, guinea-pigs or ferrets, whereas very little space is required for invertebrates
- Financial aspects – costs of housing, feeding and veterinary care. Vivarium set-ups for reptiles can be very expensive, whereas a pet hamster is very cheap to keep
- Amount of spare time available. Parrots need a lot of individual attention from an owner who is at home most of the time, whereas fish require very little attention
- Other pets already kept – some species may be incompatible or must be kept apart, such as small mammals and cats
- Human health risks – many people are allergic to the hair

Mammal	Advantages	Disadvantages
Mouse	Small, cheap, cling to handler	Smell, tend to be more active at night
Rat	Intelligent, responsive, sociable, cling to handler	
Gerbil	Odourless, active during day	Difficult to handle, easily dropped
Hamster	Odourless	Nocturnal, can bite, easily dropped
Chipmunk	Active during day	Easily stressed, difficult to handle, best kept outdoors
Guinea-pig	Rarely bite, active during day	Can be nervous
Chinchilla	Extremely attractive	Destructive, often dislike being handled
Rabbit	Generally docile, good house pets	Occasionally aggressive, or nervous and difficult to handle. Larger breeds difficult for young children to handle
Ferret	Highly intelligent, responsive, entertaining	Smell, need a lot of attention, good escape artists!

Species	Advantages	Disadvantages
Birds	Very responsive, trainable, talk (psittacines) 'Guard dogs' (geese) Provide eggs (poultry)	Require a lot of attention (psittacines) Can be noisy and destructive (psittacines) Can be aggressive (geese)
Reptiles	Quiet, low maintenance once initial vivarium equipment set up, non-allergenic	Equipment expensive, some species dangerous, do not respond to owner, diet can be unpleasant to owner, some species very inactive, some species can grow very large
Amphibians	Quiet, low maintenance, non-allergenic	Handling not advised, often very inactive
Fish	Quiet, soothing to watch, low maintenance	No direct interaction

and dander of small mammals, and there are several zoonotic diseases that can be passed on to owners from pets, such as psittacosis from parrots and pigeons, and salmonellosis from reptiles.

For specific information on the advantages and disadvantages of individual species as pets, and their care requirements, refer to the sections on 'Popular exotic pets' and 'General care'.

Popular exotic pets

When choosing a pet, it is useful to consider the advantages and disadvantages of the species available (Figures 4.2 and 4.3).

Mammals

Mice

- Small and easy to keep
- Good climbers and cling on to the handler, therefore unlikely to be dropped by small children
- Male mice have a distinctive strong smell, which can be unpleasant
- Although they are social animals, male mice often fight if kept together, so a breeding pair or harem, or two or more females, should be kept
- More active at night
- Can bite if not handled frequently.

Rats

- Increasingly popular pets, among adults as well as children (Figure 4.4)
- Like mice, they cling on to the handler and so are unlikely to be dropped
- Sociable, highly intelligent and responsive and will learn to recognize their owner
- Most are very docile and rarely bite
- Naturally more active at night, but if handled frequently they often adapt to their owner's timetable.

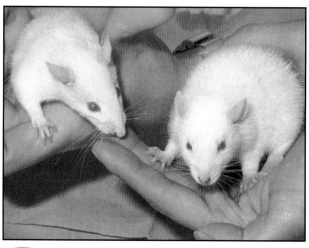

4.4 *Rats are becoming increasingly popular as pets. Courtesy of Dr P. Flecknell.*

Gerbils

- Attractive and entertaining
- Active in the day, when they are constantly arranging and rearranging their bedding, digging and gnawing
- Produce very little urine and are almost odourless
- Social animals and form monogamous pairs
- Two males can be kept together if litter-mates, otherwise a breeding pair or two females should be kept
- Rarely bite, but can be difficult to handle, and can leap vertically in the air if startled
- Do not cling to the handler and can easily be dropped
- Incorrect handling can lead to sloughing of the tail skin (see 'Handling and sexing').

Hamsters

Golden or Syrian hamster

- Many varieties exist, including long-haired and satin-coated
- Solitary, and should be kept singly
- Mainly nocturnal
- Can often bite, especially if roused from a deep sleep during the day
- Easily dropped and injured
- Hibernate at temperatures below about 5°C, and will become torpid (aestivation) at very high temperatures.

Russian (dwarf) hamster

- About half the size of Syrian hamsters, with a very round body shape
- Naturally a grey coat with black tips to the hairs, a dark stripe down the back and a pale underside, although different varieties now exist (e.g. albino). The tail is very short
- Can be very aggressive if not handled frequently and are easily dropped
- Social animals and, unlike Syrian hamsters, should be kept in female groups or breeding pairs or harems
- Do not hibernate.

Chinese (dwarf) hamsters

- Similar to Russian hamsters, but with a longer tail and more elongated body shape
- Social and do not hibernate.

Chipmunks

- Best kept in large aviary-type wire enclosures outside, as they are easily stressed and develop stereotypic repetitive behaviour in small cages

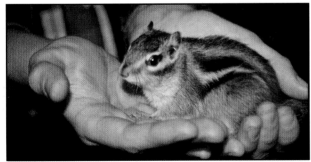

4.5   *A chipmunk.*
Photo: Anna Meredith.

- Presence of electrical equipment such as television sets and computers is very stressful – it is thought that the ultrasonic frequencies emitted when these appliances are in use are very distressing to chipmunks
- Remain essentially wild in captivity and are very nervous; can be difficult to handle unless they have been hand-reared (Figure 4.5)
- Will hibernate for short periods in very cold weather.

Guinea-pigs

- Three main types of guinea-pig kept as pets, although a huge number of breeds and varieties exists
- The English has a short smooth coat (Figure 4.6)
- The Abyssinian a longer rough 'rosetted' coat
- The Peruvian is long-haired, requires daily grooming and is mainly kept for showing purposes
- Generally very docile and almost never bite, but tend to be nervous and easily startled
- Highly sociable animals and should not be kept singly. Groups of females can be kept together, or two or more males, as long as they are not within sight, sound or smell of females. Males can be castrated or vasectomized and females spayed.

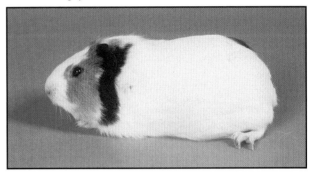

4.6   *An English guinea-pig.*
Courtesy of Dr P. Flecknell.

Chinchillas

- Very attractive with beautiful soft fur, fluffy tail and large whiskers (Figure 4.7)
- Often resent being handled
- Mainly nocturnal
- Have a tendency to gnaw and be very destructive.

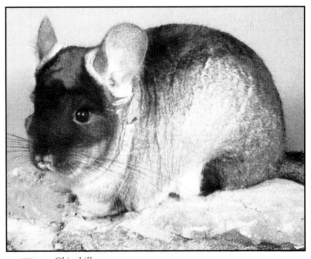

4.7   *Chinchilla.*
Photo: Anna Meredith.

Rabbits

- Over 80 breeds or varieties of rabbit, ranging in size from 1 kg to 10 kg or more
- Traditionally kept outside, but do make very good house pets
- Highly sociable, but two males (bucks) will fight
- Diurnal
- Generally docile if handled regularly. Large rabbits can be difficult for young children to handle; and incorrect handling can damage their spine
- Rabbits should be vaccinated annually against myxomatosis and viral haemorrhagic disease, and routine neutering is also advised. This expense should be born in mind before purchase.

Ferrets

- Originally domesticated and bred for hunting rabbits
- Highly intelligent and entertaining pets that require a lot of attention from and interaction with their owner and regular exercise
- Have the disadvantage of a very distinctive smell that many people find unpleasant. This is particularly strong in the male, and although neutering will decrease the odour slightly, it is a myth that a ferret can be 'descented', as the odour is from the sebaceous gland secretions rather than the anal sacs.

Birds

Psittacines

The term psittacine is generally used to refer to members of the Order Psittaciformes.
- Popular species include the budgerigar, cockatiel, lovebird, parrots and cockatoos
- Psittacines are kept indoors in or out of cages as pets, or outdoors in aviaries as breeding or exhibition specimens
- All psittacines are highly intelligent and social, and can be very destructive
- Some species, including budgerigars, African Grey parrots (Figure 4.8) and Amazon parrots, can be taught to talk

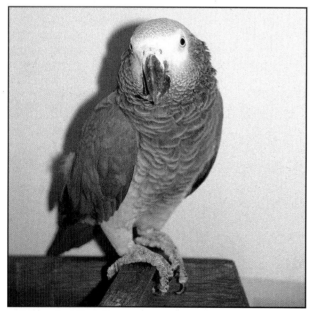

4.8 *An African Grey parrot.*
Photo: Sharon Redrobe.

- The larger species in particular make very demanding pets, require a great deal of attention and companionship, and should not be left alone for long periods. They are therefore not suitable pets for people who go out to work all day
- The larger species of parrot can live for 40 to 50 years or longer
- Hand-reared British birds make the best pets. Birds that are not hand-reared can be very difficult to tame and can inflict a painful bite
- Pet parrots kept singly often form a strong pair-bond with one member of the household and become aggressive towards other family members.

Passerines

Passerines are the perching birds, which include canaries and finches.

- Male canaries are kept for their attractive singing
- Other finches are best kept in pairs or in flocks in aviaries
- These birds are rarely very tame.

Domestic fowl

Chickens, ducks and geese are sometimes kept as pets.

- These species must be kept outside, with a secure house or pen to protect them from predators at night
- Geese can be used as guard animals, and are very long-lived (20 years or more)
- Ducks and geese will require access to water to swim on
- All three species have the advantage of providing eggs for consumption.

Reptiles

Reptiles can be divided into three main groups: snakes (Figure 4.9), lizards (Figure 4.10) and chelonians (tortoises, turtles and terrapins (Figure 4.11)). In general tortoises are terrestrial, terrapins are semi-aquatic and turtles are aquatic. There are exceptions to this; for example, the Americans tend to refer to all chelonians as turtles.

- Reptiles have very specialized husbandry requirements (see 'General care') which can be expensive
- While many people find reptiles very attractive and fascinating, they are not interactive or 'cuddly' pets, and only tolerate being handled
- Although some owners would claim to have a strong relationship with their reptile, this is largely anthropomorphism, but in some species in particular (such as tortoises) distinct personalities can be observed
- Strict attention to hygiene must be observed if reptiles are kept as pets, as they can carry salmonella in their faeces
- Some species can grow very large. For example, the green iguana when mature can be up to 1.8 m in length, and the larger snakes can grow to about 4.6 m (e.g. Burmese python). These facts must be born in mind when buying a small juvenile, especially in terms of the size of the housing they will require
- Some people find the dietary requirements of reptiles unpleasant to deal with: for example, dead rodents for snakes, insects for lizards
- Large lizards can inflict deep scratches with their claws and can lash out with their tail. Large snakes can constrict around a handler's limbs or neck. All reptiles can bite.

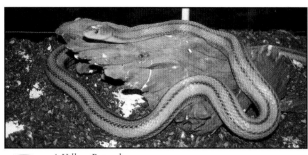

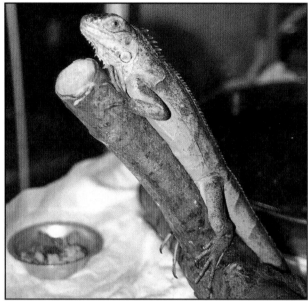

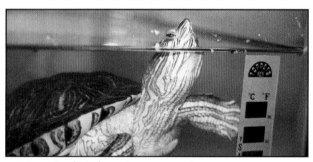

Amphibians

Frogs, toads, salamanders, newts and axolotls are all kept as pets.

- Amphibians have delicate moist permeable skin that is easily damaged, so these animals should not be handled on a regular basis
- They need a vivarium tank and some species will need special heating and lighting and water filtration arrangements.

Fish

Fish are not very interactive pets, but many people find them soothing and therapeutic to watch.

- Fish are low maintenance pets and relatively easy to keep, as long as the water quality is good
- Freshwater species, such as goldfish, and many species of tropical fish are widely available.

Anatomy and physiology

Mammals

The mammals are haired endothermic ('warm-blooded') animals that bear live young and suckle them. The small mammals kept as exotic pets share the basic mammalian features of the dog and cat, with some important differences, especially in dentition, gastrointestinal tract and female reproductive tract anatomy. Figure 4.12 gives basic biological data for small mammal pets.

Rodents

The Order Rodentia can be divided into three suborders:

- Myomorphs (mice, rats, hamsters, gerbils)
- Hystricomorphs (guinea-pigs and chinchillas)
- Sciuromorphs (chipmunks, squirrels).

All share many anatomical features.

Teeth and jaws

- Rodents are gnawing mammals, and they possess chisel-shaped curving incisors for gnawing and flat cheek teeth for chewing
- The temporomandibular joint is adapted so that the mandible can move forward and back to allow either

4.12   Small mammals: biological data

Species	Average lifespan (years)	Maturity	Oestrus	Gestation (days)	Average litter size	Weaning age	Adult weight	Body temperature (°C)
Mouse	2–2.5	3–4 weeks	every 4–5 days	19-21	5–10	18 days	20–40g	37.5
Rat	3	6 weeks	every 4–5 days	20–22	6–12	21 days	250–600g	38
Hamster	1.5–2	6–10 weeks	every 4 days	15–18[a] 19–22[b]	3–7	21–28 days	100–150g[a] 20–40g[b]	38
Gerbil	2–3	10–12 weeks	every 4–6 days	24–26	3–6	21–28 days	70–120g	38
Guinea-pig	4–7	8–10 weeks (♂) 4–5 weeks (♀)	every 15–16 days	60–72 (av. 65)	2–6	3–3½ weeks	750–1000g	38–39
Chinchilla	10–15	8 months	every 30–35 days (Nov–May)	111	2–3	6–8 weeks	350–500g	38–39
Chipmunk	3–5	1 year	every 14 days (Mar–Sep)	28–32	2–6	6–7 weeks	100–150g	38
Rabbit	6–8	3–6 months	induced ovulation (Jan-Oct)	28–32	2–7	6 weeks	1–10kg	38.5
Ferret	5–7	6–9 months	induced ovualtion (Feb–Sep)	42	2–6	8 weeks	0.5–2kg	38.8

[a] Syrian
[b] Russian/Chinese

gnawing or chewing, and from side to side

- In the myomorphs the dental formula is 1/1, 0/0, 0/0, 3/3, and the enamel covering the front surface of the incisors is orange-yellow to reddish in colour
- In the guinea-pig and chinchilla, the dental formula is 1/1, 0/0, 1/1, 3/3 and the enamel is creamy-white in colour
- The lower mandible is wider than the upper maxilla
- The gap between the incisor teeth and the molar teeth is called the diastema (Figure 4.13). Narrow cheek folds are drawn across this to separate the front and the back parts of the mouth
- The incisors have open roots and grow continuously throughout life. The cheek teeth are also open rooted and grow continuously, although this is very slow in the myomorphs
- The upper lip is cleft.

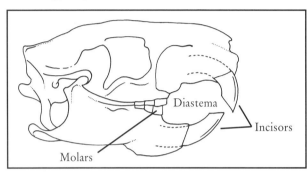

4.13 *A simplified rodent skull. The 'dental formula' of an animal shows the number of incisors, canines, premolars and molars in the upper and lower jaws. The dental formula here is 1/1, 0/0, 0/0, 3/3.*

Digestive tract

The digestive tract of rodents consists of a simple stomach, long small intestine, large caecum (which is sacculated in the hystricomorphs and is where breakdown of plant material occurs) and a long colon.

- The rat does not possess a gall bladder, but the other species do
- Mice, rats and chipmunks are omnivores, whereas the other species are mainly herbivorous
- All rodents practise coprophagy (the eating of faeces), which enhances the uptake of vitamins B and K.

Reproductive system

Female rodents have separate vaginal and urethral openings (Figure 4.14).

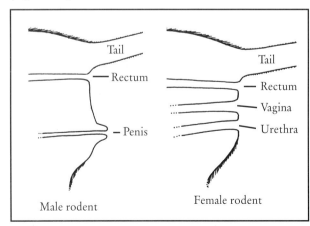

4.14 *Perineal openings in male and femal rodents.*

The vaginal opening is usually only patent when the animal is in oestrus
- After mating, a vaginal plug is formed. This is visible in the rat, mouse, guinea-pig and chinchilla and persists for 1–2 days. Its presence is used by breeders to show if mating has taken place.

In the myomorphs, only females have nipples (five or six pairs), whereas in the hystricomorphs both the males and females have two inguinal nipples. All male rodents have an open inguinal ring and can retract the testicles into the abdomen.

Toes
The myomorphs have four toes on the forefeet and five toes on the hind feet. Guinea-pigs have four toes on the forefeet and three toes on the hind feet, and chinchillas have five toes on the forefeet and four toes on the hindfeet.

Other features
Other features of individual species are:

- Hamsters have large cheek pouches
- Hamsters have scent glands on their flank which are often pigmented and become hairless with age
- Gerbils have a large hairless scent gland on the ventral abdomen (more obvious in males)
- Guinea-pigs have a glandular area in the midline above the tail which produces a greasy secretion.

Rabbits
Rabbits belong to the Order Lagomorpha, which has distinct anatomical differences from the Rodentia.

Teeth and jaws

- Lagomorphs have a second small pair of incisors ('peg teeth') directly behind the first pair in the upper jaw. The dental formula is 2/1, 0/0, 3/2, 3/3
- Rabbit teeth are not pigmented and the enamel should appear smooth and creamy-white in colour
- The upper incisors possess a single vertical groove
- As in rodents, the large diastema has cheek folds drawn across it
- Both incisors and cheek teeth are open rooted and grow constantly throughout life.

Skeleton
The rabbit skeleton is lightweight, making up only 7–8% of body weight (compared with 12–13% in dogs and cats).

Limbs and feet
The hindlegs are long and the metatarsal area is in contact with the ground at rest. The feet have no bare footpads and are completely covered in hair. There are four toes and a dewclaw on the forefeet and four toes on the hindfeet.

Tail and ears
The tail or 'scut' is short and curves upwards over the rump. The ears are large and upright, except in lop breeds. Female rabbits develop a large fold of skin under the chin, known as the dewlap.

Digestive tract
The rabbit's digestive tract has a simple large stomach, a long small intestine, a very large sacculated caecum and a long colon.

- Rabbits produce two types of faeces: soft mucus-covered caecal pellets (caecotrophs), which are produced at night or in the early morning and eaten directly from the anus (coprophagy); and hard dry faecal pellets, which are not eaten
- Rabbits excrete excess dietary calcium in the urine and it is normal for the urine to contain crystals
- Normal urine can vary in appearance from thick and turbid to clear, and range in colour from pale creamy-yellow through to a deep red, depending on the diet of the rabbit
- Reddish urine is often mistaken as containing blood; a urine dipstick will test for the actual presence of blood.

Ferrets

Ferrets are carnivores and belong to the Order Mustelidae. They have a typical carnivorous dentition similar to cats and dogs. The dental formula is 3/3, 1/1, 3/3, 1/2.

Ferrets have long backs, small rounded furred ears, short legs and a medium-length furred tail. All four feet have five toes. The digestive system is similar to other carnivores, with a simple stomach and no caecum. Ferrets possess a pair of anal sacs which secrete an unpleasant smelling liquid.

Birds

Birds are vertebrate endothermic animals with a high metabolic rate and body temperature (40–42°C). They are adapted for flight in several ways:

- The presence of feathers
- A lightweight skeleton (Figure 4.15) – the bones have thin cortices and some contain an air sac (pneumatic bones). The skull weight is reduced by containing air-filled sinuses and having no teeth
- Fusion of some of the vertebrae to provide body rigidity. The neck remains flexible to allow the bird to reach all parts of its body with the beak
- A large sternum (keel) for attachment of powerful flight muscles.

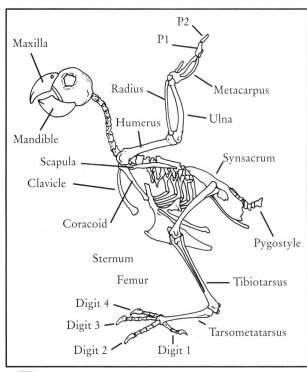

4.15   *A simplified bird skeleton.*

Feathers

Feathers (Figure 4.16) are made of keratin and can be divided into:

- Flight feathers on the wings and tail, which are rigid and long
- Contour feathers on the body, neck and head, which are short
- Down feathers and filoplumes that lie under the contour feathers and provide insulation.

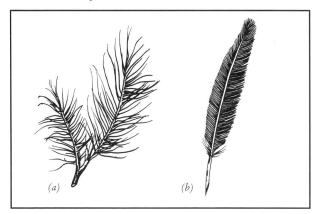

4.16   *Birds have two basic types of feather: (a) down; (b) contour, or flight.*

Feathers are moulted and replaced usually once a year in most species, but up to three times a year in some (e.g. budgerigars). Growing feathers contain a blood vessel in the shaft and are protected by a keratin sheath.

Pelvis

The pelvis of birds has an open pubis rather than a symphysis, to allow passage of a large egg.

Beak

The beak consists of bone covered in cornified keratin. In psittacines there is a hinge joint (craniofacial hinge) between the upper beak and the skull, allowing greater movement of the upper beak in relation to the lower than in other species.

Ear

Birds have no external ear.

Feet

Birds have four digits on their feet:

- In psittacines, the outer two point backward and the middle two point forward
- In most other species the outer three digits point forward and the inner digit points backward
- In ducks and geese the three forward-pointing digits are webbed
- Cockerels have a sharp, backward-pointing, horny spur above the foot which is used in fighting.

Digestive tract

There are two significant features of the bird digestive system (Figure 4.17) that are different from mammals:

- The crop, which is used to store food; it is present in some species, like psittacines and pigeons, and absent in others
- The gizzard, which has a thick muscular wall and is used for grinding food.

Bird droppings consist of three portions: brown-green faeces, white urates and liquid urine (Figure 4.18). The colour of the faeces depends on the diet of the bird.

Respiratory system

The avian respiratory system (Figure 4.19) is much more efficient than that of mammals and consists of paired lungs plus a system of air sacs that act as 'bellows'. This allows oxygenated air to flow through the lungs in both inspiration and expiration.

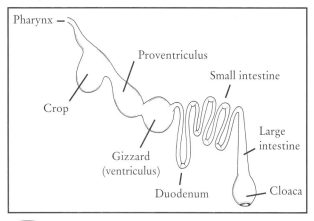

4.17 *The digestive tract of a bird.*

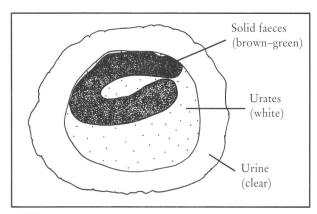

4.18 *The parts of a normal bird dropping.*

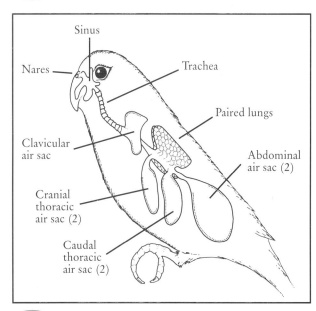

4.19 *The respiratory system of a bird*

Reptiles

Reptiles differ significantly from mammals and birds in that they are ectothermic ('cold-blooded'). This means they are unable to generate body heat and rely on an external heat source and behavioural means to regulate their body temperature.

Reptiles have a dry skin that is folded into scales (Figure 4.20). All reptiles shed their skin periodically in a process known as ecdysis. The pattern of shedding depends on the species.

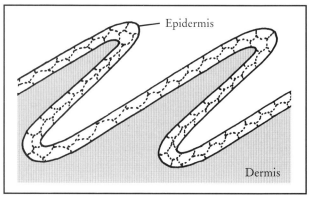

4.20 *The epidermis of a reptile is folded to form the characteristic scales.*

The cloaca is the common opening of the digestive, reproductive and urinary tracts. Reptiles produce droppings with three components: faeces, white urates and, in some species, urine.

Snakes

Snakes have an elongated slender body shape (Figure 4.21).

- They have no visible limbs. Some species have vestigial skeletal pelvic girdles and hindlimbs (e.g. boas, pythons)
- Snakes have from 150 to 400 vertebrae, each articulating with a pair of ribs as far as the cloaca. In the tail the ribs are small and fused to the vertebrae
- Snakes have no sternum
- The lower jaw has no mandibular symphysis and the upper and lower jaw are only loosely connected, enabling a snake to have a very large gape and swallow prey that is larger than its head
- Snakes have backward-pointing teeth. Only venomous snakes have fangs
- Snakes have no eyelids but have a clear scale of skin over the surface of the eye known as the spectacle.

Snakes shed their skin all in one piece, including the spectacles, starting at the head. About 4–7 days before shedding they will appear dull and cloudy, as a layer of milky fluid is secreted between the old and new layers of skin.

Lizards

The lizard skeleton follows the basic vertebrate pattern, with four limbs in most species and a tail.

- Some lizards are able to shed their tail (autotomy) as an escape mechanism, and can grow a new one. The replacement does not contain bony vertebrae, only cartilage, and will be dull in colour and have smaller scales than the rest of the body
- Lizards shed their skin in large pieces, and will often eat the dead skin

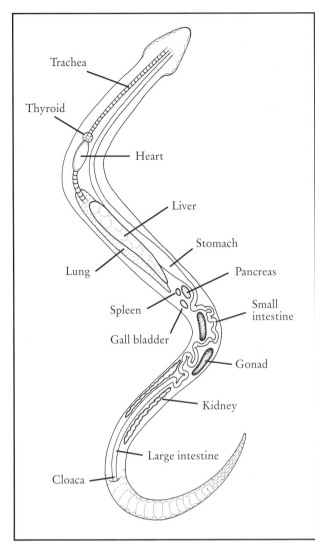

The internal organs of a snake.

All amphibians require water to breed. Their life cycle involves a larval tadpole stage with gills, which undergoes metamorphosis into the adult form. Axolotls are unique in that they remain and can become sexually mature in the larval stage, although they can metamorphose under certain conditions.

Fish

Fish are ectothermic. They possess gills which extract oxygen from the water as it flows over them.

- The skin is covered with scales
- Fish have no eyelids
- The digestive system is simple and has intestinal (pyloric) caeca
- The swim bladder connects to the digestive tract in most species (Figure 4.22).

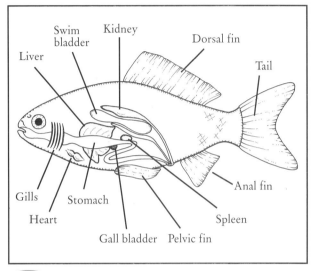

4.22 *External features and internal organs of a fish.*

- The structure of the digestive system varies depending on the diet. For example, herbivorous lizards such as the green iguana have a large caecum
- Lizards have simple teeth.

Chelonians

The body of the chelonian consists of a bony box or 'shell'. The upper shell is the carapace; the lower shell is the plastron.

- All chelonians shed the skin on the limbs, neck and head, in small pieces
- Only terrapins shed scales or 'scutes' from their shell
- Chelonians possess a hard horny 'beak' and do not have teeth.

Contrary to popular belief, it is not possible to age a tortoise from the rings on its shell. These rings correspond to periods of rapid growth, which are not necessarily annual.

Amphibians

Amphibians have a basic vertebrate skeleton.

- Frogs and toads are tailless and have long hindlegs, whereas newts and salamanders have tails
- All have moist permeable skin across which oxygen is absorbed
- Some species (e.g. toads) have skin glands that secrete toxins.

Handling and sexing

Small mammals

Male and female small mammals can be told apart by the anogenital distance, which is greater in the male.

Mice

Mice are often not used to being handled and so care should be taken not to get bitten.

- The mouse should be grasped firmly by the base of the tail and lifted out of the cage or box (Figure 4.23a)
- It can then be placed on a rough surface such as a towel or the sleeve
- If gentle traction is maintained on the tail the animal grips the rough surface and tries to pull away, making it remain stationary and enabling a visual examination to be undertaken
- For additional restraint, such as for injection, the scruff is grasped between the thumb and forefinger of either the same hand or the other hand (Figure 4.23b). Sufficient scruff must be grasped to prevent the mouse turning its head to bite.

Sexing is by anogenital distance (greater in the male), and the presence of nipples in the female.

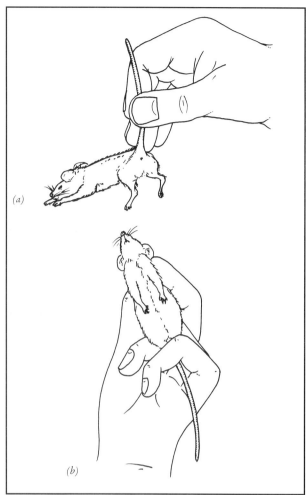

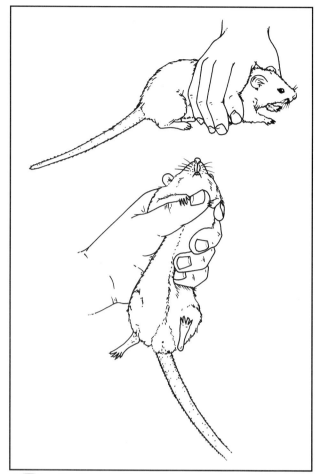

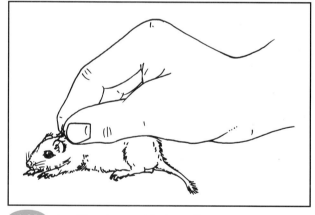

4.23 *Handling a mouse (a) Grasping the base of the tail.*
(b) Grasping the scruff.

4.24 *Handling a rat. The thumb is placed under the mandible to prevent biting.*

Rats

Most pet rats are very docile and used to being handled.

- They can be picked up by grasping gently around the shoulders and lifting out of the cage or box, with the thumb placed under the mandible to prevent biting (Figure 4.24).
- If the animal is large or pregnant the body weight should be supported with the other hand, and the tail can be held with the other hand to steady the animal – for example, if an intraperitoneal injection is to be given
- A fractious animal can be scruffed as described for the smaller rodents, but many rats resent this if they are not used to it, and vocalize
- Rats can also be lifted on to the sleeve by grasping the very base of the tail and lifting gently. They should not, however, be suspended by the tail.

Sexing is by anogenital distance and the presence of nipples in the female.

Gerbils

Gerbils must *never* be held by the tail as the skin is very delicate and can easily be pulled off. To restrain a gerbil, first capture it using cupped hands, or place the whole hand over the back of the gerbil and hold it gently around the shoulders, with the thumb under the mandible. Gerbils do not tend to bite. Alternatively, grasp the scruff as for the mouse (Figure 4.25).

Sexing is by anogenital distance.

4.25 *A gerbil can be grasped by the scruff.*

Hamsters

Make sure the hamster is awake, or gently wake it up before handling, otherwise it may be startled and bite. Some hamsters resent being handled and can be quite aggressive, especially Russian and Chinese hamsters.

- A docile hamster can be cupped between two hands (Figure 4.26) and gently lifted and rolled on to its back if necessary
- For true restraint, the loose scruff should be firmly grasped between the thumb and forefinger. (It is a myth that scruffing a hamster tightly will cause its eyes to pop out!)
- There is a lot of loose skin around the scruff in hamsters due to the presence of cheek pouches. If insufficient skin is grasped the hamster will be able to turn its head and bite

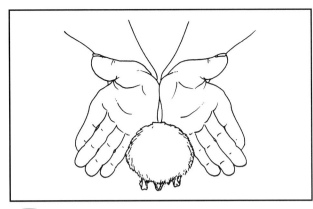

4.26 *A docile hamster can be cupped between two hands.*

- The body weight can be supported with the other hand in large or pregnant individuals.

The mature male has very large obvious testicles. Otherwise anogenital distance can be used to sex hamsters.

Chipmunks
Most chipmunks are not used to being handled and resent it. They should be grasped firmly but gently around the shoulders with the thumb under the chin to prevent biting.
Sexing is by anogenital distance.

Guinea-pigs
Guinea-pigs are often nervous and easily startled, so a rapid, smooth approach to handling should be adopted.

- The guinea-pig should be grasped around the shoulders and lifted clear of the cage or box (Figure 4.27)
- The hindquarters should be supported with the other hand (Figure 4.27)
- Guinea-pigs very rarely bite.

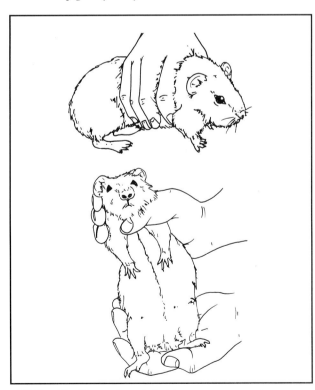

4.27 *Handling a guinea-pig. It is important to support the hindquarters.*

To sex guinea-pigs, look at the conformation of the genital opening. In the male (boar) a circle of tissue is present through which, when pressure is exerted above it, the penis can be extruded. The female (sow) has a Y-shaped opening. The anogenital distance is similar in males and females. Both sexes have two inguinal nipples.

Chinchillas
Chinchillas often dislike being handled, and wriggle violently when restrained.

- They should be grasped gently but firmly around the shoulders, and the body weight supported with the other hand
- Rough handling can lead to a condition known as 'fur-slip', where large chunks of fur fall out.

Sexing chinchillas is by anogenital distance. Confusion can arise, as female chinchillas have a large urethral process which can be confused with a penis.

Rabbits
Rabbits should never be picked up by the ears.

- The correct way to handle a rabbit is to grasp the scruff of the neck firmly with one hand and use the other hand to support the body, either by placing it along the underside of the body, or by placing it over the rump and holding the rabbit against the handler's body
- The rabbit's head can be tucked into the crook of the arm (Figure 4.28)
- Incorrect handling may allow the rabbit to kick out or twist, which can result in damage to its spine
- When putting a rabbit down, the hind end should be placed down first and the scruff released last.

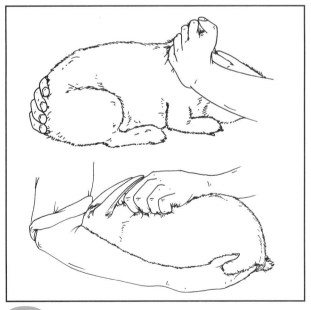

4.28 *Handling a rabbit. It is important to support the body.*

The anogenital distance is similar in male and female rabbits. To sex a rabbit, look at the shape of the genital opening – it is round in the male (buck) and the penis can be protruded with gentle pressure from above. After sexual maturity the testicles in the male can easily be seen lying either side of the penis in scrotal sacs. In the female (doe) the vulva is a V-shaped slit.

Ferrets

Tame ferrets can be held around the shoulders, with the other hand supporting the body weight (Figure 4.29).

Fractious or aggressive animals can be grasped by the tail and drawn backwards. At the same time they are grasped firmly around the shoulders, with the thumb under the chin and the forelegs crossed to prevent biting.

Male ferrets (hobs) have the preputial opening on the underbelly, as in the dog. The testicles are obvious in the breeding season (February–September). In the females (jill) the vulva is present just below the tail.

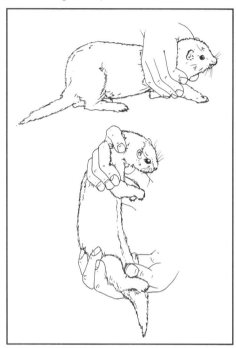

A tame ferret can be grasped around the shoulders with the other hand supporting the body. Additional measures are required for aggressive animals (see text).

Birds

Handling birds

All birds are more easily handled in dim light. Always make sure that all windows and doors are closed before the cage or box is opened. Remove toys and perches from the cage if possible. The use of thick gloves should be avoided as the handler's sense of touch is diminished and too much force can be exerted. However, thin cloths or towels are very useful to mask the hand and wrap the wings to prevent flapping. If the bird is in a cage it is often easier to approach the bird from the bottom, by tilting the cage off its base, rather than put the hand in through the small side door. Caught birds must never be squeezed as restriction of movement of the sternum and abdomen can result in asphyxiation.

> Never hold a bird around the chest, as this can hinder its respiration.

- Small birds can be grasped in one hand, with the head between the second and third finger (Figure 4.30)
- Larger psittacines should be grasped firmly from behind, using a towel or cloth, around the mandible and neck. Tilting of the cage usually makes the bird grab on to the side with its beak, making this procedure easier. With the other hand wrap the towel around the body
- Domestic fowl can be lifted around the body, holding the wings against the body, and then supporting the neck below the head.

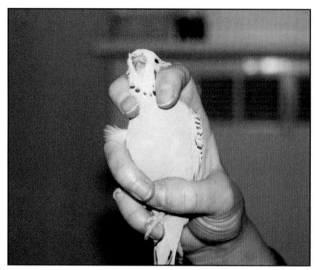

 Holding a budgerigar in one hand. Photo: Sharon Redrobe.

Sexing birds

Many species are monomorphic, i.e. the male and female look the same. For these species determination of sex is carried out either surgically, by visualizing the internal gonads via an endoscope, or by DNA analysis of a blood sample or plucked feather. Most psittacines have to be sexed in this way.

- In the budgerigar, the cere can be used to distinguish the sexes. The cere is a fleshy structure at the base of the upper beak, containing the nares. The male has a blue cere and the female a pinkish-brown cere
- In the cockatiel, the male has brighter red cheek patches and the female has pale bars on the underside of the tail feathers.

These differences are only reliable in the wild-type variety of these species. Alternatively, in some species behavioural differences can be used. For example, male canaries sing. Other birds show sexual dimorphism.

Reptiles

Reptiles should always be transported in an insulated, warm, dark and secure box or bag.

Snakes

- Snakes should be grasped by the head first, with thumb and second finger behind the occiput and the forefinger on top of the head (Figure 4.31)
- The body must then be supported. Never lift the head and let the body weight dangle, as snakes have a single occiput which can be easily dislocated
- Avoid squeezing the body too hard, as bruising can lead to debility or even death. The ribs of snakes are easily broken.

The teeth of a snake are angled caudally, so resist pulling rostrally if bitten. Pulling the hand out of the snake's mouth can result in a deeper bite or loss of the snake's teeth into the wound. This can lead to a foreign body reaction in the handler or osteomyelitis of the jaw in the snake.

> Snakes should never be placed around the neck. This is bad practice and can be dangerous – even fairly small specimens can constrict strongly.

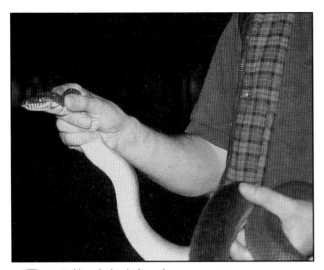

 Holding the head of a snake. Photo: Anna Meredith.

⚠️ Always handle large snakes with the help of an assistant.

Several methods can be used to sex snakes:

- Sexual dimorphism (rare)
- Length of tail – longer in the male
- Probing
- Popping (hatchlings) – the finger is rolled gently up the tail towards the cloaca to evert the hemipene(s).

The most reliable of these methods is probing. An aseptic lubricated probe is passed gently into the cloaca, pointing towards the end of the tail. In the male the probe passes into the hemipene (Figure 4.32) to a length of six to eight subcaudal scales. In the female it will only pass to a length of two to four scales. It is important to check both hemipene orifices: a plug of smegma may sometimes block them, preventing the probe from entering.

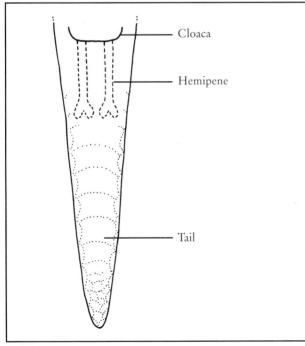

4.32 *The tail of a male snake, showing the position of the hemipenes.*

Lizards

- Lizards should be held around the neck and pelvic girdle with one hand, with the other around the pelvis and hindlimbs (Figure 4.33)
- For further restraint and to prevent being scratched, the limbs can be held down against the body. The limbs should be held near the top: if held down by the feet, violent struggling could result in a fracture, especially if the lizard has metabolic bone disease
- A soft cloth may be used to catch the delicate-skinned geckos
- Never handle a lizard by the tail – some species shed them.

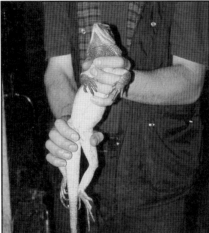

4.33 *Holding a large iguana. Photo: Anna Meredith.*

Lizards can be sexed in several ways:

- Femoral pores on the medial aspects of the hindlimbs are more obvious in males than in females (Figure 4.34)
- Some males have head ornamentation
- Hemipenes can be seen as bulges at the base of the tail in sexually mature males
- Radiography of certain monitor species will reveal the os penis.

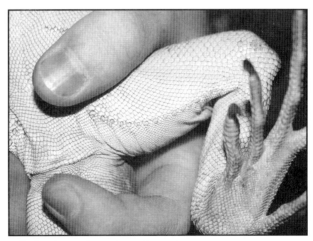

4.34 *Femoral pores in a male green iguana. Photo: Sharon Redrobe.*

Chelonians

Chelonians are easily handled by holding the shell between the fore- and hindlimbs or around the back of the shell between the hindlimbs (Figure 4.35).

In chelonians, the single hemipenis in the male makes the tail larger and longer, and the cloaca is further away from the plastron than in the female (Figure 4.36).

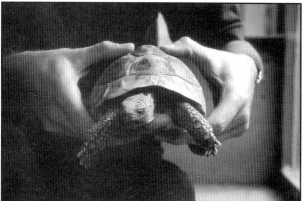

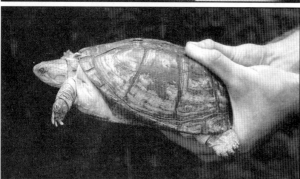

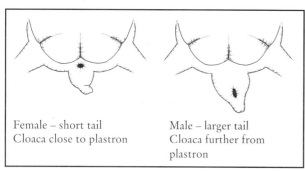

4.35 *Alternative methods of handling a tortoise.*
Photos: Anna Meredith.

 Always wash your hands after handling reptiles – they can carry *Salmonella* in their faeces.

- In some species the plastron is concave in the male, but this is not always reliable as some older female tortoises can develop a concavity also
- In the terrapin, the male has longer forelimb claws (used in courtship).

Female – short tail
Cloaca close to plastron

Male – larger tail
Cloaca further from plastron

4.36 *Sexing tortoises.*

Amphibians

Because of their delicate skin, amphibians should only be handled if absolutely necessary. Hands should be wet before handling, or wet surgical gloves can be worn.

- Aquatic species such as newts should be picked up using a soft fine-meshed net
- Amphibians can be coaxed into a small clear plastic box or bag, which will allow close inspection without the need to handle them directly

- When handling frogs and toads, care should be taken to ensure that they do not leap out of the hand. Placing the animal's head between the first two fingers, with its back lying against the palm of the hand, will restrain them.

Sexing of newts and salamanders involves looking at the cloaca, which has more swollen edges in the male. In the breeding season, the males of these species often become brighter coloured and develop crests, and the females swell with eggs. Male frogs and toads develop swellings called nuptial pads on their forelegs and are more vocal than the female during the breeding season.

Fish

Fish can be moved from tank to tank by using a soft fine-meshed net. Time spent out if the water must be kept to an absolute minimum.

General care and breeding

Mammals

For reproductive data, see Figure 4.12.

Rats, mice, hamsters and gerbils

- Mice, rats, gerbils and Russian and Chinese hamsters are highly social animals so should be kept as single sex groups (females best, as males may fight), breeding pairs or harems
- Syrian hamsters should be kept singly
- Syrian hamsters will hibernate at temperatures below 5°C and aestivate at very high temperatures, so are best kept at 19–23°C.

Housing

- Commercial metal cages and glass or plastic tanks are suitable for all small rodents
- Tough plastic modular systems are also available, with living spaces connected by tubes, mimicking burrows
- Wooden cages should be avoided, as all these species will gnaw
- Cage mesh must be small enough to prevent escape of young if breeding animals are kept (one wire/cm for mice; one wire/1.5 cm for rats)
- Cages should always be as large as possible, and enough space should be provided for cage furniture – for example, branches, tubes, ladders, exercise wheels (solid rather than open, to prevent tail injuries)
- A nest box should be provided. A deep layer of wood shavings makes suitable bedding, plus shredded paper, hay or straw as nesting material. Cotton wool-type bedding should be avoided, as it can become impacted in the stomach if ingested and in the cheek pouches of hamsters.

Gerbils can be kept in a 'gerbilarium' – a glass or plastic tank with a close-fitting wire mesh lid or plastic cover, half-filled with a mixture of peat and sawdust or shavings. Sand, although 'natural', is not a good substrate as it causes abrasions to the nose.

- Provide some nest material and wood for gerbils to gnaw
- Insides of toilet rolls and other pieces of cardboard are also gnawed with relish
- Keep the tank out of direct sunlight, as it can overheat.

The gerbils will spend all their time creating a system of burrows that they will constantly rearrange. This system only needs to be cleaned out two or three times a year, as very little urine is produced. The only disadvantage with a gerbilarium is that the occupants can be difficult to catch.

Feeding

- Rats and mice are omnivorous opportunists. A commercial rodent mix makes a suitable diet, consisting of carbohydrate type seeds/grains (wheat, maize, oats, barley) and higher fat type seeds and nuts (sunflower, peanuts) plus biscuit, locust bean and dried rolled peas. This can be supplemented with fruit and vegetables, household scraps and dog biscuits
- Gerbils and hamsters are largely herbivorous, although they may take the occasional insect in the wild. They should be fed a commercial rodent mix supplemented with small amounts of fresh fruit and vegetables. Hamsters tend to hoard food in the nest box, so perishable items must be removed regularly
- Water should be provided ad lib from a water bottle with nipple, attached to the side or roof of the cage.

Breeding

Oestrus occurs approximately every 4 days (see Figure 4.12).

In most rodents, a vaginal plug is formed after mating. This acts to prevent mating by another male, and prevents leakage of semen. Vaginal plugs are easily visible in rats and mice.

- Mice – vaginal plug can persist for up to 2 days
- Rats – vaginal plug falls out in 12–24 hours.

Newborn rats, mice, hamsters and gerbils are blind and naked (altricial). The mother should not be disturbed for the first 2–3 days after parturition or she may eat the young. All rodents have a post-partum oestrus, and so can become pregnant almost immediately after parturition.

- Breeding in rats, mice, gerbils and Russian and Chinese hamsters is easily achieved simply by placing male and female together, or keeping them as a pair or harem. The vaginal opening is patent when the female is in oestrus. Mating invariably occurs at night
- Golden hamsters usually need supervision, as the female can be very aggressive towards the male. A neutral cage can be used, or else the female can be placed in the male's cage
- Gerbils form monogamous pairs and the male will assist with the rearing of the young.

Males can be castrated to prevent breeding or enable males to be kept together.

Guinea-pigs

Guinea-pigs are highly social grassland dwellers and should be kept in single sex groups, pairs or harems. They are not hardy animals and cannot tolerate wet weather well.

Housing

A wide range of wooden hutch designs is available.

- The best types have two compartments – one mesh-fronted, and one solid-fronted for a nesting area
- Wood shavings and hay or straw are ideal bedding

- To avoid damp, hutches should be raised off the ground if outside
- Guinea-pigs need exercise and the opportunity to graze:
  - In summer a movable run or ark should be provided; this should be covered to prevent predation and should have a shelter (the hutch, a box or an old piece of drain pipe) to give a bolt-hole if the animal is startled
  - In winter the hutch should be moved indoors or into a garage and an indoor run with wood shavings can be provided.

Feeding

Guinea-pigs have an absolute dietary requirement for vitamin C. They need 10 mg/kg body weight per day, rising to three times this in pregnancy. Commercial guinea-pig diets are often supplemented with vitamin C, but the shelf life is short, and cool dark storage conditions must be provided.

- A commercial mix or pellet should be fed, well supplemented with good quality hay and a variety of greenfoods – groundsel, fresh grass, dandelion, cow parsley, broccoli, etc.
- Roughage or fibre in the form of hay or grass is essential for dental and gastrointestinal health
- Ad lib water should be provided from a drinking bottle.

Breeding

Female guinea-pigs come into oestrus every 15–17 days, and will arch their back (lordosis) when receptive. An obvious vaginal plug is present after mating.

At birth, the young are fully furred and have eyes and ears open (precocious).

It is essential to breed female guinea-pigs young, ideally at about 12 weeks old. After the age of 1 year, the pubic symphysis fuses and if guinea-pigs are bred for the first time after this they will experience difficulty in giving birth (dystocia): an emergency Caesarian operation may be required.

Approaching parturition can be detected by feeling separation of the pubic symphysis. The gap widens to approximately 2 cm 24–36 hours before birth.

Chinchillas

Female chinchillas are aggressive to each other and so they should be kept singly, or as half of a breeding pair.

Housing

Housing for chinchillas must be indoors.

- Wire cages are best as chinchillas will gnaw through other materials
- Cages should be as large as possible (at least 2 m x 2 m x 1 m)
- A nest box must be provided and plenty of branches to gnaw
- Chinchillas must have a daily dustbath in order to keep the fur in good condition.

Feeding

Chinchillas are essentially grassland dwellers and should be fed grass-based chinchilla pellets and good quality hay, supplemented with vegetables. High-sugar treats such as raisins should be avoided as these can cause tooth decay.

Breeding

Chinchillas will form monogamous pairs, or can be kept in a harem system with a male having access to several separate females. Oestrus occurs every 30–50 days, and is shown by an open vulva and mucoid vaginal discharge. A large vaginal plug is present after mating. The young are precocious.

Chipmunks

Chipmunks are social animals, so pairs or harems should be kept. Two males will fight.

Housing

Chipmunks do not make suitable house pets, and most commercial rodent cages are far too small.

- Housing is best outside in large aviary-like enclosures
- Chipmunks are very active and will exhibit stereotypic behaviour in small cages
- Nest boxes, branches, pipes, rocks, etc. should be provided and a soil, sand or bark-chipping floor
- A double safety door on the enclosure is advisable as they are very fast movers
- If kept indoors, it must be away from television sets, as the sound frequencies emitted causes intense stress and even death.

Feeding

Chipmunks are omnivorous and will eat seeds, grains, nuts, eggs, fruit, vegetables and insects. They will eat any mice that venture into their enclosure. They possess large cheek pouches and hoard food. Pregnant or lactating females can be given supplementary protein – for example, commercial baby food and milk, or cooked chicken.

Breeding

Males have a visible penis, and the scrotum is enlarged during the breeding season from March to September. Females are in oestrus every 13–14 days and will chirp to the male. Young are altricial and very vocal in the first 2 weeks of life. The mother will abandon the young if stressed. Chipmunks do not show a post-partum oestrus.

Rabbits

Rabbits are social animals: they should never be kept singly. They can be kept in small groups – but not bucks together as they will fight. Rabbits and guinea-pigs should not be kept together as rabbits tend to 'bully' guinea-pigs. Many rabbits are now kept as house pets, and they can be trained to use a litter tray.

Housing

Rabbits are generally hardy animals but need protection from extremes of weather. Most pet rabbits are housed in commercial or home-made wooden hutches, but these are often far too small.

- A hutch should be high enough for the rabbit to stand upright on its hindlegs and long enough to allow the rabbit to perform three hops from end to end
- A separate solid-fronted nesting area and a mesh-fronted day living area should be provided, bedded with wood shavings and hay or straw
- The hutch should be raised off the ground
- If it is outside, a waterproof roof and a louvred panel to cover the mesh-fronted area in bad weather should be provided
- Rabbits need the opportunity to exercise and to graze. Hutch-kept rabbits frequently suffer from osteoporosis due to inactivity. The hutch should be placed within an enclosure, or a separate ark or run should be provided
- Rabbits will burrow, so precautions should be taken to prevent escape
- When outside, a shelter or drain-pipe should be provided as a bolt-hole. Rabbits are susceptible to overheating and stress.

Feeding

Rabbits are grazing herbivores, designed to eat a low quality, high fibre diet. Small amounts of a good quality high fibre rabbit mix or pellets should be fed (not ad lib), plus large amounts of good quality hay, greenstuff (dandelion, groundsel, chickweed) and grass (never lawnmower clippings). Root and other vegetables are also enjoyed. Avoid sudden changes in diet as this can lead to diarrhoea.

Breeding

Does do not have regular oestrous cycles, but can show long periods of oestrus when ovarian follicles are constantly developing and regressing. The vulva is purple and congested when in oestrus.

Rabbits are reflex ovulators, i.e. ovulation is triggered by copulation, or sometimes if mounted by another doe. A non-fertile mating results in a pseudo-pregnancy of about 17 days. Breeding is simple – take a receptive doe to the buck and mating will rapidly occur.

The young are altricial, and it is normal for the doe to enter the nest box only once or twice a day to nurse them.

Ferrets

Ferrets are solitary in the wild, but single-sex pairs and groups or breeding pairs can be kept.

Housing

Ferrets can be kept outside in a hutch, pen or shed, or inside as a house pet.

- If kept outside, they must be sheltered from direct sun in the summer as they are very prone to heat stress. In the winter a garage or shed is more suitable
- If kept inside, they must still have a secure pen or cage where they should be secured when the owner is out of the house – ferrets are very inquisitive and destructive
- Bedding of woodshavings and straw is suitable
- Ferrets are very clean, despite their strong odour, and will use a litter tray.

Ferrets need a lot of attention and regular exercise. They can be trained to be taken for walks on a harness and lead.

Feeding

Ferrets are true carnivores and diet should consist of a good quality cat food – both wet and dry foods are readily accepted. Commercial dry ferret foods are also available. Dry diets lead to less skin odour. The diet can be supplemented with fresh dead mice, rabbits or chicks if available.

Breeding

The breeding season in ferrets is from spring to autumn. Jills in oestrus will have a swollen vulva. Mating can appear quite violent and last for up to 3 hours.

Ferrets are reflex ovulators. If unmated they will stay in oestrus for many months and this can lead to health problems such as anaemia and hair loss. It is best to spay non-breeding jills, or mate them to a vasectomized hob (known as a hobble). Treatment can be given for persistent oestrus with an injection of a progestagen or chorionic gonadotrophin.

Birds

 The Wildlife and Countryside Act 1981 requires that a bird cage must be of sufficient size to allow any captive bird to stretch its wings fully.

 Do not expose birds to:

- Cigarette smoke
- Overheated teflon
- Perches covered with sandpaper
- Chains
- Sources of zinc or lead.

Passerines

Housing
Most commercially available cages for birds are far too small. All birds are fitter if kept in aviaries.

- Mixed species can be kept together in an enclosed outdoor or covered flying area with a shed for shelter
- Aviaries should have a double safety door
- Suitable plants in pots encourage insect life
- Perches of different heights and diameters should be provided, and natural branches are best
- Shallow (1 cm) water bowls for bathing should be provided early in the day. Some aviculturalists fit timed sprinkler systems in their aviaries
- Water for drinking should be provided in column containers to prevent contamination
- Food containers should be above floor level and never under perches
- Healthy birds can withstand a wide range of ambient temperatures as long as fluctuations are not rapid.

Many passerines are kept indoors in cages (e.g. male canaries, which sing well) and these should always be as large as possible.

- Minimum dimensions must allow full extension of the wings, and the tail should be clear of the floor when perching. Cages should be as large as possible to allow horizontal flight between perches
- Sand-covered perches should be avoided, as these predispose to foot problems and do nothing to keep nails worn down
- Cages should be placed well above ground level, preferably at human head height
- Birds only feed during daylight and so artificial light should be provided to prevent reduced food intake on short winter days. A 12-hour light period is suitable.

All housing, whether cage or aviary, must be easily cleaned:

- Perches should be kept scrupulously clean, using soap and water, mild disinfectant solution or dilute chlorine bleach, and thoroughly rinsed
- Cage bottom coverings and food and water containers should be cleaned daily
- The whole cage or aviary should be thoroughly cleaned once a month.

Feeding
Birds are conservative feeders and will only eat foods they recognize or on which they have become imprinted. Therefore changes in diet must be introduced gradually.

Finches and canaries are seed-eaters. Seed of appropriate size should be provided, i.e. millet, canary seed, rape seed and hemp. Husks should be removed daily. Grit must be available at all times to ensure proper functioning of the gizzard. Grit must be of appropriate size and consist of two types: soluble (oyster shell, egg shell) and insoluble (quartz, igneous stone).

Variety is essential in providing a good balanced diet for passerine species, and lack of variety is the most common cause of malnutrition.

- At least six different food items should be offered daily
- As well as many different seed varieties as possible, green food (lettuce, watercress, alfalfa, chickweed, dandelion, parsley), sprouted seeds, vegetables and fruit should be offered
- 'Softfood', 'eggfood' and 'condition' or 'tonic' food are commercially available and can be fed at a ratio of 1:3 with the seed mixture
- 'Complete' diets are now widely available, and inexperienced owners often find these diets easier to use.

Insectivores (e.g. mynahs) usually need live food such as mealworms, crickets and fruit flies. Commercial insectivore preparations are available.

Frugivores (fruit-eaters) and nectar feeders (e.g. toucans, sunbirds and hummingbirds) need a variety of ripe fruit and/or syrupy fluids such as evaporated milk and honey with added vitamins, minerals and a little animal protein. Commercial liquid diets are also available.

Psittacines
Most psittacines should be kept in breeding pairs. A single hand-reared bird makes the best pet, however.

Housing: aviary
A garden aviary should be in a quiet secluded location, facing the sun, with shelter from prevailing wind.

- Minimum dimensions for a flight should be 1.8 m long by 1.8 m high by 0.9 m wide
- Height should be as great as possible, to minimize stress on the birds, and width must allow two birds to pass each other easily in flight
- Welded mesh of appropriate size on a treated wooden or metal framework is ideal
- Earth floors should be avoided and concrete flooring should be used for ease of cleaning. Shingle or bark chippings are also suitable
- Shallow baths or a misting system are provided for bathing
- If multiple flights are placed side by side, double mesh is essential to prevent pairs fighting.

An inside shelter must always be accessible. This can be a box-like structure at the top half of the back section of the flight, or a full indoor shed.

- To encourage roosting at night, perches in the shelter should be higher than those in the flight
- Birds only feed during daylight. To avoid reduced food intake on short winter days, artificial light should be provided to give a 12-hour light period.

Housing: cage

Even if an indoor bird is allowed free run of the house, it will need a cage to provide a territorial area where it feels safe and in which it can be secured when the owners are not present.

- A cage should be large enough to allow the bird to beat its outstretched wings and to have its tail clear of the floor when perching (this is required by law under the Wildlife and Countryside Act 1981)
- At least two perches, of differing sizes, should be provided. Any deciduous tree branches (e.g. fruit trees or willow) are ideal and the bird will enjoy stripping the bark
- Avoid sandpaper-covered perches
- The cage should be situated at or above human head height, away from strong sunlight and excessive draughts
- Birds should also be kept away from cigarette smoke and overheated teflon pans, as these fumes can kill.

Psittacines are highly intelligent, inquisitive and social birds and require a lot of attention if kept singly.

- Toys can be provided but should not be so densely packed as to interfere with the bird's movement around the cage
- Male budgerigars can become sexually bonded to one toy, or to their own reflection in a mirror
- Chains are to be avoided, as the animal can get caught and suffer serious injury.

Cages should be cleaned daily. A bath in the form of a shallow dish or a daily misting encourages preening and good feather condition and is greatly enjoyed.

Feeding

Malnutrition is the commonest cause of disease in caged psittacines. The most important thing is to feed as varied a diet as possible. Psittacines can be very fussy and conservative eaters: it is important to mix different food items in one bowl so that preferential selection of one item (e.g. sunflower seeds or peanuts) is minimized. These high fat seeds are nutritionally unbalanced, and eating only these items can lead to serious nutritional disease (hypovitaminosis A, metabolic bone disease).

- Feed several times a day
- Removing food and replacing it later stimulates interest and relieves boredom
- To avoid faecal contamination, food bowls must be placed higher than perches
- At least three types of vegetables, three types of fruit and five types of seed should be offered daily
- Treats can be offered occasionally (e.g. fruit cake, biscuits, brown bread, breakfast cereal).

Suitable food items are listed in Figure 4.37.

Alternatively, complete pelleted diets are now available for many species. These are a useful option for owners who have many birds to feed, or who do not have the time to prepare a home-made diet. However, they are expensive and lacking in variety for the bird.

Breeding

Provision of an appropriate nest box will stimulate breeding behaviour in most species. In a flock situation, sufficient nest boxes must be provided for every pair – and preferably more

4.37 Suitable food items for psittacine birds

Type	Examples
Seed mixture	Wheat, oats, canary seed, millet, buckwheat, groats Millet sprays are often preferred during the moult and by debilitated birds Budgerigars should be fed a good proprietary seed mixture containing an iodine supplement
Oil seeds	Sunflower seed, linseed, rape seed, hemp seed These should be rationed and should not exceed 20–30% of the diet, or else obesity and nutritional deficiency will occur
Fruit	Any fruit except avocado Birds will have their favourite type
Vegetables and greenfood	Carrots, celery, beetroot, alfalfa, broccoli, watercress, lettuce, groundsel, chickweed, dandelion, dock
Pulses	Haricot beans, soya beans, green peas, mung beans, chick peas, black-eyed beans, fed soaked, cooked or sprouted
Peanuts	Must be fit for human consumption, and form only a small part of the diet
Bones and household scraps	Often enjoyed as an occasional treat by larger species
Rawhide chews	Enjoyed by larger species
Cuttlefish bone	Ignored by some species and enjoyed by others A good source of calcium
Vitamin/mineral supplements	A good avian supplement will prevent any deficiencies, but over-zealous use can cause damaging excesses

than this so that the birds have a choice of box.

- Increasing day length in the spring is the normal stimulus to breeding behaviour, but some species will breed all year round
- Pairs of birds kept in cages without a nest box rarely breed
- Psittacines form strong pair bonds, especially the larger species
- The most common reason for failure to breed is that the pair is of the same sex.

Eggs are generally laid daily, or every other day, until the clutch is complete. Removal of the eggs will stimulate the laying of another clutch.

Reptiles

Reptiles are not social animals and most pet species are best kept singly, as the presence of other reptiles can be stressful if insufficient space is provided.

Environmental stress (including inadequate husbandry) predisposes an animal to infection, by immunosuppression. Thus a knowledge of the reptile's basic environmental requirements is vital in the prevention of many diseases. Most diseases of reptiles in the UK are caused by an incorrect diet or incorrect housing conditions.

Housing

Figure 4.38 shows a typical vivarium set-up for a reptile. The exact configuration will depend on the species.

Vivarium dimensions vary with species:

- Arboreal species require height
- Terrestrial species require floor area
- Aquatic species require water and basking platforms.

Items that can be ingested (e.g. small stones, gravel, corncob bedding) should be avoided. Newspaper is perhaps the best substrate as it is digestible, cheap and disposable. Other options include washable carpet squares or artificial turf.

A few items of safe cage furniture might include large stones, stable 'caves' or hides, secured branches that can take the weight of the reptile, and non-toxic non-injurious plants.

Water

A body of water is required for aquatic and semi-aquatic species with adequate filtration and heating.

Drinking water should always be available to all reptiles in a form that is acceptable to them. For example, chameleons will only lick droplets, but tortoises need to immerse their mouth and nose and so should be placed in shallow water three times a week.

Temperature

To be able to thermoregulate, reptiles require the provision of a range of temperatures. This range is known as the preferred optimum temperature zone, or POTZ. The preferred body temperature (PBT) is the optimum temperature for the functioning of the reptile's systems (e.g. movement, feeding, digestion, reproduction, immunocompetence).

The two types of heat source are:

- Primary – for background/ambient heat (this should not be a light source). A heat pad or ceramic heater (attached to a thermostat) is used.
- Secondary – specific 'hot spot' areas with a higher temperature for basking or to provide a temperature gradient. An overhead incandescent bulb, a ceramic heater or an infrared bulb is used.

Monitoring is vital to check the range of temperatures. Maximum/minimum thermometers and thermostats are essential.

Lighting

Timers are required for the maintenance of a stable photoperiod. Suitable photoperiods (light/dark) are:

- Tropical species – summer 13 h/11 h; winter 11 h/13 h
- Temperate species –summer 15 h/9 h; spring/autumn 12 h/12 h; winter 9 h/15 h.

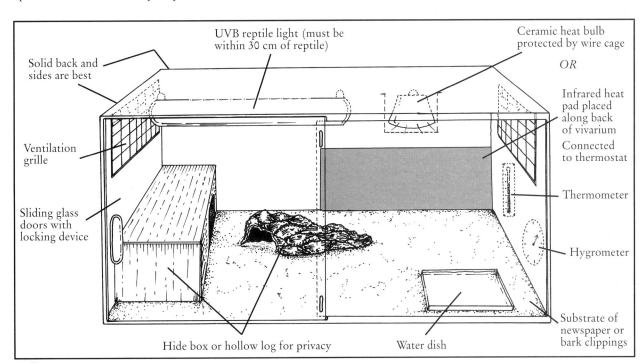

4.38 *A vivarium suitable for a reptile.*

UVB reptile light (must be within 30 cm of reptile)

Ceramic heat bulb protected by wire cage

OR

Solid back and sides are best

Infrared heat pad placed along back of vivarium Connected to thermostat

Ventilation grille

Thermometer

Sliding glass doors with locking device

Hygrometer

Hide box or hollow log for privacy

Water dish

Substrate of newspaper or bark clippings

The wavelength of the light is also a factor:

- UVA (320–400 nm) stimulates agonistic and reproductive behaviour in lizards
- UVB (290–320 nm) is important for the conversion of provitamin D_3 to previtamin D_3 in the reptile skin, and is therefore important for calcium metabolism.

 The broad-spectrum light must be placed within 30 cm of the reptile in order to expose the animal to sufficient UVB. UVB output is generally lost after 6 months, so the bulb must be regularly replaced even if the visible light appears normal.

Humidity

- A relative humidity of 50–70% is tolerated by most species. Some, such as iguanas, require higher humidity
- A humid chamber may be provided for ecdysis
- Humidity should not be increased at the expense of ventilation.

Feeding

Preferred food items for various species of reptile are shown in Figure 4.39.

- A calcium:phosphorus ratio of 1.5:1 plus vitamin D_3 is essential
- It is illegal and inhumane to feed live vertebrate prey, even to an anorexic animal. Food may be bloodied, warmed and wiggled to encourage feeding
- Insectivores may be offered live crickets, waxworms, etc. coated with a reptile mineral/vitamin supplement. Ensure that the insects themselves have been fed (nutrient-loaded) before being offered to the reptile
- Reptiles should not be handled when they have recently eaten as they may regurgitate
- Aquatic species (which feed in water) should be fed in a separate feeding tank to prevent water fouling
- Some snakes (e.g. constrictors) prefer to eat in a small dark box
- For lizards and chelonians, all food (except complete pelleted commercial diets) should be dusted with a reptile vitamin/mineral supplement.

As a guide to feeding frequency:

- Small snakes and lizards – once or twice a week
- Young of boas and pythons – three times a week
- Herbivores (e.g. iguana) – daily
- Large snake – once every 2–4 weeks.

Breeding

Many pet reptiles are still wild-caught or imported (e.g. green iguanas) but many species can be bred relatively easily in captivity (e.g. cornsnakes).

Reptile species can be divided into:

- Viviparous or live-bearing (e.g. boas, garter snakes)
- Oviparous or egg-laying (e.g. pythons, tortoises, iguanas).

Incubation facilities will be required for reptile eggs. The eggs have soft shells and require a high humidity. Incubation temperature can affect the sex of the hatchling in some species (e.g. crocodilians, chelonians, lizards).

Amphibians

Housing

Vivaria or fish tanks are suitable for housing amphibians.

- High humidity (75–95%) is required
- Some species will live in water all the time (e.g. newts, xenopus toads)
- Additional heating is required for tropical species (21–29°C)
- Temperatures are generally lower than those for reptiles
- Moist bark chippings and moss make a suitable substrate
- An ultraviolet light should be provided, as for reptiles.

Feeding

All invertebrate food items should be nutrient-loaded or dusted with a vitamin/mineral supplement.

- Frogs and toads – crickets, mealworms, waxworms, pinkies
- Salamanders – earthworms, mealworms, waxworms, crickets.

4.39 Preferred foods for reptiles

Reptiles	Families	Preferred foods
Snakes	Boas, pythons, rat snakes, gopher snakes, bull snakes, vipers Garter and water snakes Racers and vine snakes	Warm-blooded prey, e.g. rodents and birds Fish, frogs, earthworms, slugs Lizards (fed killed)
Lizards	Horned lizards Green iguanas Monitors Geckos, anoles, skinks, chameleons	Ants (small crickets) Dandelions, watercress, alfalfa, etc. Raw eggs, pinkies, rodents, birds, fish Appropriate sized crickets, fruit flies, wax worms
Chelonians	Turtles and terrapins Tortoises	Earthworms, small whole fish, pinkies, green vegetables Flowers, succulents, grass, cucumber, frozen mixed vegetables, fresh fruit

Fish

Housing: the aquarium

- The tank should be sited away from heaters, draughts and direct sunlight, and near sources of water and power
- A firm level base must be provided
- Consideration should be given to the weight of the tank when full – 1 litre of water weighs 1 kg
- Exposure to tobacco smoke and paint fumes must be avoided: these can dissolve in the water and harm the fish.

The larger the tank, the better, but the most important factor is to provide a large surface area for good oxygenation. For this reason, the traditional goldfish bowl is completely unsuitable. The best type of tank is all-plastic or stainless steel with glass sides.

For tanks that are not artificially aerated, the stocking density should be 75 cm^2 surface area for each 2.5 cm body length of fish. This can be increased up to a point if aeration is provided. Cold-water tanks can be stocked more densely than a tropical tank of similar size, due to the higher oxygen content of the colder water. Cold-water fish require an average temperature of 15°C.

- Tropical fish will require a heater and thermostat. These are generally sold as a combined unit, plugging directly into the mains electricity supply
- There are three main types of mechanical filtration available, and these systems aerate the water as well as removing particulate matter from it:
  - Bottom filter – this is hidden below the gravel and works as a simple slit system
  - Inside filter box – this is suspended in the water, usually in a corner of the tank, and contains nylon or gravel plus activated charcoal, which need to be changed regularly
  - Outside filter box – similar to the inside box but situated outside the tank.
- Biological filters are also available – these break down metabolic waste products
- Extra aeration is seldom required in a good tank (i.e. one that is not overcrowded and is well filtered, with a good surface area) but is often needed to stock smaller tanks at densities that aquarists find aesthetically pleasing. Aeration (diffuser) blocks are often used, but some fish dislike violent aeration. Excessive aeration can lead to 'gas bubble disease', seen on the skin and fins
- Light is essential for a healthy aquarium – it ensures plant survival, and is necessary to display the fish well.
  - In the wild, light enters from the surface only. It is unnatural for fish to receive light from all sides, as they do in a tank
  - Fish have no eyelids and need shelter (e.g. plants) to avoid too much light
  - Fish need dark periods in order to rest – a 12 h light/dark cycle is adequate (at least 9 h light is necessary) – Artificial light is essential as sunlight is unpredictable, warms the water and promotes algal growth. White fluorescent strip lighting is best
- Other aquarium equipment might include:
  - Gravel and rocks
  - Plants for oxygenation, decoration, shelter and food
  - Dipping nets for catching fish
  - Scraper for removing algae.

Setting up an aquarium is detailed in Figure 4.40. The aquarium must be set up for at least 5 days before fish are added.

Feeding

Commercial fish diets are often fed to exclusion, but fish require a varied diet, and live food is essential, especially for tropical fish.

- Dried diets are made of meat and cereal, with added vitamins and minerals
- Dried *Daphnia* (water fleas) and tubifex worms are also available. Home-made additions include brown bread crumbs and grated cheese. Ant eggs should only be given occasionally
- Live food should be fed regularly. *Daphnia* can be added direct to the tank but tubifex worms should be thoroughly washed first in running water, as they are reared in detritus
- Overfeeding and giving too much dry food are common mistakes. They result in fouling of the water and constipation of the fish (trailing faeces)
- Feed *once daily* at a regular time and place. Either sprinkle

---

4.40 **Setting up an aquarium**

1. Clean the tank and all fittings thoroughly with dilute detergent and rinse thoroughly.
2. Place in a suitable position. Once in place, the tank should not be moved.
3. Wash the gravel and rocks several times in running water and lay them at the bottom of the tank to a depth of 5 cm, sloping up towards the back of the tank. Position any rocks. (If a bottom filter is being used this will have to be in place first and gravel should be level.)
4. To minimize gravel disturbance during water-pouring, place brown paper or a plastic sheet over the gravel. Fill the tank with conditioned water (water can be conditioned artificially by adding a conditioning solution, or by allowing it to stand for a few days to allow for the chlorine gas to evaporate). Remove the paper or plastic sheet.
5. Plant the plants in the gravel, with the tallest at the rear and sides.
6. Place the thermometer into position.
7. Set up lighting, heater and thermostat, pump, aerators and filters.
8. Put on top cover or, if not available, a sheet of glass supported by four corks or pads. This keeps dust out but allows free entry of air.
9. Run the tank with no fish for a few days, checking that the thermostat and heater are working.
10. Add the fish, contained in the plastic bag in which they were purchased, to the tank. After 15 minutes, when the temperatures of the bag water and the tank water have equilibrated, gently tip the fish into the tank. Allow them to settle for a day before feeding.

the food on the surface or use a plastic floating feeding ring. A pinch as large as the eye of the fish is a good rule for the amount to feed per fish. After 10 minutes, or when the fish show no interest, remove the excess with a siphon or pipette
- Outdoor fish eat less in the winter than in the summer.

Signs of pain or disease in exotic pets

Signs of disease in exotic pets are listed in Figure 4.41. The following points should be noted:

- Birds are very good at hiding signs of disease. This phenomenon is sometimes called the 'preservation reflex': a sick bird in the wild would be predated, or harassed by other members of the flock. It is only when the bird can no longer compensate that an owner actually recognizes that something is wrong, and at this stage any disease process may be very advanced. It is for this reason that signs of illness, however slight, must be taken seriously in a bird and veterinary advice sought promptly
- If a fish is thought to be ill, it should be isolated immediately in a separate tank, filled with water from the main tank to avoid further stressing the fish. The rest of the original tank should be quarantined and the advice of an experienced aquarist or veterinary surgeon should be sought.

Administration of medicines and general nursing

Mammals

Administration of medicines

Injections
Details for giving injections to small mammals are shown in Figure 4.42.

Oral administration
Oral administration can be achieved:

- Via the drinking-water (inaccurate)
- By mixing with small amounts of food (e.g. injected into jelly cubes for rats)
- By syringe or dropper, if palatable
- By gavage, using a polyethylene catheter or commercial gavage needle and gag.

Further information on administration of medicines is available in the BSAVA *Manual of Advanced Veterinary Nursing*.

Nursing the sick small mammal
The general principles are:

- Provision of warmth – especially with the smaller species, due to their large ratio of surface area to body weight. A

4.41 **Signs of disease in exotic pets**

Class	Signs
Small mammals	Lack of interest in surroundings Isolation from group Hunched posture Inactivity/reluctance to move Inappetence Unexpected aggression or docility Tooth-grinding Unkempt staring coat Pale extremities 'Square' tail (prominent vertebral processes) Self-trauma Hair loss Discharge from eyes and/or nose (red in rodents) 'Rattling' respiration or sneezing Diarrhoea Lameness Abnormal masses anywhere on body Wounds/bleeding Excessive salivation
Birds	Discharge from the eyes Closing of the eyes Swelling around the eyes Discharge from the nostrils Obstruction of the nostrils Sneezing Change or loss of vocalization Open-mouth breathing at rest Tail bobbing/pumping at rest Fluffed up feathers Inactivity Reduced or no appetite Weight loss Inability to perch Equilibrium problems Muscle tremors Lameness or non-weightbearing limb Swollen feet or joints Change in quality/quantity of droppings Lumps or masses Abdominal distension Bleeding
Reptiles	Loss of appetite/anorexia Weight loss Inability to support body weight Muscle tremors/twitching Loss of righting reflex Mouth breathing Reddening under scales/scutes Dysecdysis Discharge from nose or mouth Swelling around eyes Skin or shell ulceration Lumps or masses Abdominal distension
Amphibians	Loss of appetite Reddening of the skin Skin lesions – fungus or pinpoint foci Abdominal swelling
Fish	Loss of appetite Cloudy, spotted or ragged fins Hollow sides or underparts Fins folded or not erect Dull eyes Poor skin colour Blood under scales Loss of scales Lumps/masses/growths anywhere on body Cuts/wounds/ulcers Sluggish swimming Hanging on the bottom or motionless below the surface Staying near aerator Unusual swimming action (e.g. jerkiness, imbalance) Rubbing on stones or ornaments

Site of injection and maximum volume for small mammals

Species	Subcutaneous	Intramuscular	Intraperitoneal	Intravenous
Mouse	Scruff 2–3 ml		2–3 ml	Lateral tail vein
Hamster/gerbil	Scruff 3–4 ml		3–4 ml	Not practicable
Rat	Scruff, flank 5–10 ml		10–15 ml	Lateral tail vein
Guinea-pig/chinchilla	Scruff, flank 5–10 ml	Quadriceps 0.3 ml	10–15 ml	Ear vein, jugular vein, saphenous vein
Rabbit	Scruff, flank 30–50 ml	Quadriceps, lumbar muscles 0.5–1 ml	50–100 ml	Marginal ear vein, cephalic vein, jugular vein saphenous vein
Ferret	Scruff, flank 10–20 ml	Quadriceps, lumbar muscles 0.5 ml	10–15 ml	Jugular vein, cephalic vein

temperature of 25–30°C is needed for adult animals and 35–37°C for neonates
- Comfortable bedding, such as tissue paper or fleece, should be provided – not sawdust, which can stick to eyes and nose
- A quiet environment out of sight of potential predators
- Subdued lighting or a nest box should be provided
- Guinea-pigs require at least 10 mg vitamin C/kg body weight per day
- Provision of fibre, in the form of hay, is vital for rabbits, guinea-pigs and chinchillas
- Avoid sudden changes in the normal diet
- Monitor hydration status and provide fluids if necessary
- Monitor for signs of diarrhoea, especially if receiving antibiotics
- The use of probiotics is advised in rabbits, guinea-pigs and chinchillas.

Force feeding and fluid therapy
Most rodents and rabbits have a strong chewing reflex and will readily take palatable liquid food from a syringe inserted gently at the side of the mouth. Baby foods (cereal, vegetable, fruit) are suitable, and powdered probiotics can be added to this. Ferrets can be offered liquidized cat food. Gavage is possible with care, using a gag and a polyethylene catheter. Nasogastric tubes can be used in the rabbit.

- Fluid requirements of small mammals are 40–80 ml/kg/day
- Percentage dehydration can be assessed as for larger mammals (skin turgor, etc.) and fluid deficit and ongoing requirements calculated
- Fluids can be administered by the oral, subcutaneous, intraperitoneal or intraosseous route
- The intravenous route can be used in the rabbit and ferret.

Further information is available in the *BSAVA Manual of Advanced Veterinary Nursing.*

Birds

Administration of medicines
Tablets or liquids can be incorporated into the food, but additions are often detected and uneaten, and accurate dosing is difficult. Figure 4.43 suggests routes of administration.

Gavage or crop tubing

- An assistant restrains the bird
- Place a gag between the upper and lower beak
- Insert a flexible tube or rigid metal tube with a rounded tip from the left side of the beak and down the oesophagus on the right side of the neck, into the crop.

Routes of administration of medicines in birds

Route	Site
Oral	By tube into crop
Subcutaneous	Axilla, lateral flank, interscapular area Avoid large volumes
Intramuscular	Pectoral muscles
Intravenous	Jugular, brachial, medial metatarsal vein Care with haemostasis after withdrawal of needle
Intraosseous	Distal ulna, proximal tibia Avoid pneumatic bones
Nebulization	Bird placed in tank with nebulizer attached For treatment of respiratory disease

Further details are available in the *BSAVA Manual of Advanced Veterinary Nursing.*

Nursing the sick bird

- Sick birds should be maintained at a high ambient temperature (approximately 28°C), without draughts
- Incubators are very useful – additional oxygen should be provided for birds with severe respiratory disease or those in shock
- Perches should be lowered
- Perching birds feel most secure if the cage is at shoulder height
- Dim lighting and a quiet environment reduce stress
- Birds should never be in visual contact with potential predators (e.g. cats)
- Very tame species (e.g. parrots) will respond to TLC, but wild birds should be handled and disturbed as little as possible.

Force feeding and fluid therapy
Birds have a high metabolic rate and must be force fed if not eating voluntarily. It should be remembered that birds will only eat when it is light: at least 12 h light per day needs to be provided to ensure that a bird is eating sufficiently to fulfil its metabolic requirements.

- Force feeding is achieved by crop tubing (as described above for administration of medicines, and in more detail in the *BSAVA Manual of Advanced Veterinary Nursing*)
- Commercial enteral nutrition products are available
- Commercial dog or cat liquid diets can be used for carnivorous species

- Vegetable baby foods or human high calorie invalid formulas are suitable for seed and fruit eaters
- Low fat products are preferable if hepatic function is compromised (for method, see 'Oral dosing')
- Probiotics are very useful in sick or stressed birds
- Baby birds will require feeding every 1–2 h, or whenever the crop is empty
- Do not overfeed baby birds, as crop stretching or stasis will occur.

Suggested volumes and frequencies for common species are shown in Figure 4.44.

4.44 Volume and frequency for force feeding birds

Species	Amount per feed (ml)	Times/day
Finch	0.1–0.3	Six
Budgerigar	0.5–1.0	Four
Cockatiel	1.0–2.5	Four
Amazon parrot	5.0–8.0	Two

4.45 Routes of administration of medicines in reptiles

Route	Reptile	Site
Subcutaneous	Snake/lizard	Loose skin over ribs
Intramuscular	Snake	Intercostal muscles of body
	Lizard	Fore/hindleg, tail muscles (care)
	Chelonian	As lizard, plus pectoral muscle mass at angle of forelimb and neck
	In patients weighing less than 100 g, no more than 0.2 ml should be given at any one site	
Intracoelomic	Snake	Off midline, cranial to cloaca
	Lizard	Off midline caudal to ribs, cranial to pelvis
	Chelonian	Cranial to hindlimb in fossa
	Large volumes should not be given by this route, as respiration may be impaired	
Intravenous	Snake	Ventral tail vein, jugular vein, intracardiac
	Lizard	Ventral tail vein
	Chelonian	Dorsal tail vein, jugular vein
Intraosseous	Lizard/chelonian	Femur, tibia

Force feeding

- Stomach volume in reptiles is 10 ml/kg body weight
- Some reptiles will accept liquid food being placed in the mouth via syringe
- Carnivorous and insectivorous species should be given a meat-based liquid diet
- Herbivorous species should be given a vegetable-based diet
- Commercial critical care formulae are available.

Methods of tube-feeding reptiles are given in Figure 4.46.

Fluid therapy

- Most sick reptiles will present at least 10–15% dehydrated, requiring fluid therapy
- Give oral fluids (e.g. lactated Ringer's), daily equal to 4–10% body weight if reptile is not drinking
- Oral fluids are given by stomach tube (see above)
- Warm the fluids to reptile's preferred body temperature before administration

Fluid therapy

- The daily fluid requirements of birds are a minimum of 50 ml/kg/day (5% body weight)
- Birds tolerate blood loss much better than mammals, and similarly can tolerate bolus treatment of relatively large volumes of fluid
- Percentage dehydration can be difficult to gauge in birds, but it can safely be assumed that any sick bird will be 10% dehydrated
- Fluids must always be warmed to 30–35°C.

Further details of fluid therapy are available in the *BSAVA Manual of Advanced Veterinary Nursing.*

Reptiles

Administration of medicines
Reptiles have a renal portal venous circulation, which means that injections into the hindlimb musculature may be eliminated via the kidneys before reaching the rest of the body. There is still debate as to whether this system significantly affects drug distribution.

Suggested routes of administration of medicines in reptiles are given in Figure 4.45.

- Fluids can be given by the subcutaneous, intracoelomic, intravenous or intraosseous route.

Further details are available in the *BSAVA Manual of Advanced Veterinary Nursing.*

Amphibians

Administration of medicines
Drugs for amphibians can be administered:

- Orally, by syringe into the mouth
- Topically – but beware toxicity, as the drug will be systemically absorbed
- In water, as for fish (see below).

Force feeding and fluid therapy
Small rubber tubes or catheters can be used as feeding tubes for amphibians. Great care must be taken when opening the mouth, to avoid damage to the delicate mandible. Some animals will swallow food items placed directly in the mouth.

4.46 How to tube-feed reptiles

Species	Method
Snake	1. Manually restrain animal, open mouth and insert gag 2. Hold anterior of snake vertically 3. Insert well lubricated end of feeding tube into oesophagus to level of stomach (approximately one-third down length of snake) 4. Syringe in fluids/food slowly 5. Hold snake vertically for 2–3 minutes to avoid regurgitation 6. After several feedings of liquid diet with no regurgitation, the snake can be force fed whole animals or given liquidized whole animals by tube feeding
Lizard	1. Stomach is positioned just behind caudal edge of ribs 2. Proceed as for snake
Chelonian	1. Stomach is positioned midway down plastron 2. Measure stomach tube from mouth to caudal end of abdominal shield to just beyond gular notch 3. Hold chelonian upright 4. Extend neck and hold head behind mandible 5. Prise open mouth and hold open with a gag 6. Proceed as above

Fish

Administration of medicines

Fish are not covered by the Veterinary Surgeons Act; therefore owners are able to diagnose disease, obtain non-prescription drugs and administer them. Unfortunately, diagnosis is often inaccurate and fish may have been treated with numerous over-the-counter preparations before presentation to a veterinary surgeon.

In-feed medication

Medicated feed is commercially available for farmed fish, and may be used where large numbers are kept (e.g. Koi carp). Medicated pellets can be home-made by mixing the drug with softened diet pellets and allowing them to dry.

Intramuscular injection

This is possible with larger individual fish. Commonly used sites are the base of the tail or in front of the dorsal fin.

In-water medication

Liquids or soluble powders may be added to the water. Calculation of the water volume is essential for accurate dosing. A separate treatment tank should be used.

General care of wildlife casualties

For most species of wildlife, the principles of care and management are those that apply to their domestic counterparts (Figure 4.47).

An immediate decision should be made whether to treat or euthanase wild species. Euthanasia is often the most humane option for wild animals. Factors to consider are:

- Is the animal so ill or badly injured that it is unlikely to survive?
- Is the animal in severe pain?

4.47 Management of wildlife

Species	Husbandry	Handling	Diet
Badger	Strong, escape-proof kennel (especially by digging) Dim light (nocturnal) Provide nest box	Crush cage, dog-catcher, pin down head with broom. Take great care – can inflict serious bite. Move by guiding with solid boards	Commercial dog food
Fox	Strong, escape-proof kennel Dim light Provide nest box	As for badger	Commercial dog food Rodents Rabbit
Hedgehog	Small box or kennel Dim light Provide nest material (straw) and/or nest box	With gloves Need anaesthesia to unroll in most cases	Commercial insectivore/hedgehog diet Worms, snails Small amounts dog food (take care: dental tartar)
Rabbit	Small box, cage or kennel Out of view of predator species	As domestic counterparts	As domestic counterparts
Bird	Box or cage Avoid visual contact with prey/predator species	As domestic counterparts	Mimic natural diet as far as possible Carnivores: commercial dog or insectivore diet, small rodents, chicks, worms, etc. depending on species Herbivores: seeds, grains, commercial diets where available, e.g. poultry rations

- Will the animal be able to be returned to the wild once recovered?
- If unable to be rehabilitated to the wild, will it have a reasonable quality of life?
- Does the benefit of intervention and treatment outweigh the stress that this will cause?

General principles when caring for wildlife are:

 Return to the wild in a fit state as quickly as possible must always be the aim, and in most cases is a legal requirement

- Avoid handling wherever possible and minimize all human contact
- Keep in visual seclusion wherever possible
- Keep in dim lighting conditions
- Assess progress daily and review possible outcome, to justify either continuation of treatment or euthanasia
- Be aware of legal requirements for particular species (see Chapter 10).

Further reading

Beynon PH and Cooper JE (1991) *BSAVA Manual of Exotic Pets.* British Small Animal Veterinary Association, Cheltenham

Beynon PH, Forbes NA and Lawton MPC (1996) *BSAVA Manual of Psittacine Birds.* British Small Animal Veterinary Association, Cheltenham

Beynon PH, Lawton MPC and Cooper JE (1992) *BSAVA Manual of Reptiles.* British Small Animal Veterinary Association, Cheltenham

Butcher (1992) *BSAVA Manual of Ornamental Fish.* British Small Animal Veterinary Association, Cheltenham

5 Management of animal housing

Margaret C. Moore

This chapter is designed to give information on:

- The legal licensing requirements for boarding and breeding establishments
- The considerations required when constructing or updating permanent or temporary animal accommodation
- Appropriate accommodation for different categories of animals (for example boarding, hospitalized)
- The monitoring and control of environmental conditions in animal accommodation to suit animals' requirements
- Selection of the most suitable bedding and floor-base materials for animals
- Selection of the most effective cleaning, disinfecting and antiseptic substance for a specific task
- Methods of disposal of clinical waste and other refuse
- Items classified as clinical waste and sharps
- The most recent quarantine regulations

Legal requirements for licensing

Boarding and breeding kennels and catteries operate under strict legal requirements. Licensing laws relating to such establishments should be monitored and upheld by the local authority.

Boarding kennels and catteries

Animal Boarding Establishments Act 1963
This requires that a licence be obtained annually. The licensing authority is the local authority; a veterinary surgeon may be appointed by the local authority to carry this out on its behalf.

The Act only relates to the boarding of dogs and cats; establishments boarding species other than cats and dogs do not require a licence.

There are national guidelines with recommendations for boarding. Separate documents on the cat and dog ('Model Licensing Conditions for Cat/Dog Boarding Establishments') are available from the Chartered Institute of Environmental Health. For specific local licensing conditions, the local authority's environmental department should be contacted.

Breeding establishments

Breeding of Dogs Act 1973
This requires that a licence be obtained where there are two or more bitches kept which are being bred for profit. This applies to all premises, including residential private dwellings. The licensing authority is the local authority and the Act requires that the licensing authority must check the accommodation, bedding, feeding, watering and exercise arrangements for the dogs. The licence must be obtained annually and the licensing authority must make satisfactory inspections at least yearly before the licence is granted. The recommendation is that these checks should be made several times a year at regular intervals in order to ensure that all conditions specified in the licence are being met.

Breeding of Dogs Act 1991
This gives powers of entry to local authorities to any unlicensed dog breeding establishment: it allows local authority officials (and veterinary surgeons appointed by them) to apply for a warrant to inspect such premises.

Construction of animal housing

Animal housing can be constructed from a variety of materials (Figure 5.1) and most are a mixture of two or more different types.

It is likely that most personnel employed to care for animals will simply be working with the housing that is already in place, and trying to maintain a level of comfort and hygiene for the occupants within the limitations of an existing system. Areas within a system that may be altered, such as the ideal temperature and the most desirable bedding and disinfectants to use with existing housing, will be considered later within this section.

It is also possible that, at some stage during a career of working with animals, a carer may have the opportunity to become involved with the design, purchase and construction of a totally new unit. Figure 5.1 then becomes useful as a basic guide when comparing the four parameters in the chart. When building new units, it is an excellent opportunity to look at such a project from every perspective rather than just those related to the construction materials.

Considerations

The major considerations should be species and purpose, though it is likely that choice will also be restricted by having to work within a budget. It can be seen that each of these considerations must be looked at from several angles before a final choice can be made.

Species

The small companion animal species are frequently kept and many more of these animals are held in long-term confinement, compared with dogs and cats. They include birds and small mammals in cages, reptiles in vivaria and rabbits in hutches. Poorly designed housing in terms of, say, building materials and living/sleeping space and day-to-day management of that housing can lead to many behavioural and medical problems.

Purpose

The purpose of the housing will probably be the greatest factor in determining its structure and size.

Companion or pet animals can be loosely classified into two groups:

- Large companion animals (e.g. dog, cat)
- Small companion animals (e.g. small mammals, birds, reptiles).

It can immediately be seen that, although all of these may be regarded as 'household pets', they will not all necessarily be roaming freely about the house.

Healthy animals

Wherever healthy active animals are kept in a cage or limited space, either permanently or for long periods, then the maximum size of unit possible will be the chief consideration, along with comfort, hygiene, strength and durability, and the cost of the construction materials.

5.1 Construction material for animal housing

Material	Comfort	Hygiene	Strength/durability	Relative cost
Concrete	Cold	Easy to scrub or hose Cracks may harbour parasites/bacteria	Excellent, especially for dogs and destructive mammals or birds	Cheap
Bricks or breeze blocks	Cold	Easy to scrub or hose Cracks may harbour parasites/bacteria	Excellent, especially for dogs and destructive mammals or birds	Expensive
Wood	Warm	Difficult to clean and slow to dry Cracks may harbour parasites/bacteria	Easily destroyed by chewing or scratching	Average
Stainless steel	Cold	Easy to clean and disinfect Small cages can even be sterilized	Excellent, especially for dogs and destructive mammals or birds	Expensive
Galvanized steel	Cold	Reasonably easy unless rust spots	As for stainless steel Rust spots can develop if cracked or drilled	Average
Fibreglass	Cold unless indoors	Easy to clean and disinfect	Good for small or non-destructive mammals	Average
Polypropylene	Cold unless indoors	Easy to clean and disinfect Small cages can even be sterilized	Good for small or non-destructive mammals	Average
Plastic	Cold unless indoors	Easy to clean and disinfect	Good for small or non-destructive mammals	Cheap
Glass	Cold unless indoors	Easy to clean and disinfect	Good for small or non-destructive mammals	Cheap

Healthy active animals may be caged:

- For boarding, working, showing, breeding
- As rescues or strays
- Under quarantine.

Hospitalized animals

When the purpose of housing is related to the requirements of a veterinary practice, the priorities that determine the type of housing are different.

Animals will be hospitalized because they are clinically ill, injured or pre- or postoperative. Consequently, such animals are likely to be less active. They may also need to have normal activity curtailed as part of a prescribed therapy. Maximum housing size and the choice of construction materials will therefore be different.

Other considerations

Further considerations, especially for housing materials, must take into account certain features of the animal:

- Size
- Strength
- Temperament
- Breed.

Other construction considerations include the detailed design of:

- Size of individual kennel or cattery units
- Ventilation
- Heating
- Lighting.

plus needs in relation to:

- Feeding
- Cleaning
- Safety regimes
- Noise control.

Housing requirements for dogs and cats

The housing requirements of small pets and exotic species are discussed in Chapter 4.

As the housing requirements of dogs and cats are very different in boarding and breeding establishments, compared with veterinary practices, these both will be given consideration.

The building and construction of new kennel and cattery blocks:

- Require planning permission from the local authority
- Must be built to specified national construction requirements (i.e. the building regulations standards).

Construction standards

All kennel and cattery blocks (Figures 5.2 and 5.3) must be built to building regulations standards. These will include, for example, specifications in relation to damp-proof coursing, insulation and ventilation.

Construction recommendations by local authorities also include the following.

Wood

Where wood is used, it should be protected with a suitable wood preservative such as Cuprinol or be tanalized.

Protection

Phenol-based substances should *not* be used, as they are toxic to cats.

Interiors

All interior surfaces should be waterproof, in order to allow thorough cleaning and disinfection and prevent the harbouring of parasites and infectious disease.

Flooring

Flooring should be of a material that is impervious to liquids.

Walls

- Walls should be solid to a height of
  - 1200 mm minimum between individual kennel units (Figure 5.4)
  - 1800 mm full height between individual cattery units (to act as a sneeze and hygiene barrier)
- Walls should be of materials that are impervious to liquids, or should be painted to this effect, to a minimum of 1200 mm high
- Curving is desirable where walls meet floors

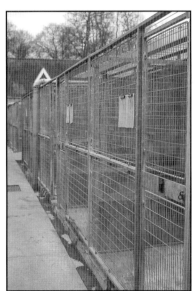

 5.2 *A typical kennel block.*

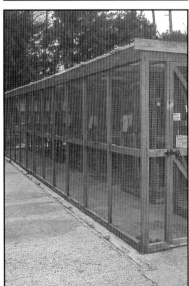

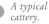 **5.3** *A typical cattery.*

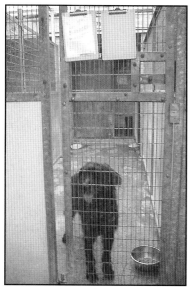

5.4 *Individual dog kennel and run. Note height of solid walls to help to prevent direct contact between adjacent animals.*

- If curving is not an option, joints should be sealed with waterproof grouting to prevent liquids, bacteria and parasites from entering.

Drainage

Floors of new units (kennel or cattery) should slope to a minimum fall of 1 in 80, towards a shallow drainage channel.

Wire

- Cattery: weldmesh (16 gauge minimum, 25 mm hole size maximum)
- Kennels: metal bars and frames (10–12 mm minimum spacing – adequate to prevent escape or entrapment).

Doors

Doors (Figure 5.5) must:

- Be strong enough to resist impact and scratching
- Be able to be secured effectively
- Open into a secure corridor.

Windows

- Windows must be escape-proof at all times
- Suitable wire (as above) should be added to allow opening for ventilation if necessary.

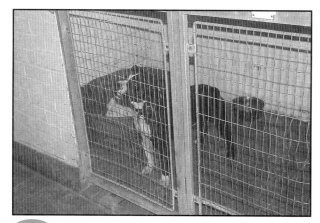

5.5 *Indoor kennel of solid construction.*

Ventilation

Ventilation is necessary to:

- Ensure that there is an adequate supply of oxygen
- Remove stale air (which contains carbon dioxide, water vapour from respiration and ammonia and methane from excretions)
- Prevent respiratory ailments caused by high humidity levels
- Reduce the spread of airborne infections
- Remove unpleasant odours
- Prevent an excessive temperature rise during hot weather.

Ventilation rate

The degree of ventilation taking place within a building is normally expressed in terms of air changes per hour, i.e. how many times all the air is replaced in an hour.

- In the case of a typical enclosed kennel block, a ventilation rate of about six air changes per hour is required
- During periods of hot weather a full kennel building is likely to need double that amount
- Conversely, the same building operating at 50% occupancy during cold weather would only require one or two air changes per hour.

Methods of ventilation

Passive ventilation

Passive systems normally rely on controlling the air flow by means of adjustable vents and opening windows and doors. Sometimes additional ridge vents are placed on the roof in order to aid the removal of hot stale air, which will naturally rise towards the roof.

Such systems are inexpensive to install and operate. They are in common use, especially in buildings that are not used to house a large number of animals. The chief drawbacks of passive systems are:

- There is very little control over the ventilation rate and movement of air within the building
- Overventilation and the production of draughts and cold zones are likely during cold weather
- Inadequate ventilation can occur during periods of hot weather, especially if they coincide with periods of low wind speed
- Frequent adjustment of the vents and windows is required.

Active ventilation

Active ventilation systems rely on the use of fans either to pull stale air out of a building, or to force fresh clean air into it. The fans are normally mounted within special housings, located on the rooftop.

There are numerous different layouts for active ventilation systems, but they are all designed to create maximum control over the ventilation rate and pattern of air flow within the building.

Many active systems are designed to reduce the danger of spreading airborne diseases by passing fresh air over individual animals, and then extracting it from the building before it can be inhaled by other animals. Such systems are often employed in veterinary hospitals and quarantine kennels.

Active ventilation systems are normally controlled by adjusting the speed of the fans and the size and angle of the vents. Often the fans are controlled by thermostats; thus the system can be regarded as semi-automatic.

The effect that the different fan speeds and vent sizes have on the ventilation rate and air flow pattern should be understood by the staff involved.

Figure 5.6 lists common ventilation problems.

5.6 Common ventilation problems

Problem	Possible causes
Overventilation	Fan speed too fast
	Thermostat setting too low
Underventilation	Fan speed too low
	Thermostat setting too high
Unsatisfactory airflow pattern	Fan speed too high or low
	Air inlet vents set at incorrect size or angle
	Windows or doors left open
Draughts or cold spots	Fan speed too fast
	Air inlet vent size set too small or air deflectors set at incorrect angle
Excessive noise	Worn fan motor
	Distorted fan blades

Heating

Kennel buildings require heating to:

- Provide a comfortable environment for the animals (this is particularly important in the case of hospitalized animals)
- Reduce the time taken for the kennels to dry after they have been washed and disinfected
- Lower the risk of respiratory diseases by reducing condensation
- Reduce the risk of frost damage during cold weather
- Improve the working environment for staff.

The common methods of heating animal accommodation are compared in Figure 5.7.

Temperature range

Figure 5.8 shows the temperature requirements of animal housing as stated in the Animal Boarding Establishments Act 1963 and the Breeding of Dogs Act 1973. Temperature considerations for the dog and cat within the required ranges depend principally on the health status and age of the animal.

Temperature measurement

There can be a considerable variation between the

5.7 Comparison of heating systems

System	Advantages	Potential problems	Safety considerations
Hot water central heating, gas or oil powered	Clean, safe and easily controlled	Supplementary heat may be required in individual kennels	
Underfloor, water-filled, gas or oil powered	Clean Animals benefit from heated floor	Expensive to repair Difficult to remove dried-onbody fluids and excrement	
Underfloor, electrically powered	Clean Animals benefit from heated floor	Expensive to repair Difficult to remove dried-on-body fluids and excrement	
Individual electric fan heaters	Can be controlled individually Heat can be directed towards animals	Noisy Spread of airborne diseases Can cause overheating of individual animals	Small fire risk Cables must be protected from interference by animals Switches should be waterproof Socket outlets should be: – waterproof – fitted with covers when not in use
Infra-red dull emitter lamp	Good source of local heat Can be controlled by adjusting distance of lamp from the animal	Can cause overheating and burning if: – too close to the animal – not thermostatically controlled	Cables must be protected from interference by animals Switches should be waterproof Socket outlets should be: – waterproof – fitted with covers when not in use
Electric oil–filled radiators	Clean Mobile	Surface temperature can be high enough to injure staff and animals	Cables must be protected from interference by animals Switches should be waterproof Socket outlets should be: – waterproof – fitted with covers when not in use

5.8 Temperature range in housing for dogs and cats

Healthy dogs and cats in boarding establishments
Sleeping area: 10–26°C
Exercise area: same as local environmental
                   temperature, as usually open-air

Healthy dogs and cats in breeding establishments
Parturition area: 10–21°C
Neonates: 26–29°C

Hospitalized dogs and cats
Hospital cage: 18–23°C

temperature of individual kennels; therefore it is important that each one is monitored individually with a minimum–maximum thermometer.

Conserving heat

Overventilation
In a typical kennel block, the major source of heat loss is due to overventilation, caused by doors and windows being left open or having poor seals around them.

Considerable savings in heating costs can be achieved by fitting draught-excluding seals to doors and windows and making sure that there is a policy that all staff keep doors and windows closed during cold weather.

Heat loss through the roof
The second major source of heat loss is through the roof. Further savings in heating costs can be achieved by insulating the roof with proprietary thermal board. Alternatively, it could be professionally sprayed with polyurethane foam insulation, which will not only reduce heat loss from the building, but will also render the roof more stormproof and help to make the building soundproof.

Lighting
Good lighting in kennels is necessary in order to:

* Create a safe working environment for the staff
* Allow the animals to be observed properly
* Stimulate the animals to expect an 'activity phase' – e.g. waking, feeding – when the light intensity increases.

Natural light
This is the cheapest light to provide and in general is a beneficial option for the animals. However, the following points must be considered.

* Natural light can only be a serious option for a boarding establishment, where there are healthy animals
* Should an animal fall ill and need attention during the hours of darkness, natural lighting alone may raise welfare and safety issues
* It will reduce the length of the working day considerably in the winter months, which may be inconvenient and may upset cleaning, feeding regimens and other routines
* Sleeping areas need reduced light levels, and therefore need to be sited away from a window or skylight

* Screens may need to be placed at the windows, otherwise:
  – Animals may become restless too early in the morning
  – Direct sunlight entering a kennel area may cause overheating during the summer months.

Artificial light
Even in buildings where maximum use is made of natural light, it is usually necessary to provide additional artificial lighting.

In corridors, lighting normally consists of fluorescent tubes, which are fitted with diffusers in order to protect them from physical damage and to create a more uniform shadowless light.

Additional lighting may need to be provided in each kennel. This is usually only found in a boarding or breeding establishment – mainly because animal housing in veterinary practices tends to be smaller and so light fittings could easily be reached and destroyed.

The Chartered Institute of Environmental Health recommends that artificial lighting is provided in the sleeping areas of kennels and catteries for boarding animals, in case an animal needs to be checked during the night. Exercise areas should also have adequate lighting, if the animals are using these areas out of daylight hours.

If lighting is necessary in these larger kennels, the safest method is to fit bulkhead lights, in which the bulbs are fitted behind a thick glass or plastic cover. These lights are located on the ceiling or high on the walls so that dogs cannot reach them. Operating costs can be reduced by fitting energy-saving bulbs.

Safety considerations

* Electricity is dangerous when used in damp environments
* Bulkhead lights should be waterproof
* All light switches within a kennel area should be waterproof as they may:
  – Become wet during cleaning procedures
  – Be touched by staff with wet hands
* Faulty fluorescent lights that flicker should not be used: they can induce fits in epileptic animals or staff
* Lights must be turned off before they are cleaned or serviced. In the case of lights operated by two-way switches it is advisable to turn off the whole light circuit
* Professional advice should be obtained before a bulb is replaced with one of a higher wattage – it may overheat the fitting and cause a fire. This is important in the case of bulkhead lights.

Size of individual accommodation for boarding

It is recognized by the Chartered Institute of Environmental Health that existing kennels and catteries may not fulfil all the requirements that it recommends. Establishments with smaller accommodation and more basic facilities are being encouraged to phase these out where possible and replace them with housing that meets the model guidelines (Figures 5.9 and 5.10).

Size of dogs (housed individually – more than one dog if same owner, with written consent)	Height of unit	Exercise area (floor area)	Sleeping area (floor area)
Up to 60 cm at shoulder	1.85 m	2.46 m²	1.9 m²
Over 50 cm at shoulder	1.85 m	3.35 m²	1.9 m²

5.10 Recommended size of individual cattery units

Number of cats	Height of unit	Exercise area (floor area)	Sleeping area (floor area)
One cat only	1.85 m	1.7 m²	0.85 m²
Three cats maximum (if same owner, with written consent)	1.85 m	3.0 m²	1.50 m²

Tiered cages

Tiered cages for boarding and breeding establishments are not recommended and should have been phased out by now. It is also recognized that if cages are small enough to be tiered then they are of a size that is too confined for the boarding of healthy animals. Cats or small dogs kept in such situations would not be able to exercise or stretch out properly and are more likely to pass airborne infections easily when using the same air space.

Food preparation area

All animal housing should have a separate kitchen or food preparation area. This area should:

- Be close enough to the accommodation for convenience of feeding and watering regimens
- Have enough room for the storage of not only food but also feed bowls and utensils
- Have deep sinks for washing and soaking feed bowls and utensils
- Be rodent-proof (but as a precaution any dried foods should be stored in large rodent-proof containers)
- Have a freezer to store moist foods, or, in a veterinary practice, a refrigerator to store soft convalescent foods or made-up oral rehydrants.

Bedding considerations

Beds

Whether animals are kept in a free-roaming situation in the home or are caged for short or long periods, they require a bedding area for warmth, comfort and security.

There are many different types of 'bed' on the market – for example, nest-shaped and igloo-shaped ones made of materials such as moulded plastic, covered foam, wood and wicker. Of these, the first two types are probably the easiest to clean.

In a commercial kennel or cattery the bed area is just as likely to be a raised area within the main housing. This area may also be locally heated from a source above or below.

In a veterinary practice, because animals may be undergoing treatment that prevents them from stepping up to or into beds, bedding material is usually put straight on to the floor base of the hospital cage. This also assists the high levels of hygiene that have to be maintained in such an environment, where a patient's bedding may need changing many times during the day because of (say) incontinence or vomiting.

Veterinary practices also have many individual cages, which are likely to be too small to have a separate area as a bed or to have the bedding contained (rather than laid on the floor base of the cage). Generally there is a smaller floor area available for caging in veterinary practices, but there are several other good reasons for this:

- Animals tend to be confined for shorter periods – many are only day-patients
- Long-term patients kept in reasonably small areas may have been prescribed cage rest – following a fractured pelvis, for example. Such a patient may need to have its movement restricted and therefore be encouraged to lie down and rest
- Large cages that are deep but not 'walk-in' make regular treatment of the animal difficult, because it is uncomfortable for staff to lean in and may block the light
- Leaning in is also dangerous for the staff: it is a very threatening posture to an animal and may cause it to respond aggressively.

Bedding materials

Whatever the arrangements are for the actual bed area, the animal will still need to be provided with bedding material. This is even more important when an animal is confined and therefore often obliged to lie down for long periods.

With regard to the choice of bedding, the primary factor should be the animal itself. Account should be taken of:

- Species
- Size and weight
- Health status.

Figures 5.11 and 5.12 show other related factors that subsequently need to be considered.

5.11 Bedding materials for the dog and cat

Bedding	Comfort	Insulation	Absorbency	Wash/dry	Harbours parasites	Cost	Comments
Acrylic bedding	Reasonable for the healthy animal	Reasonable	Very good – urine, etc. soaks through	Easy care	No	Expensive initially, but long lasting	More durable than most bedding material
Beanbags (filled with polystyrene balls or chips)	Excellent – thick and conform to body shape	Excellent – allows very little heat loss by conduction	Easily saturated	Difficult to wash and dry	Not easily	Expensive	Polystyrene flattens over time, reducing comfort & insulation value
Foam-filled (either chips or wedges) Bags filled with acrylic wadding	Both excellent – thick and conform to body shape	Both excellent – allow very little heat loss by conduction	Both easily saturated, especially foam	Both difficult to wash and dry	Foam – no when new, but yes when foam begins to crumble Acrylic wadding – no	Both good value	Dogs can easily destroy foam-filled beds
Duvets	Excellent – thick and conform to body shape	Excellent – allow very little heat loss by conduction	Easily saturated	Easy to wash in machine Long time to dry naturally	Potentially	Expensive	Dogs can easily destroy
Blankets	Reasonable for the healthy animal. Several layers needed	Good if several layers used	Easily saturated	Easy to wash in machine Long time to dry naturally	Potentially	Expensive to purchase but often donated	Dogs can easily destroy
Towelling	Reasonable for the healthy animal. Several layers needed	Reasonable if several layers used	Easily saturated	Easy to wash in machine Long time to dry naturally	Potentially	Good value Often donated	Dogs can easily destroy

5.12 Bedding materials for small pets

Bedding	Comfort	Insulation	Absorbency	Disposable	Harbours parasites	Cost	Comments
Shredded paper	Good	Reasonable	Good, unless 'office' paper (which is not very absorbent)	Yes	Not if changed daily	Usually free of charge in small amounts	If produced from shredded office paper, remove paper clips and staples and any acetate and polythene materials first
Straw	Excellent	Excellent	Not very good	Yes	Yes	Relatively expensive in small amounts	Can contain *Aspergillus* (mould) spores, which can cause respiratory problems in small mammals, tortoises, etc.
Hay	Excellent	Excellent	Not very good	Yes	Yes	Relatively expensive in small amounts	Can contain *Aspergillus* (mould) spores, which can cause respiratory problems in small mammals, tortoises, etc.
Acrylic/nylon wadding	Excellent	Excellent	Not very good	Yes	No	Relatively expensive in small amounts	Can easily wrap around limbs of small mammals, cutting off blood supply to lower limb causing necrosis and gangrene
Polystyrene chips or balls	Reasonable	Excellent	Not very good	Yes	No	Can be free of charge (e.g. discarded packing material)	Small rodents may eat it – causes constipation, and can cause death if blockage results Risk of fumes, which can be toxic to small rodents and when used for hibernating tortoises

Species

Small mammals that like to 'nest' (e.g. hamsters) need bedding material that they can get in amongst and can move about in easily, such as shredded paper. Conversely, mammals that like to burrow (e.g. gerbils, jirds) prefer a few inches of peat in which they can dig out their own bedding area.

It is essential that those who look after animals find out at least the basics regarding an animal's natural habits. Only then is it possible to provide the ideal bedding material for that particular species, in order to create a feeling of security as well as comfort.

There are two main exceptions to this rule:

- Hospitalized animals – where comfort is still paramount but hygiene is of equal importance for the recumbent patient and where wound and surgical sites need to be kept clean and dry
- Reptiles – especially those kept in vivaria, where heat and humidity are usually high.

The introduction of natural bedding material into such vivarium conditions can:

- Encourage the growth of dangerous moulds (e.g. *Aspergillus* spp.) that can cause disease of the respiratory system
- Bring scale mites into the environment, which can cause anaemia and secondary anorexia.

Size and weight

Although cats, dogs and many other species may prefer to sleep curled up, the chosen material should be of sufficient area to allow all animals to lie out flat whilst keeping the whole body surface on the bedding.

The bedding should be pliable and of sufficient depth so that it still gives substantial insulation from the floor or containing-bed or basket even when the whole weight of the animal is on it. The material must also be soft and supportive enough to prevent bedsores from developing at pressure points on the body.

Health status

Categories of animals likely to need to lie out flat are:

- Pregnant and lactating (and possibly those undergoing parturition)
- Geriatric
- Surgical and trauma cases
- Clinical cases associated with pain (e.g. pancreatitis, tumours)
- Suffering from a raised body temperature (many possible causes).

Floor-base materials

The floors of large kennels and catteries for boarding and other categories of long-stay animals are usually made of concrete or hard impervious material. Because of the greater floor areas involved, they rarely have extra materials added as a floor-base.

Floor-base materials tend to be used where animals are confined in small areas, such as those that are hospitalized, or for small pets kept in cages or tanks, and they help to absorb urine and aid cleaning out.

The different types of floor-base materials in general use, and their advantages and disadvantages, are considered in Figure 5.13.

5.13 Floor-base materials for caging

Material	Comfort	Insulation	Absorbency	Disposable	Harbours parasites	Cost	Comments
Newspaper	Good if shredded but not if layered in pages	Reasonable	Very good, especially if used multilayered or shredded into deep piles. Urine or vomit produced in one corner can be absorbed and drawn across newspaper, making it difficult for the animal to avoid	Yes	Not if changed daily	Usually free of charge	Excellent for hospitalized animals that need floor-base material changed frequently. Can hinder procedures such as endoscopy and associated radiography, as confined dogs and some rodents will often eat it
Sawdust	Excellent – small mammals can dig into it	Excellent	Excellent, especially if used in a thick layer. Urine produced in one corner remains localized if used in a thick layer	Yes	Yes	Relatively expensive especially in small quantities	Good for caging or tanks containing small healthy mammals. Digging through this material provides a more stimulating environment than newspaper. Impractical for any hospitalized animal – as expensive and slow to change several times a day. Would lodge in wounds and interfere with healing

Figure 5.13 continues ▶

Material	Comfort	Insulation	Absorbency	Disposable	Harbours parasites	Cost	Comments
Pre-sterilized peat	Excellent, small mammals can dig into it	Good	Excellent, especially if used in a thick layer Very useful for small mammals – reduces ammonia in excreted urine, which can build up to toxic levels near cage floors Reduces cage smells caused by ammonia, therefore excellent for mammals housed indoors and for pungent animals such as ferrets	Yes	Not easily if changed regularly	Expensive, especially in small quantities, though wet areas can be changed daily and a full change made every 2 weeks	Excellent for cages or tanks containing small healthy mammals and birds Digging into this material provides a more stimulating environment than newspaper Impractical for any hospitalized animal – expensive and slow to change several times a day Would lodge in wounds and interfere with healing

Quarantine

Rabies is a viral disease of the central nervous system for which there is no known cure. It is endemic in animals in many parts of the world. It is maintained in particular host species, the dog being the host in many parts of the developing world. It is the canine strain that is responsible for the deaths of many thousands of people world-wide.

The UK has been free from indigenous animal rabies since 1902, except for a brief period between the years 1918–1922, and no case has occurred outside quarantine since 1970 (although a case of the related European bat lyssavirus occurred in 1996).

Despite a massive growth in international travel for commerce and leisure the UK has remained free from rabies. The fact that it is surrounded by water has contributed significantly to the preservation of the status quo. However, there is no doubt that the rigid enforcement of the quarantine regulations has been the greatest single factor responsible for preventing the reintroduction of the disease. It should be noted that rabies, although the most notorious, is not the only disease against which the quarantine system has helped to protect the UK.

Until recently, the advisers of successive governments have held the view that there was no alternative to the existing quarantine regulations. The most salient points of these regulations are:

- A licence must be obtained from the relevant Department of Agriculture before a pet can be imported
- The pet can only be transported into the country by a carrier authorized by the country's Department of Agriculture
- All dogs and cats entering the UK have to be held for a period of 6 months in official accommodation, which is under the daily supervision of a veterinary surgeon
- The veterinary surgeon, who is known as the Veterinary Superintendent, is appointed by and responsible to the Minister of Agriculture, Fisheries and Food (or the Secretary of State for Scotland or Wales)
- The Veterinary Superintendent (or an official deputy)

must visit the quarantine accommodation daily from Monday to Saturday and also on Sundays when necessary
- The Veterinary Superintendent must visually inspect every animal at least twice a week and examine every imported animal on the day of its arrival at the quarantine premises and within 2 days prior to its release
- It is also the duty of the Veterinary Superintendent to report the arrival of imported animals as soon as possible to the Ministry
- Newly imported animals must be vaccinated against rabies at their owner's expense within 48 hours of their arrival. The vaccine used must be approved for the purpose by the Ministry and can only be given by the Veterinary Superintendent or their deputy. Should the vaccination have to be postponed for reasons such as illness of the animal, the agreement of the Divisional Veterinary Officer must be obtained
- The only persons allowed access to quarantined animals are:
  - The Veterinary Superintendent or deputy
  - The owner of the premises and their staff
  - A Ministry Veterinary Officer
  - Someone authorized by and assisting any of the above
  - Someone visiting an animal with the permission of the owner of the premises
- All visitors must be accompanied by the owner of the premises or a nominated member of their staff, unless the visitor agrees to being locked in with the animal that they are visiting.

Exception from quarantine

Although pet animals are required to be quarantined, a specific exception from the quarantine regulations was introduced in 1994 for dogs and cats being moved in trade from other EU member states. This exception is known as the Balai arrangements. The very few animals imported under these arrangements are subject to alternative safeguards.

Quarantine accommodation

Construction of the accommodation must conform to strict regulations, which will ensure that no animal can possibly escape. These regulations also state that provision must be made to prevent nose or paw contact between two or more animals unless they are being housed in the same unit (Figure 5.14). Shared accommodation in the same unit is only allowable when animals under the same ownership enter quarantine at the same time; and even then the agreement of the Veterinary Superintendent must be obtained. Furthermore, the maximum number of animals allowed to share a unit is three and they must be of the same species, i.e. dogs or cats.

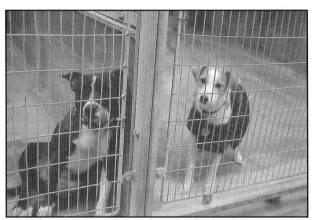

5.14 *Two kennels with solid division to prevent contact between noses, mouths or paws of adjacent animals.*

Suitable alternative accommodation must be available at all times in case animals need to be separated at short notice. The alternative accommodation has to be of the same standard as the main units.

In order to reduce the risk of spreading disease, quarantine kennels should be built in small self-contained groups of units. In the event of an outbreak of rabies or other infectious diseases, the implementation of the necessary special restrictions is made much easier when the accommodation is split into small groups in this way.

Proposed changes to the quarantine regulations

It is stressful for owners to be forced to place their animals in quarantine and there has been growing public pressure to have the quarantine regulations re-examined in the light of recent advances in preventive veterinary medicine and the technology of animal identification.

In 1994 the House of Commons Agriculture Select Committee published a report on the import controls for live animals. In brief it recommended that the 6-month quarantine requirements should be replaced for dogs and cats being imported from certain 'approved' countries (EU member states and all other countries internationally recognized to be rabies-free and carrying out policies to maintain their rabies-free status, Figure 5.15) by a new system.

In 1998 the Kennedy Group recommended that the quarantine regulations should be changed and proposed a new approach, which adopted many of the 1994 Select Committee's recommendations. There was overwhelming public support for the proposed changes and on 26 March 1999 the Government stated formally that the quarantine regulations would be radically changed and that the new

system would be introduced by April 2001, with a pilot scheme operational within 12 months.

Early in August 1999 the Government made a further announcement about the pilot for the 'Pet Travel Scheme', in which it was declared that it would be in place in the early months of the year 2000.

The pilot scheme:

- Only applies to dogs and cats
- Is limited to those animals entering the UK from countries listed in Figure 5.15
- Will only operate on specified rail, sea and air routes to England.

5.15	Countries qualifying to participate in the pet travel scheme

Andorra	Austria	Belgium	Denmark
Finland	France[a]	Germany	Gibraltar
Greece	Iceland	Italy	Liechtenstein
Luxembourg	Monaco	Netherlands	Norway[b]
Portugal[c]	San Marino	Spain[d]	Sweden
Switzerland	Vatican		

a Not including French Overseas Departments and Territories.
b Excludes Spitzbergen
c Includes the Azores and Madeira
d Includes the Canary Islands but not Ceuta and Melilla.

The salient points of the new system apply to animals that have been continuously resident in a 'qualifying' country (see the 1994 Select Committee recommendations above) for at least 6 months. These animals will have to be:

- Microchipped with an electronic permanent number identification chip (Figure 5.16). It is recommended that a microchip is used which conforms to the International Standards Organisation standard 11784 or to Annex A to 11785, otherwise it may not be readable by the standard microchip reader, when the animal is checked before travelling

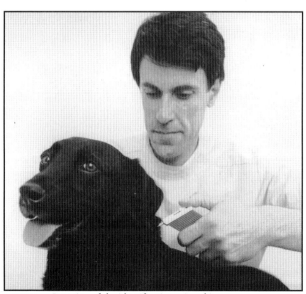

5.16 *Insertion of the identification microchip. Reproduced with permission of Animalcare Ltd.*

- Vaccinated against rabies using a MAFF-approved inactivated adjuvanted vaccine, but only *after* the animal has had a microchip fitted. At vaccination, a record card must be filled out by the administering veterinary surgeon to show: the date of the vaccination, vaccine product name and batch number, date of the next vaccination (or booster), microchip number and the animal's age and/or date of birth (it must be a minimum of 3 months old before vaccination)
- Blood tested at a laboratory approved by MAFF. The test must show that the required antibody titre level has been achieved following vaccination
- Brought into the UK only after 6 months have elapsed from the blood test. The exception will be animals which are normally resident in the British Isles (including the Irish Republic) that are microchipped, vaccinated and blood tested before the pilot scheme comes into operation. These pets can re-enter the UK after a trip abroad, without having to wait 6 months
- Issued with an official Health Certificate for the Pet Travel Scheme which contains details of the animal itself, plus the details recorded by the veterinary surgeon on the vaccination record card. In the UK, only Local Veterinary Inspectors (LVIs) who have been trained and approved by the Animal Health Office may issue Pet Health Certificates
- Treated against specified parasites, that is *Echinococcus multilocularis* (the fox tapeworm) and ticks, to prevent the spread of serious zoonotic diseases currently not present in the UK. The pet must be accompanied by a certificate signed by an official veterinary surgeon to the effect that this treatment has been carried out 24–48 hours before the animal enters the UK.

It was proposed by the Select Committee that pre-entry checks on the travelling animals should be carried out by transport operators approved by the Government, but this is being challenged by the veterinary profession. Transport Companies offering the Pet Travel Scheme will be subject to MAFF spot tests and stringent auditing. Pets failing to meet all the conditions will have to be quarantined if they are re-entering the UK or return to their country of origin if not normally resident in the UK.

The existing quarantine regulations will continue to be enforced for animals being imported from non-qualifying countries and this is likely to be the case for the foreseeable future. However, it is hoped that, as Australia and New Zealand are rabies-free, eventually Guide and Hearing dogs may be allowed to travel between the UK and these countries if all relevant authorities agree.

Antiseptics and disinfectants

Understanding the terminology
Before the most effective cleaning method can be chosen to remove and destroy microorganisms, the related terminology must be understood.

Sterilization
Sterilization is defined as the destruction of all microorganisms – including the most resilient part of some bacteria, i.e. the bacterial spores.

In veterinary practice, sterilization is usually carried out by:

- Moist heat, under pressure (autoclaving)
- High temperatures, at atmospheric pressure (hot air oven)
- Chemical methods (ethylene oxide or formaldehyde gas, or glutaraldehyde solution). These are not reliable. In hospitals for humans, chemical sterilization has been unacceptable to the Department of Health for over 20 years
- Disinfectants. These *cannot* produce sterilization; manufacturers who state that their disinfectants are 'sterilizing' are making a false claim. Disinfectants will not remove bacterial spores.

Disinfection
Disinfection is defined as the destruction or reduction of microorganisms that are pathogenic. Transient and less harmful bacteria are also reduced in number or removed. Bacterial spores are not usually destroyed.
Methods of disinfection are:

- Boiling (the maximum effect is achieved after 15 minutes contact from the time boiling begins)
- Chemical disinfection (to be effective, recommended exposure or contact times must be adhered to)
- Mechanical movement (cleaning – e.g. scrubbing, mopping, wiping).

Antisepsis
Antisepsis is the opposite of sepsis or toxicity and is the destruction of microorganisms *on living tissue*. The delicate nature of tissue means that methods used for antisepsis cannot destroy bacterial spores.

Antisepsis is achieved with the use of antiseptics. Many antiseptics are a weak solution of the disinfectants used on non-living objects, and when used as an antiseptic they can be referred to as skin disinfectants. Not all disinfectants are safe to use on tissue and even at a very low concentration some disinfectants can destroy living tissue.

Deodorizers
Deodorizers do exactly what the name implies – they simply mask smells. They are not a substitute for thorough cleaning and disinfection.

Bactericides and bacteriostats
Bactericides destroy or kill bacteria – the suffix -'cide' indicates killing, rather than simply preventing an increase in the numbers of bacteria.

Bacteriostats slow down or stop bacterial growth (multiplication of their numbers) – the suffix -'stat' indicates no growth or increase.

Therefore bactericides are more useful, as bacteriostats may only slow down bacterial action for a short period.

Viricides
Viricides are disinfectants used to destroy viruses.

One of the most useful groups for this is the hypochlorites (bleaches): they release the gas chlorine, which is a powerful viricide. Viruses have a core of either DNA or RNA, which are acids and therefore most are easily neutralized and destroyed by the alkaline nature of hypochlorites.

Viruses that are more difficult to neutralize, such as parvovirus, need to be destroyed with disinfectants containing an aldehyde or formaldehyde base. Extreme caution should be exercised when using such compounds.

Fungicides

Fungicides are disinfectants used to destroy fungi and their spores. Most disinfectants will destroy these, though one exception to this is the quaternary ammonium compound group.

Disinfectants and their use

Disinfectants are classified into different compound groups, each developed for specific uses (Figure 5.17).

Before any inanimate object or area is disinfected, it should first be cleaned with soap or detergent to remove any organic material and then rinsed thoroughly with plain water in order to avoid inactivating the disinfectant (Figure 5.18). Before using any disinfectant, manufacturer's instructions and COSHH regulations should be checked.

5.17 Disinfectants and their use

Disinfectant use	Examples of disinfectant	Dilution strength (in water)	Compound classification	Active against	Effectiveness
Initial washing of inanimate objects (food bowls, cages, work surfaces, floors) to make clinically clean (clean to the naked eye)	Teepol Flash Liquid	12 ml in 1 litre 12 ml in 1 litre	Anionic detergent Anionic + non-anionic detergent	B, F B, F	Both: B, average F, good
General disinfection of inanimate objects	Domestos, i.e. bleach	12–24 ml in 1 litre	Hypochlorite (halogen base group)	B, F, V	B, F, V, excellent
Floors, kennel runs, sinks, drains (Not near cats – even fumes from the phenol group are toxic to them)	Jeyes Fluid Izal Stericol	All: 10–20ml in 1 litre for floors and runs Undiluted for sink/drains	Black phenol White phenol Clear phenol	B, F	All: B, F, very good
Kennel or cattery (especially useful in veterinary practice)	Parvocide Cidex Formula-H Vetcide	Follow manufacturers' instructions for dilution (will depend on microorganisms present)	Glutaraldehyde/Aldehyde group	B, F, V (especially resistant viruses, e.g. Parvovirus)	B, F, V, excellent but slow to work
Antiseptic: skin scrub – for 'scrubbing-up' prior to surgical procedures	Pevidine Hibiscrub Hibitane Phisohex	No need to dilute any of these disinfectants. Use direct on to palm of hands, enough to create lather when warm water added	Iodophore (halogen base group) Chlorhexidine + added detergent Chlorhexidine Chlorinated phenol	B, F (may irritate or stain) B, F B, F	B, F, excellent Both: B, average F, good
Antiseptic: operation site preparation wound cleaning (as appropriate)	Pevidine Hibiscrub Hibitane	Both: Op. site: can be undiluted Wound: 1 ml in 100 ml	Iodophor (halogen base group) Chlorhexidine + added detergent Chlorhexidine	B, F (may irritate or stain B, F	B, F, excellent B, F, average
Antiseptic: general skin cleansing Disinfectant: food preparation surfaces	Dettol, Ibcol Cetavlon, Roccal, Marinol Blue Savlon	Antiseptic: 60 ml in 568 ml Disinfectant: 27 ml in 568 ml Antiseptic: 1–2 ml in 100 ml Disinfectant: 10 ml in 100 ml Antiseptic: 1 ml in 100ml Skin cleaning: 5 ml in 100 ml Disinfectant: 10 ml in 100 ml	Chlorinated phenol QAC (quaternary ammonium compound) QAC plus a diguanide to aid destruction of bacteria	B, F B B	B, average F, good B, good if solution fresh B, good if solution fresh

B = bacteria, F = fungal spores, V = viruses.

Inactivating material	Disinfectant compound groups inactivated
Organic material, e.g. faeces, urine, vomit, pus, food	Chlorhexidine, hypochlorites (bleaches)
Organic material, e.g. wood, wool, cotton, cork	Chlorhexidine
Plastics (some) and rubber – significant when choosing buckets and bowls for cleaning regimens	Chlorhexidine, phenols
Soaps	Chlorhexidine, Quaternary Ammonium Compounds (QACs)
Detergents that are cationic (includes QACs)	Hypochlorites, phenols
Hard water	Chlorhexidine, chlorinated phenols
Bacteria *Pseudomonas* bacteria actively grow in QAC solutions. Such solutions should therefore be discarded and replaced regularly, ideally every 6 hours; maximum time as a made-up solution no longer than 12 hours	Quaternary ammonium compounds
Cotton wool QACs inactivated over the course of a day when diluted as an antiseptic and cotton wool dipped into the solution, or a bottle containing the solution is regularly inverted on to cotton wool. After one day, only coloured water remains	Quaternary ammonium compounds

Waste disposal

Since the introduction of the Environmental Protection Act 1990, any business generating waste has a 'duty of care' to dispose of waste safely and in line with the requirements of the law.

It is therefore the legal responsibility of the employer or the self-employed practitioner to develop a system for waste disposal and to ensure that all employees are familiar with it and follow procedures for the safe disposal of waste. Any establishments that are found not to be carrying out such measures are subject to prosecution.

The type of waste generated by veterinary practices and commercial boarding or breeding establishments would be classified initially as industrial waste. Much of the waste from these sources will also be further classified as clinical waste.

A refrigerated room, a freezer or a specifically designated area, suitable for the volume and type of waste, is a requirement for storage of clinical waste.

Controlled Waste Regulations Act 1992
This Act clearly defines clinical waste, for veterinary practice and other establishments housing animals, as:

- Animal tissue
- Body excretions
- Body fluids, including blood
- Dressings and swabs from wounds
- Pharmaceutical products
- Syringes, needles or other similar sharps
- Any other waste arising from nursing, veterinary, pharmaceutical or similar practice, treatment or care (this also includes similar waste generated by the collection of blood for transfusion, which may carry pathogens that can infect humans)
- Any of the aforementioned waste that may arise from related teaching or research.

The Act also states that all of this must be made safe, or it is considered to be hazardous to anybody who comes into contact with it.

Hazard groups
How clinical waste is managed is based on further classification into different hazard groups. There are five groups of clinical waste. For each group, Figure 5.19 shows the potentially hazardous waste that may be produced by veterinary practices. It should be noted that these groups

5.19 Categorization of clinical waste

Waste group	Type of clinical waste
Group A	Includes the following items where the risk assessment by the Health and Safety Executive indicates a risk to staff handling them: • Blood, animal carcasses and tissue from veterinary centres or laboratories • Soiled surgical dressings, swabs and other similar soiled waste • Other waste materials where the assessment indicates a risk to staff handling them (for example, from infectious disease cases)
Group B	Discarded syringe needles, broken glass and any other contaminated disposable sharp instruments or items
Group C	Microbiological cultures and potentially infected waste from pathology departments (laboratory and post-mortem rooms) and other clinical or research laboratories
Group D	Certain pharmaceutical products and chemical wastes
Group E	Items used to dispose of urine, faeces and other bodily secretions or excretions which do not fall within Group A

Adapted from Health and Safety Executive Regulations

are not set out in order of the level of risk from clinical waste, as the risk level will vary within the groups themselves.

Clinical waste disposal (Groups A–E)

UN-type approved containers

The actual practicalities of clinical waste disposal in a veterinary practice, or other establishment likely to produce such waste, mean that under current legislation it is recommended that the different categories of clinical waste in Figure 5.19 should be placed into the correct containers Figures 5.20–5.23.

It is not a case of simply putting such waste into 'yellow sacks'. There are, for example, yellow sacks with a single black stripe down them, which denote that the waste collected in them is designated for a land-fill site. This method of disposal is illegal for clinical waste, as it may contravene the landfill site licence.

With UN-type containers and sacks, the correct one should be used for the type of clinical waste being placed in it.

When special clinical waste containers or sacks are used (Figure 5.20), they should:

- Have a UN-type 3291 number stamped on them, which will denote the *type* of clinical waste that can be put in it
- Have a UN Testing number on it, as the containers are tested to make sure that they can withstand particular types and sometimes a designated weight of clinical waste
- Be denoted by being bright yellow
- State on the outside: 'Clinical waste for incineration only'.

It is illegal to put the wrong type of clinical waste into a clinical waste container. The UN-type number and waste suitability should be checked with the disposal service being used.

It is recommended that containers and sacks without a UN-type number should not be used for clinical waste, even if they are yellow.

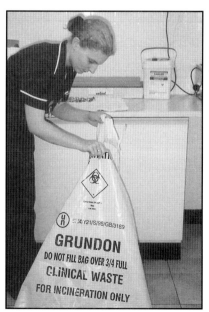

5.20 *Yellow sack with number clearly seen, to conform to UN standard.*

One-way burn bins

These should be used for clinical waste that may leak (Figures 5.21 and 5.22).

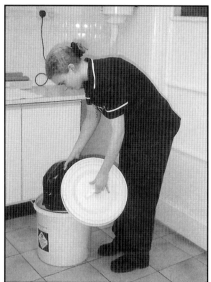

5.21 *One-way yellow burn bin (small) for body parts, tissues, dressings and other substances that may leak.*

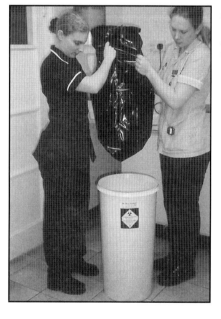

5.22 *One-way yellow burn bin large enough to take a canine cadaver.*

- This type of 'wet' clinical waste should not be put into yellow sacks
- These bins are sealed once full
- They can also be used for sharps that are classified as clinical waste, but if this occurs it is advisable to place sharps in just before sealing the bin, otherwise 'buried' sharps may cause injury (although waste of any type should not be pushed down into containers by hand)
- The bins are obtainable from commercial disposal companies who should collect them, when full, along with yellow sacks and sharps containers, for incineration at temperatures exceeding 1100°C
- European legislation recommends that from 2002 all clinical waste (including the cadavers of animals) must be placed into leak-proof one-way burn bins. The Health and Safety Executive (HSE) is currently looking at the practical implications associated with this recommendation for the UK.

Sharps (Group B)

'Sharps' should be treated as clinical waste (see Figure 5.19) and disposed of in a special UN-type sharps container to be collected with other clinical waste, once full, for incineration (Figure 5.23).

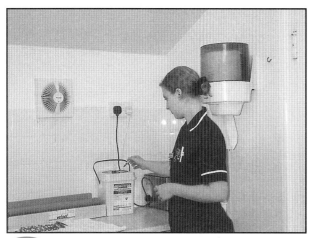

5.23 *Yellow sharps container for items such as needles and glass.*

Treated waste

If clinical waste is to be 'treated' (that is, sterilized) before it is disposed of, veterinary practices, boarding and breeding establishments could have this waste reclassified from 'clinical' to 'treated' (i.e. non-hazardous). Under environmental legislation, the establishment concerned must be able to prove to the Environment Agency or the Scottish Environment Protection Agency ('the Agencies') that the waste:

- Has been rendered safe and non-infectious
- Cannot be distinguished from other non-clinical waste of a similar type.

Special waste

The Special Waste Regulations Act 1996

This Act deems that 'special' means 'needs special arrangements', without which the waste presents a particular hazard to either human health or the environment. The transport of 'special' waste requires 'specially written' consignment notes for each movement. The Agencies' advice is that most clinical waste will not need to be considered as 'special waste'. There are exceptions that apply to veterinary practice:

- Waste that is made up of or contains prescription-only medicines (POMs) (it is recommended that all medicines, other than controlled drugs, are treated as POMs – POM waste has been classified as 'special waste' under UK legislation since 1980)
- Clinical waste contaminated with Risk 4 organisms.

The potential human health hazards associated with 'special' clinical waste have not yet been fully interpreted by the courts of law. Therefore current advice from the Agencies is that organisms fall into the risk groups shown in Figure 5.24, and that only waste from Risk Group 4 needs to be treated as 'special' clinical waste.

If there is any concern about the Risk Group of organisms arising from veterinary practice, then a 'best practice' precaution to adopt would be: if in doubt – autoclave before disposal.

Clinical waste arising from home visits

A duty of care is placed on a veterinary surgeon as an employer, or on the self-employed practitioner, to dispose safely of any clinical waste that may be generated from home visits to clients. Such waste should be disposed of as already described.

Cadavers

Veterinary surgeons have no statutory (legal) obligation to dispose of the dead bodies of animals. This is because under environmental law it is recognized that the owner of the live animal still owns the animal when it is dead. The only exception to this legality is when, for example, a badly injured wild animal or a stray is euthanased and not claimed. The body would then be classified as clinical waste and disposed of appropriately. The majority of veterinary surgeons provide this service.

There are several ways in which animal cadavers (bodies) may be safely disposed of by a veterinary practice:

5.24 Infectious substances – Risk Groups

Risk Group	Microorganisms included	Level of risk	
		Individual	Community
Risk Group 1	Unlikely to cause human or animal disease	Low	Low
Risk Group 2	Cause human or animal disease, are unlikely to spread and against which there is usually effective prophylaxis or treatment available	Moderate	Limited
Risk Group 3	Cause severe human or animal disease and may present a high risk of spreading, but against which there is usually effective prophylaxis or treatment available	High	Low
Risk Group 4	Cause severe human or animal disease and may present a high risk of spreading, and there is usually no effective prophylaxis or treatment available	High	High

 It should be noted that only Risk Group 4 organisms will classify waste as 'special' for animal health care waste will require *special waste consignment notes* from the disposal company handling waste from veterinary practices

Adapted from Health and Safety Executive Regulations

- Collection by the local authority
- Commercial disposal companies licensed for this procedure
- Individually arranged:
  - Pet cremation
  - Pet burial.

In the first two cases, the cadavers are then treated as clinical waste and incinerated at temperatures exceeding 1100°C.

Reputable companies providing a cadaver disposal service will also supply veterinary practices with strong plastic colour-coded sacks (current law does not require such cadavers to be placed in UN-type approved sacks or containers). For example:

- Yellow sacks with a green stripe to denote individual cremation
- Yellow sacks with a burgundy stripe to denote mass incineration
- Red sacks to identify bodies that are not to be collected, as the owner wants the body or it is for post mortem.

Such companies are also beginning to extend their good practices by bar-coding the sacks supplied, so that each veterinary practice has its own bar code. Bodies can then be traced back to that particular establishment if necessary.

It should also be remembered that an owner who wishes to take their pet's body for burial within their own garden is allowed to do so, as individuals are not liable to the same waste disposal legislation as commercial companies.

Notifiable diseases

Veterinary practices that treat animals suffering from a notifiable disease such as anthrax must, under the Animal Health Act, inform the Ministry of Agriculture, Fisheries and Food (MAFF). Disposal of such animal bodies then becomes MAFF's responsibility.

Chemical waste

There is a duty of care to dispose of chemicals in a safe manner. Those that are generated by establishments caring for animals include cleaning materials, disinfectants and antiseptics. These are likely to be diluted before use and so the amount of the chemicals being poured into the sewerage system would not be very great.

In veterinary practice additional chemical waste will be generated in the form of:

- Stains used in the laboratory – these are likely to be diluted before use and so the total volume of such chemicals being poured into the sewerage system would not be very great
- Chemicals associated with radiography – it is illegal to pour such chemicals into the drain, even in the diluted form in which they are used. These should be collected by a commercial disposal company with a special licence to dispose of them safely
- POM drugs – see 'Special waste disposal' section
- Controlled drugs – these should be collected by:
  - A Home Office Inspector or other authorized personnel, such as a member of the police drugs squad

- The veterinary drug supply company from which the drug was purchased (veterinary drug supply companies are authorized to carry controlled drugs, but their authorization to destroy them must be checked first).

Duty of care

It cannot be stressed enough that, legally, the duty of care to dispose safely of clinical, special and chemical waste lies with the employer or self-employed person who produces the waste. Even when an authorized disposal service is being used, the onus is still on such an employer or self-employed person to make sure that the disposal is being carried out in accordance with the law.

In law, the practicalities of this mean that the employer or self-employed person generating such waste must:

- Make sure that all staff are aware of the classification and subclassifications of the different types of waste and follow correct disposal procedures
- Arrange for the safe disposal of such waste by the methods described above
- Before signing a contract with the disposal services being used:
  - Check the driver's registration and carriage certificate, to ascertain that they are licensed for this type of haulage
  - Check that the disposal service is authorized for this type of disposal
- Regularly number waste disposal sacks and containers, then 'track' them by checking with the disposal services to find out how and when they were disposed of
- Visit the disposal service's establishment to 'track' the disposal of such waste – every six months is recommended.

It is worth noting that if any commercial disposal company was not conforming to the law, and was found to be negligent of disposing of such waste correctly, then the waste generators employing them (for example, a veterinary surgeon or owner of commercial kennels) would also, under environmental law, be found negligent. Ignorance of this law is no longer considered to be a protection against prosecution.

Further reading

Animal Boarding Establishments Act 1963. (Recommended schedule of conditions for use by local authorities.) Available from the RSPCA

Model Licence Conditions and Guidance for Dog Boarding Establishments. Chartered Institute of Environmental Health

Model Licence Conditions and Guidance for Cat Boarding Establishments. Chartered Institute of Environmental Health

Promoting Animal Welfare Through Local Authorities. RSPCA

The Commercial Breeding and Sale of Dogs and Puppies. (Working party report.) Available from the RSPCA

Indiscriminate Dog Breeding and Dealing. (Working party report.) Available from the RSPCA

Lane, DR (1989) *Jones's Animal Nursing*, 5th edn.
     Pergamon Press, Oxford. (Chapter 3: Management,
     Hygiene, Feeding – Antiseptics and Disinfectants)
Special Waste Regulations 1996. Agency Interpretation/Policy.
     Environment Agency - (frequent updates)
Safe Disposal of Clinical Waste. Cambridge Pet Crematorium

Acknowledgements

Special thanks from the author to:

- Grundon - Clinical Waste Section
- Cambridge Pet Crematorium
- Nurses at Kelperland Veterinary Surgery.

6 Introduction to healthcare

Joy Howell

This chapter is designed to give information on:

- How to perform a basic physical examination
- The regular health checks that are necessary
- The correct terminology when describing normal and abnormal conditions
- Prediction of the common behavioural characterisitics of the dog and cat, so that the most successful method of restraint will be used
- The principles of restraint, so that the animal is handled safely and without unecessary stress for either the animal or the handler
- Types of restraint equipment
- The importance of regular grooming as a part of preventive healthcare management programmes
- Types of grooming equipment
- Basic grooming techniques
- The six basic nutrients and their role in supporting life

Introduction

Early recognition of signs of ill health during the initial stages of disease is vital to ensure diagnosis and treatment. In certain conditions, this early diagnosis is likely to lead to a more satisfactory long-term response.

Preventive veterinary healthcare includes the performance of regular routine examination of animals, in order to identify abnormal states. This entails methods of handling and restraint to allow examination of the animal; in addition grooming is necessary to facilitate thorough examination of skin and to maintain coat condition. A further facet of healthcare and preventive medicine is nutrition, tailored to the animal's lifestyle and life stage.

Signs of health and disease

Regular health checks

Figure 6.1 shows the regular health checks and procedures to be used on companion animals and suggests how often they should be carried out.

In the case of elderly patients or those on long-term medication, full examination should be carried out more often, according to the animal's condition. With all health checks, including those that are not carried out on a daily basis, it is vital to be alert to any obvious signs of ill health at all times.

Physical examinations

Figure 6.2 outlines the steps in performing a physical examination. The animal needs constant reassurance throughout the examination, especially prior to invasive techniques such as temperature taking.

Some of these examinations can easily be demonstrated to the owner, for carrying out at home. More detailed explanation is required for techniques such as the taking of temperature, pulse and respiration rates and these procedures are outlined in Figure 6.3. Normal values for these measurements are shown in Figure 6.4.

History taking

A programme of regular health monitoring establishes an accurate and detailed history, which will prove invaluable to the veterinary surgeon when an animal is presented with signs of ill health. The history supplies a record of the animal's normal characteristics, and so allows any new sign that is truly abnormal to be highlighted (for example, pale mucous membranes or red conjunctiva).

6.1 Regular health checks and procedures and their suggested frequency

Daily

- Appetite
- Thirst
- Faecal production
- Urinary production
- Demeanour (bright, alert?)
- Abnormal signs evident.

Weekly

- Condition of ear canals
- Condition of teeth, gums
- Colour of mucous membranes
- Coat and skin condition
- Abnormal discharges – prepuce, vagina
- Pain on palpation/ movement of joints
- Presence and development of 'lumps'.

Monthly

- Body weight
- Nails – dew claws in particular
- Beaks – in birds and chelonia (tortoises, turtles).

Every 3–4 months

- Carry out anthelmintic (worming) protocols as recommended.

Annually

- Booster vaccinations
- Full physical examination by veterinary surgeon
- Annual blood tests may be recommended in some geriatric animals.

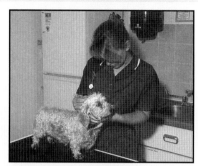
Checking ear canals

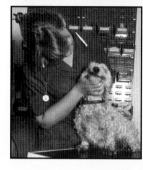
Checking teeth and gums

6.2 How to perform a basic physical examination

- Assess the animal's temperament prior to handling
- Talk in a reassuring tone
- Allow the animal to feel comfortable with your presence before undertaking an examination
- Start with the head:
  1. Examine both eyes for discharges or abnormal colour of conjunctiva
  2. Examine both nostrils for abnormal discharges
  3. Examine both ears for abnormal discharges, inflammation or smell
  4. Examine the mouth – colour of the mucous membranes, capillary refill time, dental and gum condition, abnormal-smelling breath
  5. Palpate submandibular lymph nodes
- Gradually and systematically move down the body to examine:
  - all the limbs and tail for wounds or evidence of pain on palpation or movement
  - the feet for overgrown or unevenly worn nails, evidence of inflammation or wounds, or damage to the foot pads
  - the skin for signs of inflammation, ectoparasites, lesions or poor condition
  - all areas for any abnormal swellings or lumps (compare the animal symmetrically to identify abnormalities)
- Examine the genital tract of the male animal for:
  - (unneutered) asymmetrical size or shape of testicles
  - preputial discharge
  - inflammation or swelling of scrotal sac
- Examine the genital tract of the female animal for:
  - (unneutered) evidence of being in season*
  - vaginal discharge
  - evidence of enlarged mammary glands
  - milk production
- Examine anal region for swelling, inflammation, discomfort
- Measure temperature, pulse and respiration rates (see Figure 6.3).

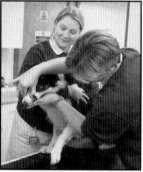
Examining the mouth

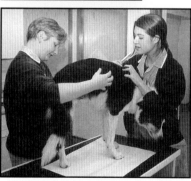
Examining the skin

> * Evidence of being 'in season':
>
> - In the bitch:
>   - swollen vulva
>   - bloody or watery vaginal discharge
>   - receptive to male advances
>   - deviation of the tail and presentation of the vulva when the lumbar region is touched
> - In the queen:
>   - persistent vocalization ('calling')
>   - arched back with vulva presented ('lordosis').

6.3 How to take temperature and check pulse and respiration rates

Taking temperature

- Make sure the patient is suitably restrained
- Using either a mercury thermometer (which requires the mercury to be shaken down to the bulb of the thermometer prior to use) or by following carefully the instructions provided with a digital thermometer:
  1. Lubricate the end of the thermometer with petroleum jelly or water soluble jelly
  2. Gently insert the thermometer into the animal's rectum, with a twisting motion. The thermometer should be directed against the upper surface of the rectum to avoid insertion into faecal material (which may alter the result)
  3. *Hold* the thermometer in the rectum for 1 minute
  4. Remove from the rectum and clean, taking care *not* to hold the tip during this procedure
  5. Now read the thermometer.

Taking the pulse

- Make sure the patient is suitably restrained
- Locate the artery with the fingers. The femoral artery, which runs down the inside of the thigh, is commonly used for this procedure
- Apply firm pressure to the artery, using at least two fingers. Take care not to occlude the vessel
- Count the pulsations for exactly 1 minute.

Observing respiration rate

- Make sure the patient is at rest but *not* sleeping or panting
- By observing movement of the chest, count *either* the breaths in *or* the breaths out (but not both) over 1 minute.

6.4 Normal ranges for vital signs

Animal	Temperature	Pulse (beats per minute)	Respiration (breaths per minute)
Dog	38.3–38.7°C	60–140 (lower part of range in large breeds, higher in small breeds)	10–30
Cat	38.0–38.5°C	110–180	20–30

When taking the history of an animal's condition, it is important to consider the following points:

- Do not lead the questioning – ensure that the owner gives accurate information, rather than being led by a series of 'yes/no' questions that may encourage an answer although the owner is actually uncertain
- Rather than vague answers, gather information about actual quantities (of fluid intake, urine production, etc.)
- Confirm the accuracy of vital information, such as the reproductive status, vaccination status and age of the patient
- Confirm whether signs such as 'nasal discharge' involve only one nostril (unilateral) or both nostrils (bilateral).

In addition to details already noted during regular health monitoring, the veterinary surgeon will need further information to assist with diagnosis. This might include:

- Temperature, pulse and respiration rates
- Sex of the animal
- Whether the animal has been neutered
- Vaccination status
- Whether the animal has eaten recently
- In the case of a female, when she was last in season.

Reporting clinical signs

Abnormal demeanour

'Demeanour' describes outward behaviour. In order to report on an animal's demeanour, it is essential to understand the normal behaviour patterns of the particular species. Owners who know their pet's character well are in a position to determine subtle changes in demeanour far earlier than an outside observer.

Examples of abnormal demeanour include:

- Reluctance to undertake normal activities – walking, playing, etc.
- Uncharacteristic aggression
- Changes in normal patterns of:
  - eating
  - drinking
  - urination
  - defecation
  - sleeping
- Unusual posture
- Withdrawal and lack of response to familiar environments, people and other animals.

Anatomical positions

It is essential to provide accurate descriptions, including precise references to anatomical positions, e.g site of pain or position of wound (Figure 6.5).

Pain

Pain is a feeling of distress or suffering caused by stimulation of specialized nerve endings. Its purpose is chiefly protective – it acts as a warning that tissues are being damaged. Recognition of the signs of pain is an essential skill of the handler.

 It must not be overlooked that certain individuals will successfully disguise the signs of pain in order not to display vulnerability.

Signs of pain include:

- Vocalization
- Abnormal posture (huddled)
- Dilated pupils

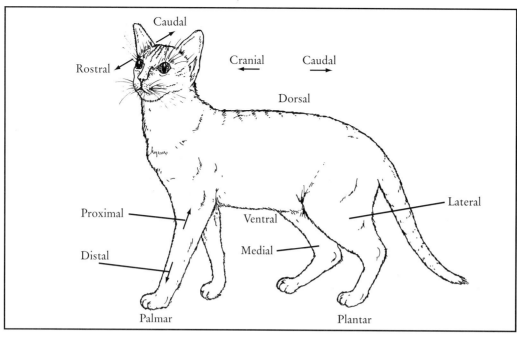

Caudal

Rostral

Cranial   Caudal

Dorsal

Proximal

Ventral

Lateral

Distal

Medial

Palmar

Plantar

6.5 *Anatomical directions and planes. Reproduced from Learning Veterinary Terminology by Douglas McBride (1996) with the permission of Mosby – Year Book, Inc.*

- Lameness
- Panting
- Tachycardia (rapid heart rate)
- Pyrexia (raised body temperature)
- Inappetence
- Shivering
- Hiding.

Information from owners

Accuracy in gaining information from owners and in reporting to the veterinary surgeon will ensure an enlightened assessment of the urgency of the case. An example of questions to ask an owner and assessment of the requirement for immediate action is given in Figure 6.6.

Describing clinical signs

Figures 6.7 to 6.15 give definitions and guidelines for describing clinical signs relating to appetite, thirst, defecation, urination, vomiting, abnormal discharges, coughing, itching and lameness.

- A *sign* is an observable physical phenomenon that is associated with a given condition frequently enough to be considered indicative of the condition's presence
- A *symptom* is any indication of disease perceived by the patient.

For this reason, changes in animals are described as signs – only humans can have symptoms.

6.6 Assessing information from owners: an example

Owner's description: 'My dog has jumped through the patio window. There's not a *lot* of blood but he has got a large deep wound on his side.'

Questions (Q) to the owner, the sequence according to the owner's answers (A) and action to be taken (boxed) might be as follows.

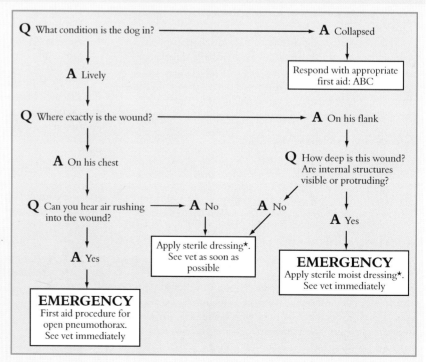

Q What condition is the dog in? ——→ **A** Collapsed

A Lively

Respond with appropriate first aid: ABC

Q Where exactly is the wound? ——→ **A** On his flank

A On his chest

Q How deep is this wound? Are internal structures visible or protruding?

Q Can you hear air rushing into the wound? ——→ **A** No   **A** No

A Yes

Apply sterile dressing*. See vet as soon as possible

A Yes

EMERGENCY
First aid procedure for open pneumothorax. See vet immediately

EMERGENCY
Apply sterile moist dressing*. See vet immediately

*With all dressings, advise regarding the possibility of embedded glass.

6.7 How to describe appetite

Definitions:

- *Polyphagia*: excessive ingestion of food
- *Anorexia* (anophagia, inappetence): lack or loss of appetite for food
- *Coprophagia*: ingestion of faeces
- *Pica*: craving for unnatural articles of food.

Questions to ask:

- What are the normal eating patterns?
- For how long has the appetite been abnormal?

6.8 How to describe thirst

Definitions:

- *Polydipsia*: increased thirst
- *Adipsia*: absence of drinking.

The histories that accompany patients are often inaccurate on this point and the following details should be recorded:

Measured water intake over 24 hours

Questions to ask:

- Has a change in feeding occurred (e.g. from tinned food to dry)?
- Have glucocorticoids or diuretics been administered?

6.9 How to describe defecation

Definitions:

- *Constipation*: failure to evacuate faeces
- *Diarrhoea*: frequent evacuation of watery faeces
- *Tenesmus*: ineffectual and painful straining (at defecation or urination).

Details to be recorded:

- Colour of faeces
- Smell of faeces
- Texture of faeces
- Volume and frequency of defecation
- Presence of blood, mucus or worms in faeces
- Recent changes in diet.

6.10 How to describe urination (micturition)

Definitions:

- *Polyuria**: excretion of a large volume of urine
- *Oliguria*: reduced output of urine
- *Anuria*: absence of urination
- *Dysuria*: painful or difficult urination
- *Haematuria*: presence of blood in the urine.

Other details to be recorded:

- Presence of urgency
- Frequency
- Tenesmus.

> * Since polyuria and polydipsia often occur together, the abbreviation PU/PD is often used to describe this syndrome.

6.11 How to describe vomiting (emesis)

Confirm whether the vomiting is:

- Projectile (vomited with great force)
- Regurgitation (casting up of undigested food with minimal effort)
- Retching (unproductive effort to vomit)
- Dry (vomiting with ejection of gas only)
- With presence of blood (haematemesis)
- With presence of bile (yellow staining).

Confirm *when* vomiting occurs:

- Immediately after eating
- If not, actual length of time after eating
- Cyclical (recurring attacks).

Describe the *product* of vomiting:

- Food
- Bile (bilious vomit)
- Blood
- Faeces (stercoraceous vomit)
- Hair
- Bones
- Other foreign material.

Confirm further details:

- Vaccination status
- Any known consumption of foreign matter (bones, toxic substances, etc.)
- Patient's overall condition, including state of hydration
- Any other presenting signs:
  - polydipsia
  - polyuria
  - diarrhoea
  - pregnancy
  - last known oestrus.

6.12 How to describe abnormal discharges

Be specific:

- Type
  - purulent (containing pus)
  - mucoid (clear, tenacious)
  - serous (watery)
  - haemorrhagic
- Colour
- Viscosity
- Origin
  - nasal
  - ocular
  - vaginal
  - rectal
  - preputial
  - aural
  - wounds
- Unilateral (affecting only one side)
- Bilateral (affecting both sides).

6.13 How to describe coughing

Clarify:

- Sounds
  - chesty/moist
  - throaty/dry ('hacking')
- Whether productive
  - from bronchi (mucus)
  - blood
- Is vomiting or regurgitation induced?
- Whether the coughing occurs:
  - first thing in the morning
  - after exercise
  - at night
- Whether any foreign materials or abrasive items have been consumed.

Confirm vaccination status, particularly for:

- Distemper
- Canine contagious respiratory disease (kennel cough)
  - canine parainfluenza virus
  - *Bordetella bronchiseptica*
- Feline upper respiratory tract disease (cat 'flu)

6.14 How to describe pruritus (itching)

Confirm whether:

- Parasite control has been undertaken and note the product and schedule used
- There are particular zones
  - ears, head and neck
  - anal region
- The skin appears inflamed or abnormal
- The animal has been exposed to products not used before
  - topical antiparasitics
  - shampoos
  - medications
  - home cleaning agents
- The signs appear worse when the animal
  - has walked among grasses
  - becomes hot
- There has been any change to the diet.

In summary

The early and successful recognition of signs of disease and ill health depends on the observation skills of the owner and (in the case of the hospitalized patient) those of the veterinary nurse in charge of in-patient care.

These observation skills depend on a thorough understanding of any deviation from the normal state.

Handling and restraint

In order to handle animals safely and skilfully it is important to appreciate the behavioural differences between various species. Handlers, including veterinary nurses, must learn to avoid rushing in without first observing the animal's body language and assessing whether any obvious injuries are evident. This will prevent causing the animal unneccessary pain and will avoid unnecessary risk to the handler.

6.15 How to describe lameness

Definitions:

- *Lame*: incapable of normal locomotion; showing deviation from the normal gait
- *Lameness*: the state of being lame
- *Gait*: the manner or style of locomotion
- Examples of abnormal gait
  - *ataxic*: unsteady uncoordinated walk
  - *spastic*: a walk in which legs move in a stiff manner, the toes seeming to drag and catch
  - *antalgic*: a limp adopted so as to avoid pain on weightbearing structures.

Clarify:

- Was a known trauma involved?
  - road traffic accident (RTA)
  - fall
- Which limb is involved?
- Chronic or acute? (This will aid in determining whether this is a fracture/dislocation that requires immediate veterinary intervention)
- Severity: partial or non-weightbearing
- Visible/palpable:
  - deformity of limb
  - swelling
  - bruising
  - heat in the region
- When is the lameness worse?
  - after exercise
  - after rest.

Dogs

Dogs are social pack animals and they look to a pack leader, in particular, to provide support and decision making. The veterinary nurse's aim is to take on the role of pack leader.

Body language is complex in the dog (Figure 6.16). Although they can signify much more than simply dominance or submission, these characteristics are the most important for a handler or veterinary nurse to recognize before approaching an unknown dog.

Training by owners

Whilst educating owners in the importance of responsible dog ownership and preventive health care, the veterinary nurse should emphasize how important it is that owners should:

- Be able to examine their animal without causing distress or aggression
- Realize the relevance of being able to examine *all* areas of the animal, including the feet, mouth and ears.

During a dog's life, it will have to be handled for many different reasons:

- Grooming and bathing
- Examination of an injury
- Administration of first aid
- Administration of drugs prescribed by the veterinary surgeon, including those that the owner will need to give
- Weekly checks.

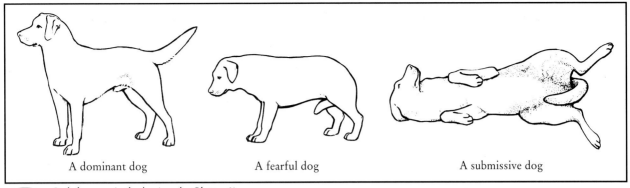

| A dominant dog | A fearful dog | A submissive dog |

Body language in the dog (see also Chapter 2).
Reproduced from Thorne (1992) The Waltham Book of Dog and Cat Behaviour with permission of the WALTHAM Centre for Pet Nutrition..

Responsible owners can prepare their animals for such handling from an early age. They can start by teaching the puppy to tolerate and even enjoy being examined. With particularly difficult areas, such as the paws and mouth, an animal that has been taught to tolerate examination will be a much easier patient for veterinary staff and owners alike.

Handling for examination

In order to be examined, the dog must be submissive. This means that the veterinary nurse needs to establish dominance over the dog. The first step is to interpret the animal's demeanour correctly. Then the dog can be approached, bearing the following guidelines in mind:

- Approach the dog quietly but confidently
- Use the dog's name
- Talk in a reassuring manner
- Lower yourself to the animal's level (in order to appear less threatening) but ensure you can escape if necessary
- Allow the dog to examine the back of your hand
- Do not appear to trap the animal in a corner, or at the back of the kennel, etc.

> ⚠ Do not make assumptions of aggression based on breed type alone. *All* types of dog can be equally aggressive.

If the dog shows signs of aggression, the handler's safety is paramount. Figure 6.17 explains how to deal with an aggressive animal.

Avoiding excessive restraint

In order to assess the need for active measures of restraint, it is important that the following considerations are made on admitting a dog to the hospital.

- Discuss with the owner the animal's temperament (e.g. kennel guarding, or 'He only likes women', etc.)
- In the case of kennel guarding and uncertain temperament, do not remove the collar and lead. Instead, extend its length with another lead or rope and leave the extension outside the cage. This will allow the handler to retrieve the lead safely and thus lead the animal out of the kennel without being bitten or distressing the animal
- Ensure that the kennel, case records and computer records are clearly marked with the details of the dog's temperament, to ensure that all staff know the patient's character
- Discuss the animal's temperament with the veterinary surgeon *prior* to administration of routine premedicant drugs, as the anaesthetic regime may need to be adapted to allow for the difficulties in restraint

- Having discussed sedative or anaesthetic protocols with the veterinary surgeon, consider allowing the owner to stay whilst the animal is sedated, prior to admission to the hospital environment.

Restraint equipment

Collars and check chains

Before taking over control from an owner or admitting a patient to the hospital, certain procedures should be carried out to prevent patient escape or injury:

- Always ensure that a check chain is fitted correctly, so that gravity ensures that the untensioned chain slackens
- Always check that a collar is fitted properly. Often they are loose fitting and the patient is able to slip its head out and escape
- Always check that clips and fastenings are in good working order. If they appear broken or likely to snap, exchange them for a hospital collar and lead
- Never leave a trailing lead (for a kennel guarder) attached to a check chain, as this could result in asphyxiation (strangulation). Either clip or tie the chain into a locked position or exchange it for a collar.

6.17 How to deal with an aggressive dog

- Personal safety is paramount – do *not* take unnecessary risks
- With a dog known to be aggressive, ask the owner to apply a muzzle before examination
- 'Kennel guarding' behaviour – secure all windows and doors and allow the dog out of the kennel before attempting to handle (this should only be attempted if it is certain that the aggression *is* kennel guarding!)
- If the owner is present, ask them to leave, which may improve the animal's behaviour
- If the owner is absent, ask them to attend the surgery to calm the animal during administration of sedation to avoid unecessary distress for the dog
- Carefully interpret body language – only use dominant behaviour (such as direct eye contact and standing over the dog) if the animal is adequately restrained
- Remember that often the aggression shown whilst the dog is injured or unwell may be uncharacteristic ('fear aggression') or an indication of pain and the animal may therefore require less dominant handling techniques or analgesia.

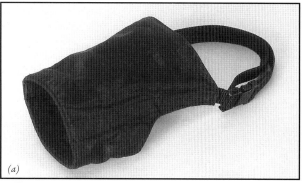

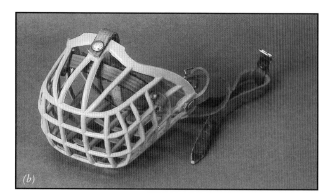

 6.18 *Types of commercial muzzle: (a) nylon; (b) box.*

6.19 How to restrain a dog for application of a muzzle

- Stand to one side of the animal, facing the same direction. Alternatively, stand astride larger dogs
- Hold the scruff of the neck securely behind each ear
- If the dog attempts to bring up its front feet to remove the muzzle, a second handler may be required to restrain its forelimbs
- If the dog attempts to walk backwards out of the muzzle, both the handler and the person applying the muzzle should move with the dog or back into a corner or up to a wall to prevent further movement.

⚠ A struggling patient can inflict injury to a handler, even if the animal is muzzled and prevented from biting. Scratch wounds from dogs can be extremely painful. Dogs may also pull against the lead with which the handler is restraining them; therefore the handler should avoid wrapping the lead around the wrist, or fingers, as this could lead to personal injury.

Muzzling
As well as protecting everyone from being bitten, a muzzle tends to distract the animal's attention.

Types of muzzle (Figure 6.18) include:

- Tape muzzle
- Commercially available nylon muzzle
- Box muzzle
- Wire muzzle.

⚠ Muzzles can be fitted to animals by their owners; however, it is vital that muzzled animals are not left unsupervised. The handler or veterinary nurse must be aware of the dangers involved should an animal vomit whilst wearing a muzzle, or the possibility of injury to the front claws (dew claws in particular) if the animal should attempt to remove the device.

Methods of handling a dog while a muzzle is being fitted are described in Figure 6.19.

If specifically designed muzzles are not available, a useful skill is that of applying a simple tape muzzle (Figure 6.20).

6.20 How to apply a tape muzzle

1. Select an adequate length of non-conforming bandage (conforming will stretch!)
2. Form a loop with a square knot
3. Direct someone to restrain the dog correctly
4. Approach from the side of the animal
5. Slip the loop over the dog's nose with the knot being quickly tightened uppermost
6. Cross the free ends under the jaw
7. Bring the ends under the lower jaw and under the ears
8. Tie in a quick-release bow around the back of the head.

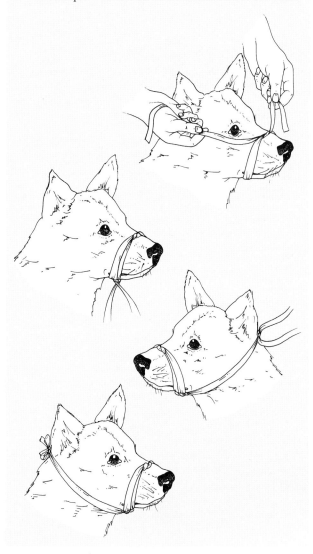

Muzzling is unsuitable for most brachycephalic (short-nosed) breeds. For small breeds such as Pug and Pekingese, a towel placed around the neck behind the ears is a suitable method of restraint that does not lead to prolapse of the eyeballs (an unfortunate risk when 'scruffing' these patients).

In larger brachycephalic breeds such as the Boxer, a specially adapted commercial muzzle is required or a modified version of the tape muzzle can be used.

Dog graspers (catchers)

The dog grasper (Figure 6.21) can be used as a last resort. However, the use of this equipment can be traumatic for both operator and animal, and alternative methods are usually considered first.

> **6.21 Dog graspers**
>
> Dog graspers (or dog catchers) vary in complexity. The simplest form consists of a long handle with a lasso loop of rope or another material at one end. The other end of the rope runs up the handle so that the size of the loop can be controlled once the loop has been placed over the dog's head.

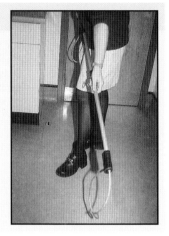

Alternative restraint techniques

The following techniques require more than one operator.

- The lead is passed through a ring on the wall, pulling the dog's head up to the wall. An assistant holds the animal's body against the wall
- The lead is passed through a doorway. Once the dog's head is through, the door is carefully held against the dog's shoulders
- The lead is wrapped around the leg of a table to restrain the dog's head
- The lead is pulled through kennel bars to restrain the dog's head.

These alternative techniques could facilitate:

- Application of a muzzle
- Injection of a sedative drug (if necessary, by means of a syringe pole – a tubular structure 1.6–1.9 m long with a fitment for a normal hypodermic syringe and needle at one end and an extended plunger at the other, thus allowing long-distance techniques).

Lifting

Once the dog has been secured (and muzzled, if required), it can be lifted. It is important to be careful when lifting, in order to prevent injury to the handler. For a larger dog, it is advisable to seek the assistance of another person (Figure 6.22). See also Chapter 9.

Holding

When handling, the hands are not the only method of restraint. Holding an animal close to the handler's body will make the patient feel more securely held and will allow better control. Animals may require restraint in particular positions and for various procedures (Figure 6.23).

> **6.22 How to lift a dog**

Unaided

- Prior to handling, determine the position of any injuries and take measures to avoid hurting the patient
- Grasp the animal around the front and rear legs
- Press the animal's body against the chest to prevent struggling
- With the knees bent and back straight, now carefully lift the patient up on to the examination table.

Small dogs can be supported by tucking the animal under the arm and supporting the barrel of the chest, without having to support the hindlimbs.

With an assistant

- One person can support the front quarters by placing one arm around the front of the animal's neck to restrain the head, whilst placing the other arm underneath the barrel of the chest
- The second person can support the hindquarters by placing one arm under the abdomen and placing the other arm around the rump
- Both handlers lift carefully and simultaneously.

> **6.23 How to restrain a dog**
>
> **For examination**
>
>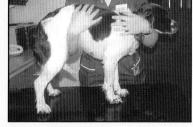
>
> 1. Lift on to a table
> 2. Stand to one side of the animal
> 3. Wrap the arm nearest to the animal's head around its neck, in order to restrain its head
> 4. The other arm can then be:
>   - either pressed against the dorsal part of the neck to assist in restraint of the head
>   - or placed underneath the chest or abdomen, to hold the animal against the handler's body to secure the patient.
>
> **On one side**
>
> **On the floor**
>
> 1. Kneel to one side of the patient (with the patient standing)
> 2. Hold the front and hind legs by placing the arms across the back and grasping the legs nearest the handler at the level of the tibia and radius
> 3. Pull the legs away from the handler, whilst rolling the dog's body gently down the handler's lap and on to the floor
> 4. Restrain by holding the limbs nearest to the floor and using the forearms and elbows to hold down the head and neck and the rump.
>
> *Figure 6.23 continues* ▶

On a table

1. Follow the same procedure as on the floor, but stand rather than kneel to one side of the patient
2. Slide the patient gently down the chest rather than across the lap.

With large dogs two handlers may be required. As with lifting, one handler takes control of the forelimbs whilst the other controls the hindquarters. Once the animal is on its side (lateral recumbency) it may be possible for one handler to hold it down in position.

For an injection

Intramuscular and subcutaneous

1. Use the technique for handling for examination
2. On the floor 'scruff' the dog, with handler's legs straddled across the animal's shoulders to secure (see Figure 6.19)
3. With an aggressive animal, dog catchers etc. can be used.

Intravenous injection or blood sampling

Cephalic vein (forelimb)

1. Stand to one side of the patient, opposite to the site of the injection
2. Patient is sitting or in sternal recumbency, handler places one arm around the neck and the other arm across the shoulders to restrain the limb used for venipuncture
3. Hold the limb extended by grasping behind the elbow, which will prevent the elbow from bending
4. Use thumb placed across top of limb to apply pressure and thus prevent venous return and achieve 'raising' of vein

Saphenous vein (lateral aspect of tarsus)
- Dog restrained in lateral recumbency with leg to be used uppermost.

Cats

Cats are agile, quick and independent by nature. This means that they may only tolerate handling for short periods. They have sharp teeth as well as four sets of claws and can inflict painful injuries to the handler.

The degree of restraint required depends on the individual cat. Most respond to a loose and gentle approach (rather than forceful restraint) gained by an unhurried but firm technique:

- Approach calmly but confidently
- Speak quietly
- If the cat is not hissing or growling, attempt to stroke its head and run a hand confidently along its back.

Take warning from aggressive behaviour such as hissing, lowered ears and swiping out with a paw.

The body language of cats is illustrated in Figure 6.24. To remove an unwilling cat from its container:

- Attempt to cover the cat's head with a towel
- Wrap the cat in the towel and gently lift it out of the container.

Avoiding excessive restraint

In general, cats respond best to light restraint (Figure 6.25). However, if the handler is acting alone, firmer restraint such as scruffing may prove necessary.

It is best to use only as much restraint as necessary, provided that firmer control can be applied rapidly if required. In some cases, once a cat has been scruffed briefly, a further attempt at a more gentle approach proves effective and can be tried if the handler is confident. It may be necessary to wrap the cat's body in a towel after scruffing, to protect the handler from the cat's claws.

To prevent the need for forceful restraint:

- Assess the patient's temperament
- If it is decided that sedative drugs will need to be administered before examination, place the cat directly into a crush cage
- To allow adaptation of sedative or anaesthetic protocols, discuss the animal's temperament with the veterinary surgeon prior to the administration of premedicant drugs.

Lifting and holding

Lifting techniques depend on the cat's body weight and temperament, and from where the cat is being lifted (Figure 6.26). Figure 6.27 describes techniques for holding a cat for examination.

Restraint equipment

In order to avoid injury to the handler, it might be necessary to wear handling gloves. A more aggressive cat might require restraining aids such as a crush cage, muzzle, cat bag or cat grasper.

- Crush cages have a movable internal wall which can be eased across gently to hold the patient against the wire side of the cage, allowing injection through the wires
- Cat muzzles are fitted in the same manner as a dog muzzle but they also cover the eyes like a blindfold, thus subduing the animal
- Cat restraining bags are specially designed zip-up bags with holes to expose the head or limbs as required
- Cat graspers are like a pair of tongs, used to grasp the animal by the neck; a towel is used to wrap up the limbs (Figure 6.28).

Cat graspers should only be used in extreme cases. It is essential that the cat's unsupported body should *never* be lifted by the neck.

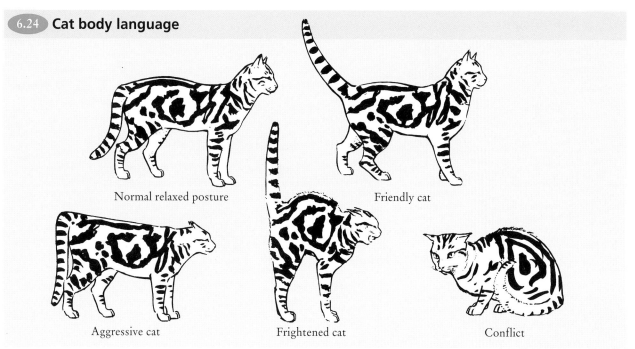

6.24 Cat body language

Normal relaxed posture

Friendly cat

Aggressive cat

Frightened cat

Conflict

Reproduced from Thorne (1992) The Waltham Book of Dog and Cat Behaviour with permission of the WALTHAM Centre for Pet Nutrition..

6.25 How to hold a cat

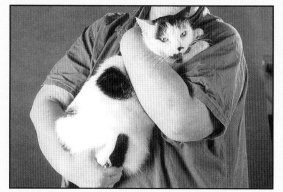

- With one hand over the chest wall and the other supporting the rump, hold firmly towards the handler's body

6.26 How to lift a cat

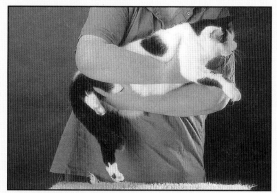

- Pass one hand over the chest wall and support the sternum, whilst the other hand supports the abdomen from the other side
- To retrieve from a basket, gently grasp both forelegs from the elbow and pull free.

6.27 How to hold a cat for examination

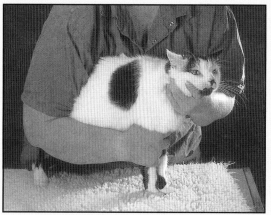

For examination of the head

- Hold the cat under the arm or against the handler's chest whilst holding the forelegs to prevent the person examining the cat from being scratched
- The free hand can be used to hold the cat's chin in order to support the head.

For examination of the body

Depending on the cat's temperament:

- Either gently hold the cat's shoulders and forelegs
- Or hold the head under the jaw and use the other hand to hold the cat against the handler's body and restrain the forelegs.

Techniques for removing an aggressive cat from its kennel are described in Figure 6.29.

Administration of injections

Cats can be restrained for injections in a similar manner to that used in dogs, but with extra precautions to prevent handler injury from claws (Figure 6.30).

6.28 Cat graspers

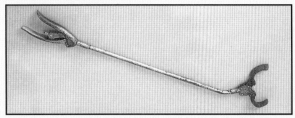

Unlike dog catchers, cat graspers do not incorporate a loop to lasso the animal but are designed like a set of tongs to grasp the cat by the neck. They should only be used in extreme cases. *Never* lift the unsupported body by the neck (use a towel to wrap up the limbs).

6.29 How to retrieve an aggressive cat from a kennel

- Attempt to cover the cat's head with a towel, wrapping the animal in the towel and gently lifting it out of the kennel
- In extreme cases the cat's head can be restrained by use of a cat grasper around the neck, to enable wrapping the animal in a towel to remove from the kennel
- Slide a cat basket into the kennel, trapping the cat between the cage back and the basket. Once the cat has entered the basket, slide a towel between the cage back and the basket to prevent escape. Now slide the cat basket out of the kennel, close the lid of the basket and withdraw the towel before fastening.

6.30 How to hold cats for injections

Cats can be restrained for injections in a similar manner to that used for dogs. However, there must be extra consideration to prevent injury to the handler from the cat's claws. A technique that can be implemented when giving an *aggressive* cat an intramuscular injection is:

- Scruff the neck with one hand
- Extend the hindlimbs with the other hand
- This stretches the cat's body and thus prevents movement.

Grooming and coat care

Reasons for grooming
Regular grooming accustoms an animal to being handled and also enables the early identification of a range of health problems. Motives for grooming include:

- To clean the coat and remove dead shedding hair
- To prevent the coat from matting or soiling with faeces, urine or discharges
- To allow regular inspection for signs of:
  - external parasites (lice, fleas) (Figure 6.31)
  - hair loss in particular regions
  - poor skin condition
  - wounds/injuries
  - abnormal swellings or lumps
  - pain or discomfort when moving or touching any part of the body
  - overgrown nails (particularly dew claws)

- To enforce dog pack hierachy and form a bond with the animal (dogs lower in the pack order submit to grooming by a more dominant member).

A carefully managed grooming protocol ensures a successful grooming session. Procedures for commencing and carrying out grooming are outlined in Figures 6.32 and 6.33.

6.31 How to examine for fleas

Fleas are notoriously difficult to see and even harder to catch. Therefore it is more appropriate to examine for the evidence of fleas in the form of flea dirt (faeces).

- Place a white sheet of paper on the floor or table top
- Mist over with water
- Stand the animal on the paper and groom with fingertips or comb
- Examine particles that have landed on the moist paper
- Flea dirt is formed from excreted blood and will stain the paper red or brown.

6.32 How to introduce grooming to a new animal

- Ideally, introduce the pet to grooming from an early age, as a continuation of the grooming administered by the animal's mother
- Start with brief grooming sessions and gradually increase
- Allow the animal to enjoy being examined, before using grooming equipment. Incorporate handling in your stroking of the animal, several times every day when it is calm and relaxed
- Initially pretend to brush, but use your hand instead of a brush
- Do not aim to cover all of the body: do a little at a time, reward the animal for being good and then stop
- Keep a titbit or toy to hand to retain the pet's interest and reward the animal with it at the end of the session. Try smearing a foodstuff (such as pâté, cheese spread, etc.) on a wall or cupboard door at nose height in front of the animal, which will lick at this while you introduce handling of feet, tail, etc.
- If a dog tries to 'mouth' you, say 'Ow!' in a very hurt way and reward them for stopping
- Gradually increase the time spent grooming and handling each day and introduce other examinations, such as:
  - examining the mouth (including opening it and looking down the throat)
  - examining the eyes
  - wiping the inside of the ears with cotton wool (do not insert cotton buds down the ear canal)
  - examining the tail and anal area
  - examining the vulva/prepuce
  - checking the pads and between the paws
- Do not try to teach tolerance of all of these procedures at once – concentrate an a different one at each session
- Always reward good behaviour – with a titbit, play session or just a cuddle and verbal praise
- Remember the independent nature of cats – it is often extremely difficult to teach them to tolerate a lot of handling or grooming and it often depends on whether they have been introduced to handling at an early age.

6.33 How to carry out grooming

- Assess the animal's temperament – is muzzling, sedation or anaesthesia indicated?
- Prepare *all* the necessary equipment to hand, including titbit rewards for the animal
- Carry out a physical inspection of the animal to ascertain that there are no wounds or injuries that need to be avoided or treated prior to grooming
- Put on an overall or apron
- Loosen dead hair, using fingertips
- Use a comb to remove tangles and further loosen dead hair in long-haired animals
- Brush the coat with the appropriate brush or hound glove required for the hair type (not all hounds require a 'hound' glove: for instance, the Saluki has long fine hair)
- After combing and brushing, a smooth or silky medium coat can be finished off by using a damp cloth, a smooth hound glove or a piece of velvet or chamois cloth
- It may also prove necessary to pluck excess hair carefully from the ear canal in breeds prone to overgrowth.

Hair growth

Unlike humans, whose hair grows continuously and therefore has to be cut, dogs and cats periodically shed their coats (moult).

The hair grows in cycles:

- Growth phase (brief)
- Resting phase
- Shedding phase.

The average rate of hair growth is 0.5 mm per day.

A number of factors can affect hair growth and moulting:

- Central heating – animals kept in centrally heated houses will often moult continuously
- Seasons
  - in the spring: summer coat produced, winter coat moulted
  - in the summer: increased sebaceous gland activity to allow air circulation through coat
  - in the autumn: winter coat produced, summer coat moulted
  - in the winter: reduced sebaceous gland activity, increased density of insulating coat
- Hormones
  - oestrogen slows hair growth (bitch on heat)
  - thyroid deficiency: slow-growing dull rough coat with bilateral flank alopecia (hair loss)
  - hormonal alopecias are also occassionally seen during pregnancy and lactation, and after neutering
- Poor diet – insufficiency of nutrients or an imbalance of nutrients such as amino acids and essential fatty acids or vitamin and mineral deficiencies such as zinc and iodine
- External parasites such as fleas, mites and lice
- Ill health – various chronic diseases may affect hair growth.

Coat types

A variety of coat types are seen in dogs and cats (Figure 6.34). The choice of grooming equipment needs to be correct for each type.

6.34 Examples of coat type

Animal	Type of coat	Breed examples
Dog	Smooth 　Short fine	Boxer Dachshund
	Intermediate or coarse dense	German Shepherd Dog
	Wire	Wire-haired terriers
	Double	Rough Collie Long-haired German Shepherd Dog
	Single 　Medium 　Long fine	Spaniels Afghan Hound
	Woolly	Poodle Irish Water Spaniel
	Corded	Hungarian Puli Komondor
Cat	Long hair	Chinchilla Persian
	Semi-long hair	Birman Maine Coon
	Short hair	Manx Siamese

Grooming equipment

Choice of equipment (Figure 6.35) depends on the coat type to be groomed.

Brushes

Brushing takes time and effort, especially when dealing with long-haired, dense or matted coats.

Pin brushes

Pin brushes have a series of pins mounted on a rubber-backed cushion, with a wooden or plastic frame. Sometimes the ends of the pins are coated in plastic to minimize scratching of the skin during grooming. A pin brush cannot break or pull out hair, so the coat must be free from knots and tangles. The main function of a pin brush is to keep the coat sleek and glossy by distributing natural coat oils from the skin.

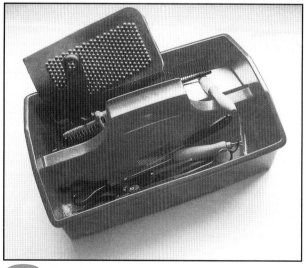

6.35 *Grooming equipment.*

Bristle brushes

Bristle brushes are very similar in design and function to the pin brush except that the grooming surface consists of either manmade or natural bristles instead of metal pins.

Slicker brushes

Slicker brushes consist of hooked wire pins mounted on a rectangular pad with a handle. Care should be taken when brushing in areas where hair cover is thin, such as axillas (arm pits). Slicker brushes are excellent for use on matted and tangled coats, as their design and shape enables them to pull out dead hair and break down mats.

Hound gloves/mittens

These brushes resemble gloves or mittens. They remove dead hair from the undercoat and give the outer coat a polish. The grooming surface of the glove consists of rubber bumps, wires or bristles. Because the glove fits the hand like a mitten, the grooming process is as easy as stroking. Gloves and mittens are especially useful and effective on smooth short-haired breeds and on short wire-haired terrier coats.

Rubber grooming devices

Available for both dogs and cats, these consist of a one-piece handheld rubber grooming device with large bumps along the grooming surface. These grooming aids are useful for short-coated breeds such as the Labrador Retriever.

Combs

The several different types of comb can be divided into two basic groups: traditional and special function combs.

Traditional combs

These are available either with or without a handle. They have rigid metal teeth that are rounded at the tip and are available in various tooth widths. The most commonly used traditional comb has coarse tooth widths at one end and fine tooth widths at the other. Traditional combs are only to be used along the lie of the hair, at an angle of 45 degrees, to remove dead hair, to groom long silky hair behind the ears and to untangle and break up mats.

Dematting comb

Designed to cut through mats without destroying too much of the coat, these combs usually consist of a series of metal teeth bladed on one side and blunt on the other.

The comb is introduced behind the mat but in front of the skin. With the sharpened side of the blade facing towards the groomer, a firm but gentle sawing motion is adopted. As the blade works through the mat it breaks it down into smaller mats, which can then be combed out. This comb allows the maximum amount of coat to be preserved once the matt is removed.

Rake comb

Rake combs have rigid metal teeth with round ends perpendicular to the handle. Care should be taken not to inflict skin trauma. Rake combs are used in dense coats for the removal of dead undercoat and the breaking up of some small mats.

Flea comb (nit comb)

Available either with or without a metal, wooden or plastic handle, these have very finely separated metal teeth. They are used to eradicate fleas, lice and their eggs (nits are lice eggs).

Untangler

This has a plastic grip with metal pin teeth that can roll, thus preventing pull on tangles.

Scissors

The routine clipping or trimming of some areas in long-haired dogs will assist in maintaining cleanliness. Clipping, hand stripping and trimming of specific breeds should be carried out by a trained groomer. However, maintenance of specific problem areas can be carried out by the veterinary nurse or owner. For example:

- Trimming between the toes, to prevent mat formation and the trapping of grass seeds during the summer and autumn
- Trimming the ears, particularly the underside, to prevent mat formation and trapping of grass seeds and to prevent soiling with food in breeds with pendulous ears
- Trimming the anal region and feathering of the tail and hindlegs to prevent mats and faecal soiling
- Trimming pregnant bitches around the vulval region and hindlegs to prevent excessive soiling during whelping.

Trimming scissors

Trimming scissors have long and very sharp blades that taper to a point. They are used to trim around the edges of ears.

Toe scissors

Scissors with short blades with blunt ends are used to trim delicate areas between toes.

Thinning scissors

Thinning scissors have either a single serrated and a single plain blade, or two serrated blades. The specialized blades cut small amounts of hair and leave an equal uncut amount at intervals. This action thins the coat without leaving 'steps' – for example, to enhance features such as the shoulder.

Clippers

Cosmetic clipping for specific breeds should be carrier out by a trained groomer. However, in the case of the elderly or difficult-to-handle patients veterinary advice is often asked for. Sedation prior to professional grooming may be required or anaesthesia may be the only course open to facilitate the dematting of a patient. In these circumstances the use of clippers (Figure 6.36) is recommended over the use of scissors, which in the inexperienced grooming hands can lead to accidental skin wounds.

6.36 How to use electric clippers

- Choose an appropriate blade size for the required clip, following manufacturer's guidelines
- Hair must be completely dry, as wet hair blunts the blades
- Do not force clippers through a thick coat or matting – use a slicker comb first to break up matts
- Allow clippers to cool down whenever they become hot during use
- Thoroughly clean and oil after each use, using only manufacturer-recommended lubricants and cleaners.

Dematting

Important points that should be borne in mind are:

- Always discuss thoroughly with the owners prior to the procedure, in order to prevent misunderstandings regarding the amount of hair that will be removed

- Avoid scissors if at all possible, as skin wounds are easily inflicted when cutting away large mats
- Depending on the weather conditions, make appropriate arrangements for the animal whilst the coat is regrowing:
  - avoid exposing shaved skin to excessive sunlight; use sunblocks
  - protect from the cold; use coats.

Bathing

Bathing is not normally carried out routinely on animals (particularly cats) without specific indications. However, it should not be overlooked as an important process in encouraging owners to check regularly every area of their pet – particularly in long-haired animals, where skin wounds and the development of swellings and lumps can easily be undetected.

Indications for bathing:

- Preparation of show animals prior to exhibition
- Ectoparasite control
- Medication of specific skin problems
- Cleaning of soiled coats
- Removal of unpleasant or unwanted odours.

Figure 6.37 gives the appropriate steps in bathing a dog.

Types of bath

- Domestic bath (not ideal, as it can often be easily damaged by claws)
- Baby bath (useful for smaller animals but can be easily tipped over)
- Metal bath or specifically designed grooming bath.

6.37 How to bath a dog

1. Apply a collar and lead, which can be used to restrain the animal whilst it is in the bath
2. Prepare all the required equipment
3. Groom the dog before bathing
4. Wear the required protective clothing (often includes impervious gloves)
5. Place the animal carefully in the bath
6. Having prepared the correct flow and temperature of the water from the shower fitment, carefully apply the water to soak the dog's coat
7. Apply shampoo and massage in
8. Follow manufacturer's guidelines regarding contact time and dosage
9. Rinse thoroughly
10. Squeeze out excess water
11. Lift dog from the bath (do *not* encourage the dog to jump out, as this may cause injury)
12. Towel dry
13. Use hair dryer
14. Now carry out final grooming and finishing.

For all types of bath, certain requirements should be considered:

- Ease of getting animal into and out of bath
- Non-slip surface (a bath mat to give additional protection)
- Shower fitment available for rinsing
- Access to adjustable water and heat controls
- Easy to clean and maintain

Dryers

Dryers range from the very cheap to the very specialized and expensive.

Types of dryer include:

- Hand-held dryers
- Floor or stand dryers
- Forced air dryers or blasters
- Cage or kennel dryers
- Cabinet dryers.

Hand-held dryers

For normal domestic or veterinary purposes the hand-held dryer is the most commonly used.

- Advantages:
  - light
  - simple
  - cheap
- Disadvantages:
  - slow when used to dry a large heavy-coated dog
  - being held, they limit the groomer to only one free hand.

Floor or stand dryers

Dryers mounted on stands are generally more powerful and larger than hand-held ones. They therefore dry the coat more quickly as well as leaving the groomer with both hands free.

Forced air dryers or blasters

These do not have a heating element as they rely on the velocity of air coming out of the nozzle to force the water and dead hair out of the coat. They are very noisy and therefore unsuitable on cats or smaller nervous dogs.

Cage or kennel dryers

These dryers are attached to the front of standard kennels, thus allowing the dog to be drying whilst the groomer is doing something else. However, the dog needs to be moved at intervals to ensure that all of the coat dries, especially the underside.

Cabinets

Heated drying cabinets in which the animals are placed are often used in the large professional grooming parlours. They must be carefully monitored to prevent the animal becoming hyperthermic (overheated). The cabinets have built-in drying elements and viewing doors. The dog stands on a false floor with integrated vents through which warm air flows.

Shampoos

There are several different types of shampoo:

- Cleansing, for general-purpose cleaning and conditioning
- Insecticidal, used for control of ectoparasites
- Medicated, for treatment of specific skin ailments.

When using shampoos, the following precautions are important:

- Follow manufacturer's directions precisely
- When using new products, carry out a 'patch test': apply to one small area, following directions, and then observe for any adverse reactions before using on the entire coat
- Particularly with medicated products, wear protective apron, gloves and masks and use in a well ventilated area, if directed to do so
- Wear non-slip footwear to avoid accidents
- Transfer shampoo from glass bottles to unbreakable receptacles in order to apply without risk of breakages
- Protect delicate areas of the animal from shampoo:
  - put cotton wool into ear canals (remember to remove later)
  - apply barrier cream to delicate anal, vulval, preputial and scrotal areas
  - take measures to prevent shampoo from running into eyes (apply non-medicated eye ointment).

Claw maintenance
The claws of a healthy animal do not normally require regular clipping. Trimming may be necessary for animals that appear not to wear down their claws naturally or for practical reasons:

- Dogs that do not have access to hard ground that would naturally wear down their nails
- Animals that are inactive (e.g. elderly)
- Paraplegic animals
- Those with disease conditions of the foot or nail that have led to abnormal growth
- Those with abnormal nail position or uneven wearing down of nails due to lameness or uneven gait
- Cats that damage furniture, (scratchposts would be a solution in the long term)
- Puppies, to prevent trauma to bitch's mammary region.

Also, regular observations must be made of the length of dew claws, though usually they are slow growing.

Nail-clipping equipment
- Suitable nail clipper for the size of the animal
- Cotton wool and a silver nitrate pencil (in case of inadvertent cutting of the quick and subsequent bleeding).

The technique for nail trimming is described in Figure 6.38.

Dental hygiene
When carrying out grooming and coat care, the opportunity arises to maintain good dental hygiene.

The teeth of dogs and cats were designed for killing prey and tearing and chewing raw flesh. With changes in feeding protocols and the consistency of many petfoods, it has become evident that regular (daily) oral hygiene is required in many pets.

As with grooming and handling, it is best to commence these techniques in young animals. However, if introduced gradually and with patience, many animals will accept dental cleaning later in life (Figure 6.39).

Other aids to oral hygiene include:

- Specifically designed dental chews
- Oral hygiene gels and pastes
- Specifically designed dental biscuits.

For optimum results oral hygiene routines should become a daily event.

6.38 How to cut claws

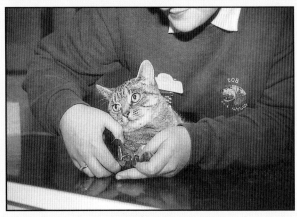

- Gather equipment together
- Suitably restrain the animal
- Hold the foot firmly and examine the claws to be trimmed
- In cats, gentle pressure to the foot will expose the normally retracted claws
- If the quick is visible, cut below the quick
- If the quick is not visible (black claws), estimate where the quick should be by examining how much claw exceeds the bottom of the pad. Cut with care, avoiding cutting too high up and causing bleeding
- If bleeding occurs, apply silver nitrate via styptic pencil and cover with cotton wool
- Continue until all claws (including dew claws) have been trimmed.

6.39 How to introduce dental hygiene

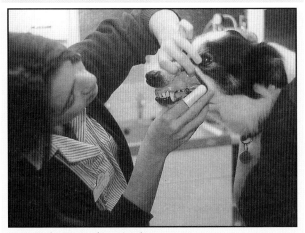

- Firstly assess the animal's temperament
- Begin by handling the animal's mouth daily for several days and praising good behaviour
- Gradually start to mimic tooth brushing with the finger alone, for several days
- Begin to apply specific canine or feline toothpaste (human preparations are unsuitable) with the finger for several days
- Now very gradually replace the finger with a toothbrush
- Once the animal has learnt to tolerate dental cleaning, it may prove possible to clean the inner surfaces of the teeth as well as the outermost (finger brushes are helpful with this).

Introduction to nutrition

In order to maintain optimal body health, it is essential that the body receives adequate nutrition. This requirement comes second only to the requirement for water and air.

It is important to have a good understanding of normal nutritional requirements before considering those specific to various life stages.

Basic nutritional requirements

During various disease states and stages of life, the nutritional and energy requirements of animals will vary. However, the basic nutritional requirements of all animals are:

- To meet energy requirements without excess
- To meet all nutrient requirements without incurring detrimental excesses.

Animals can be classified as:

- Carnivores: eating primarily flesh
- Herbivores: eating plants and plant products
- Omnivores: eating both plant and animal foods.

Although they belong to the group Carnivora, dogs are actually omnivorous. They can feed not only on animal tissue like meat, but also on vegetable matter.

Cats, however, are true carnivores and must have animal tissue in their diets. Cats cannot be vegetarians.

Meeting energy requirements

Animals eat to obtain energy and it is therefore important that all nutritional requirements are balanced to the calorific level of food, as the animal will only eat to meet calorific requirements.

The smaller an animal is, the greater is its body surface area (relative to the environment) and the higher is its energy requirement.

For example:

- A Chihuahua needs more calories per kilogram of body weight per day than a Great Dane
- A Labrador puppy is a small version of the mature Labrador and therefore needs more calories per kilogram of body weight per day (approximately twice as much).

Hunger

Hunger is a craving for food, stimulated by :

- Decrease in blood glucose
- Decrease in circulating amino acids
- Increase in gastric motility.

Nutrients

A nutrient is a substance assimilated from the gastrointestinal tract and utilized by cells of the body to support life. It may be:

- Non-essential: manufactured within the body and therefore not an essential daily dietary requirement
- Essential: must be provided in food, because the nutrient is either not synthesized by the body at all, or the rate of synthesis is too slow to meet demands.

The function of nutrients is to supply:

- Energy
- Materials for growth, repair and reproduction
- Substances that regulate the processes involved in energy production or the utilization of materials for growth, repair and reproduction.

Classes of nutrients are:

- Water
- Protein
- Fat
- Carbohydrate
- Minerals
- Vitamins.

Water

Every body cell requires a continuous water supply in order to function. In total, water makes up 70% of the animal's body weight:

- Intracellular water (inside the cells) makes up 50% of the animal's body weight
- Extracellular water (inside the body but not inside the cells) makes up 20% of the animal's body weight.

Functions of water

- Digestion: protein, fats and carbohydrates are digested by hydrolysis in water
- Transport: water-soluble materials are transported in the gut and bloodstream
- Body temperature regulation: water is an ideal medium to transfer heat.

Water intake

The body cannot store water for long periods and an intake is therefore required to meet demands. Water intake and output *must* be in balance.

Water sources

- Water drunk (as fluid)
- Water in food
- Metabolic water.

Metabolic water

When carbohydrates, proteins and fats are broken down in the body they release a certain quantity of water.

Each nutrient will yield a different amount of water from every gram that is oxidized. Fat creates more water in the body than the weight of fat actually eaten. Therefore if an animal eats a high fat diet it needs to drink less.

Water output

Water is normally lost in:

- Urine
- Faeces
- Evaporation from the skin
- Expiration from the lungs
- Milk (when a female is lactating).

Water can also be lost abnormally, in:

- Vomit
- Discharges such as pyometra
- Diarrhoea.

Protein

Proteins are very large molecules that consist of hundreds of simple single units called amino acids, joined together to form chains.

Each amino acid can be thought of as a building block used to make up a particular protein. Digestion is involved in the breakdown of this protein into its component blocks (amino acids). The body can then assimilate (rebuild) these amino acids into new proteins to form body tissue.

Functions of protein

- Production of energy
- Tissue building and maintenance
- Regulation of metabolism (enzymes and some hormones)
- Formation of antibodies.

Protein sources

- Animal sources: meat, fish, eggs, milk
- Plant sources: soya, cereals.

Protein output

- Energy production
- Utilized in the body
- Faeces
- Urine
- Hair
- Skin
- Sweat.

Protein metabolism

Digestible protein is that part which is absorbed through the gut wall into the body and not lost in faeces. This can range from as low as 50% in some cereals to over 95% for milk or egg protein.

Much protein metabolism takes place in the liver. Unlike fat and carbohydrate, protein contains nitrogen molecules and urea is one of the few safe forms in which nitrogen can be eliminated from the body. Nitrogen is converted to ammonia and eventually urea. This urea can be safely transported in the blood and excreted via the kidneys.

Amino acids

There are 23 amino acids, of which 10 are classified as essential in the dog. These amino acids must be supplied in the diet, as the animal is unable to synthesize them from other materials in sufficient quantity to meet its needs.

Non-essential amino acids can be made in the body from other raw materials.

Taurine

In cats, as well as the essential amino acids there is a nutritional requirement for taurine (an aminosulphonic acid). Taurine is only available as a dietary source from animal-derived proteins.

Protein quality

Protein quality is governed by certain characteristics. A high-quality protein should:

- Be well digested and absorbed
- Have a balanced amino acid profile.

Examples of high-quality protein include:

- Eggs
- White fish
- Meat.

Protein deficiency

Lack of one or more amino acids, or an inadequate quantity of protein, can result in deficiency diseases.

Signs of protein deficiencies include:

- Lack of appetite
- Poor growth, loss of body weight
- Impaired immune function
- Loss of coat condition
- Retinal degeneration (taurine deficiency in cats).

Fat

Fats are made up of a mixture of triglycerides and cholesterol. Each triglyceride is composed of a glycerol 'backbone' with fatty acids attached. The difference between one fat and another is mostly a result of the different combinations of fatty acids attached to this backbone. Some fatty acids are essential (must be ingested) but most can be synthesized in the body.

Fats contain 2.25 times more energy per unit of weight than either proteins or carbohydrates. Fats are therefore an extremely good source of concentrated calories.

Functions of fat

- Provides energy
- Provides essential fatty acids
- Carrier of fat-soluble vitamins (A, D, E, K)
- Increases dietary palatability.

Fat sources

- Animal sources: dairy produce, meats (variable), fish
- Plant sources: seed oils, nuts.

Fat output

- Energy production
- Faeces (a few hydrogenated fats are poorly digested)
- Haircoat condition
- Deposition in the body.

Essential fatty acids (EFAs)

- Linoleic acid: required by *all* animals
- Linolenic acid: synthesized from linoleic acid by both cats and dogs
- Arachidonic acid: essential in the cat; other species can synthesize from linoleic acid. Arachidonic acid is a constituent of animal fat and is not present in plant products of any type.

Signs of EFA deficiency include:

- Poor coat condition
- Skin lesions
- Reproductive failure.

Carbohydrate

Carbohydrates are classified as:

- Polysaccharides: starches and cellulose
- Disaccharides: paired monosaccharides (e.g. sucrose)
- Monosaccharides: simple sugars (e.g. glucose).

The long polysaccharide and short disaccharide chains have to be broken down into simple sugars in order to be digested. The polysaccharide starches are broken down into their component sugars, but cellulose (because of the way the sugars are linked) is not easily digested by single-stomached animals.

Functions of carbohydrate

Carbohydrates are not generally considered to be an essential nutrient in dogs and cats but they are a cheap source of energy.

Carbohydrate sources

- Animal: milk sugar (lactose), meat (very small amount, quickly lost after death)
- Plant: fruit sugars, cereal starches, root vegetables.

Dietary fibre

Dietary fibre describes the portion of foodstuffs that cannot be broken down by intestinal enzymes and juices of monogastric (single-stomach) animals and therefore passes through the small intestine and colon undigested. It is mainly composed of cellulose (the 'skeleton' of plants), lignin, pectin and other carbohydrates. It is essential to maintain the health of the gastrointestinal tract.

Carbohydrate deficiency

Carbohydrate deficiency is not seen in dogs and cats.

Minerals (ash)

Minerals are inorganic elements that can be divided into two groups:

- Major minerals: needed in quite large quantities (Figure 6.40)
- Trace minerals: (also know as trace elements) needed in very small amounts (Figure 6.41).

Functions of minerals

- Major structural components (e.g. calcium and phosphorus in the skeleton)
- Maintenance of fluid balance (e.g. sodium and potassium)
- Regulation of metabolism through enzyme function.

Mineral balance

It is vital to remember that the balance of minerals in the diet is as important as the quantity.

Calcium and phosphorus

The calcium to phosphorus ratio should be 1–1.5 Ca : 1 P.

Pure meat diets have an adverse calcium to phosphorus ratio of 1 Ca : 20 P.

6.40 Major minerals

Mineral	Source	Function	Deficiency	Excess
Calcium	Bones, milk, cheese	Bone formation, nerve and muscle formation	Poor growth, rickets, convulsions	Bone deformities
Phosphorus	Bones, milk	Bone formation, energy utilization	Rickets (rare)	Similar signs to calcium deficiency
Potassium	Milk, meat	Water balance, nerve function	Poor growth, paralysis, kidney and heart lesions	Muscular weakness, heart failure
Sodium	Salt, cereals	Water balance, muscle and nerve activity	Poor growth, exhaustion	Thirst, increased blood pressure
Magnesium	Cereals, bones, green vegetables	Bone formation, protein synthesis	Anorexia, vomiting, muscle weakness	Diarrhoea

6.41 Trace minerals

Mineral	Source	Function	Deficiency	Excess
Iron	Eggs, meat (liver), green vegetables	Part of haemoglobin	Anaemia	Weight loss, anorexia
Iodine	Fish, dairy produce	Part of thyroid hormone	Hair loss, apathy, drowsiness	Unknown
Copper	Meat, bones	Part of haemoglobin	Anaemia	Hepatopathy in Bedlington Terriers
Zinc	Meat, cereals	Digestion, tissue maintenance	Hair loss, skin thickening, poor growth	Diarrhoea

Supplementation

If a good quality prepared petfood is used, there is no need for supplementation in the normal healthy animal. Foods rich in calcium include milk and cheese.

 Indiscriminate supplementation with one or even several minerals is likely to be more harmful than beneficial, and is the main cause of mineral imbalances in dogs and cats.

For example, oversupplementation with calcium may lead to the development of skeletal abnormalities. It will also interfere with zinc absorption, so that the animal will become zinc deficient.

6.42 Common names for vitamins

Vitamin	Name
A	Retinol
B_1	Thiamin
B_2	Riboflavin
B_6	Pyridoxine
B_{12}	(Cyano)cobalamin
C	Ascorbic acid
D_2	Ergocalciferol
D_3	Cholecalciferol
E	Tocopherol
K_1	Phylloquinone
K_2	Menaquinone
K_3	Menadione

Vitamins

Vitamins (Figure 6.42) are complex organic molecules involved in most essential body functions. They are usually needed in only very small quantities.

Fat-soluble vitamins

Fat-soluble vitamins (Figure 6.43) require fat for their absorption, utilization and storage. Once in the body, unused fat-soluble vitamins are not excreted and are therefore potentially quite dangerous if oversupplemented. The storage ability of the fat-soluble vitamins prevents the need for a daily supply.

Water-soluble vitamins

Water-soluble vitamins (B group and vitamin C; Figure 6.44) are not stored and are therefore required on a daily basis.

Unlike humans (and guinea pigs), dogs and cats can produce vitamin C from glucose in the liver to meet their needs.

Nutrition in life stages

Gestation and lactation

The bitch

Malnourishment of the bitch before and during gestation is thought to contribute to 20–30% of neonatal deaths. However, provided that the bitch is receiving a nutritionally well balanced diet, there is no need to alter the regimen until 6 weeks into the pregnancy, when the fetuses start to grow.

6.43 Fat-soluble vitamins

Vitamin	Source	Function	Deficiency	Excess
A	Fish oil, liver, vegetables	Vision in poor light, skin maintenance	Night blindness, skin lesions	Anorexia, bone pain (malformation)
D	Cod liver oil, eggs, animal products	Calcium balance, bone growth	Rickets, osteomalacia	Anorexia, calcification of soft tissue
E	Green vegetables, vegetable oils, dairy produce	Reproduction	Infertility, anaemia, muscle weakness	Not known
K	Spinach, green vegetables, liver	Blood clotting	Haemorrhage	Not known

6.44 Water-soluble vitamins

Vitamin	Source	Function	Deficiency	Excess
B_1	Dairy products, cereals, liver and kidney	Release of energy from carbohydrate	Anorexia, vomiting, paralysis	Not known
B_2	Milk, animal tissue	Utilization of energy	Weight loss, weakness, collapse, coma	Not known
B_6	Meat, fish, eggs, cereal	Metabolism of amino acids	Anorexia, anaemia, weight loss, convulsions	Not known
B_{12}	Liver, meat, dairy produce	Division of cells in bone marrow	Anaemia	Not known
Folic acid	Offal, leafy vegetables	Division of cells in bone marrow	Anaemia, poor growth	Not known
C	Fruit, green vegetables	Synthesis of collagen, osteoblast function	Scurvy, gingival haemorrhage, anaemia, epiphyseal fractures	Not known

Figure 6.45 gives guidance on feeding pregnant or lactating bitches.

The queen

A pregnant or lactating queen should be fed in a similar manner to the bitch, except that calorie intake should increase from the 5th week of pregnancy. With a growth or lactation diet, it is recommended that the queen should be allowed free-choice feeding at all times.

Growing animals

Puppies

Weaning (separation from the mother) normally occurs at 6 weeks of age and preparation for this can start as early as 3–4 weeks of age. Specialized weaning diets are available, or milk replacements and liquidized growth diets can be used, gradually increasing the viscosity of the diet until the puppies are on solid food.

The aim is to reach a growth rate of 2–4 g/day per kilogram of anticipated adult body weight.

Mature body weight is reached at about 7–8 months of age in small breeds, but not until about 18–24 months of age in giant breeds. Therefore a Chihuahua can move straight from puppy food to adult food. Labradors and larger breeds need an interim food between puppy and adult and these are often described as junior diets.

Figure 6.46 summarizes how to feed a growing puppy.

Kittens

Kittens may be fed on a free-choice basis on a growth diet from 3 weeks of age. As with puppies, supplementation should be avoided.

Maintenance

Average maintenance requirements can be estimated and are indicated on all good quality petfoods. Some of the terms used in these estimations are:

- Basal metabolic rate (BMR; also called basal energy requirement, BER): the minimal energy expended for the maintenance of respiration, circulation, peristalsis, muscle tone, body temperature, glandular activity and other body functions
- Resting energy requirement (RER): energy required at rest
- Maintenance energy requirement (MER): energy required in an active animal.

  Factors that affect maintenance energy requirement include:

- The animal's life stage
- Pregnancy and lactation
- Illness or disease
- Environmental conditions (e.g. temperature)
- Level of activity
- Reproductive state (MER often decreases after neutering).

Obesity

It is important to realize that regular assesment of an individual's weight is required in order to prevent under- or (more commonly) overfeeding. Many commercial petfoods are now available to cater for animals prone to obesity; the foods provide reduced calories but still satisfy hunger.

- Dogs are pack hunters and therefore tend to eat voraciously whenever food is available; they are therefore prone to obesity
- Cats are solitary hunters; they eat every few hours and are therefore unlikely to overeat when offered free-choice food.

6.45 How to feed a pregnant or lactating bitch (with average litter size)

Do:

- Feed a diet formulated for growth or lactation
- Increase calorie intake by 10% weekly until whelping (from 6 weeks of pregnancy)
- Feed at frequent intervals during the last 10 days of gestation (as the stomach capacity may be limited by the enlarged uterus)
- Feed 1.5 times maintenance requirement for the first week of lactation
- Feed 2–3 times maintenance requirement during the 2nd and 3rd week or allow free-choice feeding at this stage
- Always allow free access to fresh drinking water, especially during peak lactation
- Commence weaning the puppies from 3 to 4 weeks of age by giving them supplementary feeding and thus decreasing the demand on the bitch.

Do not:

- Give supplements when feeding a good quality prepared growth/lactation diet (calcium or vitamin D supplements can cause soft tissue calcification and physical anomalies in puppies)
- Give unsupplemented meat diets, which are low in calcium
- Increase calorie intake until the 6th week of pregnancy onwards.

6.46 How to feed a growing puppy

Do:

- Commence weaning at 3–4 weeks of age
- Aim to reach a growth rate of 2–4 g/day/kg adult weight for the first 5 months of life
- Allow 20–30 minutes to eat each meal
- Offer four meals a day from 4 weeks of age
- Gradually reduce the number of meals to one or two meals per day as the animal approaches adult body weight
- Feed toy breeds 3–4 times per day until 6 months of age (they are susceptible to hypoglycaemia)
- Gradually (over 3–4 days) change from one diet to another when required.

Do not:

- Overfeed to increase growth rates – maximum growth rate is not in the best interest of the dog. Adult body size is not determined by growth rate as a puppy
- Supplement with minerals and vitamins when a suitable good quality pet food is used
- Allow the puppy to become overweight – a fat puppy becomes a fat adult
- Allow free-choice feeding until the dog has reached 80–90% of anticipated adult weight
- Allow food not eaten within 30 minutes to remain available
- Change from one diet to another rapidly, as this can lead to dietary disturbances and subsequent diarrhoea.

Working dogs

Working dogs have an increased energy requirement, as a result of their lifestyle. Depending on the level of activity, dogs may have, in general, requirements as much as 2–3 times their adult maintenance. These increased energy requirements are often met by feeding a calorie-dense high-fat diet.

Older animals

In general, older animals are less active. This can lead to energy requirements being 20% less than their previous maintenance level. For this reason, it is clear that a reduction in calorific intake is required in order to prevent obesity.

Older animals are also prone to conditions such as constipation and for this reason other nutritional considerations are made when preparing food for the ageing animal (Figure 6.47). There is now a wide range of diets available for all stages of life, including those designed for the older animal.

Further reading

Anderson RS and Edney ATB (1991) *Practical Animal Handling*. Butterworth Heinemann, Oxford.

Blood DC and Studdert VP (1990) *Baillière's Comprehensive Veterinary Dictionary*. Baillière Tindall, London.

6.47 How to feed ageing pets

- Reduce energy intake, if weight gain is evident
- Reduce fat intake, again in order to prevent obesity
- Divide total daily food allowance over two to three meals to aid digestion
- Increase fibre intake, if constipation is evident
- Feed highly palatable and easily digested foods
- Consider that alterations in the gastrointestinal tract and general metabolism may result in increased requirements for vitamins A, B_1, B_6, B_{12} and E
- Seek veterinary surgeon's advice on the need to reduce sodium, phosphorus and protein levels if clinical examination indicates organ failure (kidney, liver or heart for example).

Earle KE (1990) Feeding for health. *Journal of Small Animal Practice* **31**, 477–481.

Evans JM and White K (1992) *The Doglopaedia*. Henston, Guildford.

Lane DR and Cooper B (1995) *Veterinary Nursing*. Butterworth Heinemann.

O'Farrell V (1992) *Manual of Canine Behaviour*. BSAVA, Cheltenham.

7 Animal function

Judith Philipson

This chapter is designed to give information on:

- Cells, tissues and systems
- Homeostasis and internal regulation
- Temperature regulation
- Hypothermia
- Removal of wastes and osmoregulation
- Immunity and the defence against disease

Introduction

Warmblooded animals such as cats and dogs maintain a stable body temperature, despite changes in the temperature of their surroundings. Water balance (osmoregulation) and the elimination of waste materials (excretion) are mechanisms that regulate the internal environment of the animal. Without continual adjustments, the animal would soon cease to function effectively. Immunity describes some of the defence mechanisms that enable animals to resist infection and diseases.

Cells, tissues and body systems

Body systems

An animal is composed of many body systems, which perform specific functions. For example:

- The *respiratory system* takes in oxygen and eliminates waste gases
- The *digestive system* processes food, absorbs nutrients and expels wastes
- The *circulatory system* transports blood round the body, delivering oxygen and nutrients (foodstuffs) to all parts, and removes wastes such as carbon dioxide, excess water and other breakdown products
- The *excretory system* removes wastes and excess water from the blood and eliminates them from the body.

Other body systems perform other functions vital to the body. Each system is composed of a number of different organs which perform a special role. For example: the stomach is an organ of the digestive system; the lungs are organs of the respiratory system.

Tissues
The organs and body systems are composed of different tissues, such as muscular tissue, blood, bone and nerve tissue.

Cells
All tissues are composed of individual units called cells. There are many millions of cells in the body. As they are microscopic (very small), examination of them requires that specially prepared samples are stained and magnified. Some of the structures illustrated in Figure 7.1 can be seen at 400 times magnification using a microscope.

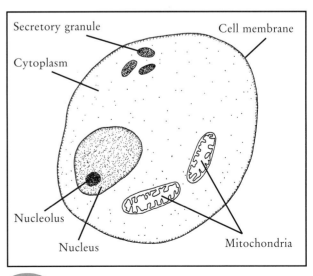

Secretory granule

Cell membrane

Cytoplasm

Nucleolus

Nucleus

Mitochondria

7.1 *The structure of a simple cell (drawing not to scale).*

Even though cells become specialized into different types of tissue with different functions, they retain the basic structures illustrated and carry out many functions to maintain the cell.

Cell structure

- The *cell membrane* forms the cell boundary and controls the movement of substances into and out of the cell. Nutrients and oxygen are taken in and wastes expelled
- The *nucleus* contains the hereditary chromosomes. It controls all the cell activities and controls cell division (the formation of daughter cells)
- The *chromosomes* contain DNA
- The *cytoplasm* is semi-fluid and contains many dissolved substances such as protein, water, salts, glucose and tiny subcellular structures called organelles
- The *mitochondria* (singular: mitochondrion) are the powerhouses of the cell. These organelles make energy for cell activities, using oxygen and glucose. Energy is stored in *ATP* (adenosine triphosphate) until required. Cells that need lots of energy, such as muscle cells, have many large mitochondria.

Figure 7.2 shows the relationship between cells, tissues, organs and body systems.

Homeostasis

Cell specialization allows many processes to continue at the same time in the animal. Cells themselves are also very efficient at carrying out many functions at once, but they can only achieve this when stable conditions are maintained in and around them.

The maintenance of stable internal conditions for the efficient functioning of all cells in the animal is called *homeostasis*. Homeostasis maintains a stable internal environment for the animal despite constant changes that can occur. Consider the following practical example.

Example

During an exercise session for a dog, a ball is thrown and the dog runs to retrieve it. This is repeated many times until the dog and its owner rest.

During exercise and immediately afterwards the dog pants, his heart beats faster, his breathing is more rapid. Within a few minutes of rest the dog's heart and breathing rate are normal again and panting has subsided.

When the dog was running, his muscle cells required more oxygen and glucose to produce energy and the heart rate and breathing rate increased to supply these demands.

This example illustrates that internal mechanisms enable the dog to obtain extra energy and oxygen when required for exercise, and to eliminate the excess heat and carbon dioxide produced. The heart and breathing rate return to normal after the exercise session. While the owner is running with the dog, similar mechanisms are active in the owner's body.

The internal environment

Cellular fluids

The living cells of the animal are kept moist. They are bathed in watery fluid called tissue fluid or *extracellular fluid* (fluid

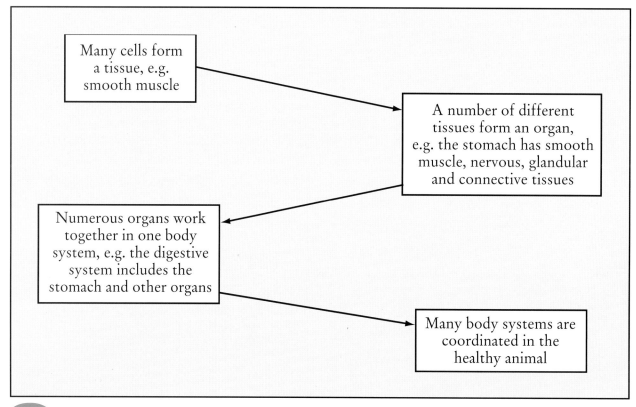

7.2 *Relationship between cells, tissues, organs and body systems in animals.*

outside the cells). There is continual movement of fluid from the tiny blood vessels of the circulatory system into the tissue fluid and from there into the cells. The watery cytoplasm inside cells contains the *intracellular fluid*.

Oxygen and nutrients (dissolved foods that cells require) are delivered to all cells of the animal via the tissue fluid. Cells require a constant supply of oxygen and nutrients, otherwise they will quickly die.

Cellular waste materials
Waste materials move from the cells where they are formed, into the tissue fluid and into the blood or the lymphatic vessels (Figure 7.3). Wastes such as carbon dioxide must be removed from the tissue fluid, otherwise they can build up to toxic levels.

Blood circulatory system
The circulatory system carries blood (which is pumped by the heart) in blood vessels – arteries, veins and capillaries.

Lymphatic system
The lymphatic system consists of lymphatic vessels and small glands. It forms a link with the general circulation as it returns tissue fluid to the blood.

The lymphatic system contains *lymph*, a whitish fluid. As lymph is at a lower pressure than blood, excess water and some wastes can move into lymphatic vessels more easily. Lymph is emptied into the blood circulation through two lymphatic ducts, which join large veins near the heart.

Effects of stress
Stress can alter the balance of the internal environment. It can be the result of high temperature, cold, shortage of oxygen or a build-up of wastes. Severe stress can be caused by an infection, high blood pressure or the effects of a major operation or injury.

The body works unconsciously to counteract stress and restore the internal balance. The greater the stress, the harder the body must work to restore homeostasis.

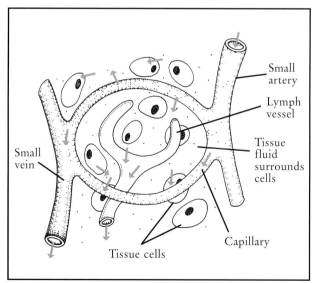

7.3 *Tissue cells and the network of blood and lymph vessels. Arrows indicate movement of fluids.*

Communication within the body
Homeostasis is controlled by the nervous system and the endocrine system. Both systems allow communication between different parts of the body.

The nervous system
The nervous system consists of the brain, spinal cord, special senses and a network of nerves. It controls homeostasis by detecting when the internal balance of the body changes and sends messages or nerve impulses to particular organs to adjust the imbalance. Nerve impulses travel extremely quickly and bring about rapid changes to the internal environment.

The part of the nervous system that regulates homeostasis is the *autonomic* (non-voluntary) *nervous system*. For example, messages from the correct branch of the autonomic nervous system can speed up or slow down the heart rate as required.

The endocrine system
The endocrine system is composed of many glands throughout the body, each of which secretes (produces) chemical messengers called *hormones*. Hormones travel in the blood and cause changes in specific cells of the body. Hormones act more slowly than nerve impulses but the effects last for longer.

The nervous system and the endocrine system work together to coordinate the regulation of the body and ensure that as far as possible, in a healthy animal, the correct balance of cell activities is maintained.

Negative feedback
Homeostasis almost always works through a negative feedback mechanism.

> **Example**
> A simple non-biological example is a domestic hot-water system.
>
> A water tank with a heater is connected to a switch and a thermostat. In this example, the thermostat is set in the range of 55°C to 65°C. When the heater is on, water is heated to 65°C. The thermostat detects when the temperature rises above 65°C and switches off the heater. Once hot water is drawn from the tank, cold water enters to fill the gap and the temperature drops below 55°C. The thermostat detects this and activates the switch to turn on the heater.
>
> Thus the temperature in the tank fluctuates around a set point. An increase in water temperature causes the thermostat to switch off the heater and the temperature gradually drops. A decrease in water temperature causes the thermostat to switch on the heater, raising the temperature.
>
> The relationship in each case is opposite or a negative to the situation in the water tank. This is known as negative feedback. The temperature fluctuates around a set point, but does not remain constant all the time. It can drop to 55°C and rise to 65°C, but is normally maintained within these limits.

In the cat, dog and other mammals, physiological processes rely on negative feedback mechanisms to maintain homeostasis. The nervous system and the endocrine system coordinate this.

Example

Glucose is an important source of energy for mammals. Blood glucose levels must be kept within narrow limits to prevent brain damage and to allow all cells to function effectively. Two hormones, insulin and glucagon, act together to maintain the blood glucose balance.

When a dog digests a meal, the blood glucose level rises. The raised level becomes a stress and the hormone *insulin* is released in greater amounts. Insulin lowers blood glucose to normal levels in a number of ways, one of which is to convert blood glucose into storage granules in the liver.

As the animal uses up the glucose for all activities requiring energy, the blood glucose level gradually drops. This low level also becomes a stress on the animal and the hormone *glucagon* is released. This brings blood glucose back within the normal range by, for example, releasing some of the stored glucose into the blood.

Maintenance of body temperature

The normal ranges of temperature for the dog and cat are:

- Dog: 38.3–38.7°C
- Cat: 38.0–38.5°C

The body temperature of a dog operates around a set point of 38.5°, with a 0.4°C range in a healthy animal. The range indicates the amount of normal fluctuation that occurs. If the temperature of the blood rises or falls, the brain detects the change and starts a series of reactions that help to bring it back to the set point. Many of the reactions are involuntary and operate through negative feedback mechanisms.

- *An increase in body temperature* in the dog stimulates reactions that result in temperature decrease.

For example, the animal's coat traps heat. The flatter the coat lies, the less body heat is trapped. Heat is a by-product of *metabolism* (chemical reactions in cells) and so metabolic processes are slowed to reduce heat production. In addition the animal will consciously seek shade and drink to slake increasing thirst and cool the body.

- *A decrease in body temperature* stimulates reactions that result in temperature increase.

For example, the muscle at the base of each hair follicle in the skin contracts, pulling each hair upright and causing the coat to stand out, which insulates the body. A cold animal may start shivering, generating heat production in the muscles, raising the temperature of the muscles and circulating blood. Other cells also increase metabolism, producing more heat. The animal may consciously seek warmth and curl up to reduce heat loss.

The temperature detector, or thermostat, in the cat and dog is situated in the brain. As blood flows through the hypothalamus in the brain, sensitive cells detect the temperature. They also receive information from thermoreceptors in the skin. Nerve impulses travel to the arrector pili muscle at the base of the hair follicle, raising or lowering each hair shaft. The result is that the animal's coat will appear bushy when cold but smoother and sleeker in a hotter environment. Blood vessels in the skin are dilated or constricted by nerve impulses to help to regulate heat loss or heat conservation.

The hormone *thyroxine* is released in greater amounts during cold weather. Thyroxine speeds up cell metabolism, thereby assisting the production of more body heat. Figure 7.4 summarizes the regulation of body temperature.

Hypothermia

Hypothermia is an abnormally low body temperature. It occurs when there is excessive heat loss or insufficient heat production and homeostatic mechanisms are unable to restore the animal's normal temperature. If the core (internal) temperature remains low for too long the animal's metabolic rate will slow, which could result in death.

Signs of hypothermia include:

- Slow pulse rate
- Subnormal rectal temperature
- Shivering
- Cold limbs
- Pallor of mucous membranes.

Causes of hypothermia are shown in Figure 7.5.

Removal of wastes and osmoregulation

It is essential that wastes are removed from the body.

Osmoregulation is the maintenance of the water and electrolyte balance of the body fluids. The systems that remove or excrete wastes and contribute to osmoregulation are:

- Respiratory system
- Digestive system
- Urinary system.

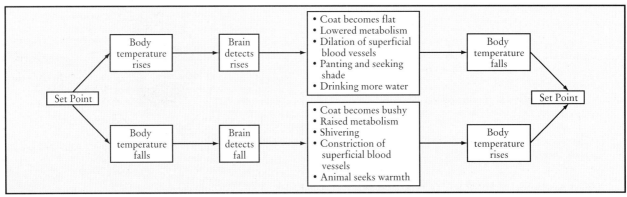

7.4 *Homeostasis: the regulation of body temperature by negative feedback.*

The respiratory system

The breathing or respiratory system allows for the exchange of gases between the animal and its environment.

External respiration is the gaseous exchange between the air and the blood. This process occurs in the lungs during breathing. Oxygen (O_2) is taken into the blood and carbon dioxide (CO_2) leaves it.

Internal or *tissue respiration* is the release of energy in the cells, using oxygen and the nutrient glucose. Carbon dioxide and water are produced as waste products.

Thus, during breathing, not only is oxygen taken in, but also the respiratory system eliminates:

- Carbon dioxide (CO_2)
- Water vapour.

The CO_2 diffuses from cells into the tissue fluid, enters the blood and is carried to the lungs. Exhaled air contains more CO_2 and water vapour than inhaled air. High levels of CO_2 in the blood increase blood acidity, which upsets the balance of homeostasis. Nervous receptors (sensitive nerve tissue) in large blood vessels detect blood acidity and send impulses to the brain, which responds by sending impulses to speed up the breathing rate. This occurs as a rapid response to increased acidity. It accounts for the increased breathing rate during exercise, when more CO_2 is produced.

Some of the water produced in cells is removed via exhaled air, and some via the urinary and digestive systems. A dog loses up to 20 ml of water per kilogram of body weight per day during breathing.

The digestive system

The main function of the digestive system is to process ingested food, so that nutrients (substances required by the animal) can be absorbed by the digestive tract and delivered to tissue cells. The digestive system secretes *enzymes* (specialized proteins) which speed up the breakdown of foods into small, easily absorbed nutrients. The faeces contain wastes, which are eliminated via the anus.

Faeces consist of:

- Undigested foodstuffs which were never absorbed
- Bacteria (useful microorganisms that live in the gut)
- Bile pigments (produced in the liver from the breakdown of old red blood cells), which colour the faeces
- Water (variable amounts).

The urinary system

The urinary system is the main excretory system. It produces *urine*, a liquid containing water, salts, urea and breakdown substances from hormones, and other chemicals that are no longer needed by the body.

The urinary system maintains homeostasis by controlling the composition, volume and pressure of the blood. By adjusting the amount of water in urine it maintains osmoregulation (water balance) of the body.

The excretion of wastes prevents substances from accumulating to toxic levels. The urinary system excretes acids and alkalis; this regulates the blood's acid/alkali balance (also called the acid/base balance).

The system consists of:

- Two kidneys, which filter blood to produce urine
- Two ureters, which carry urine from the kidneys
- One bladder, which stores urine
- The urethra, which leads from the bladder to the outside.

The kidneys lie against the dorsal wall of the animal, partially protected by the vertebrae and the ribs. The bladder enlarges as urine drains into it and eventually the animal becomes aware of the pressure. The process of urinating is an involuntary reflex, although house-trained animals can consciously control muscles at the exterior sphincter (circular opening) of the bladder and control the time of urination.

The kidney

The internal appearance of each kidney shows a granular, dark reddish cortex which surrounds the more striated medulla. The medullary region converges into pyramids – funnel-shaped regions which drain fluid into the pelvis of the kidney. The ureter, blood vessels and nerves enter or leave at the hilus (Figure 7.6).

The nephron

The medulla and cortex of each kidney are composed of many thousands of microscopic units called nephrons (Figure 7.7), which filter the blood as it passes through the kidney.

The *Bowman's capsule* or renal capsule receives an afferent (carrying towards) blood vessel from a branch of the renal artery. This forms a *glomerulus* (knot) of tiny blood vessels. The efferent vessel leaves the glomerulus and forms a network of blood capillaries surrounding the nephron. This network drains into a branch of the renal vein, which leaves the kidney at the hilus.

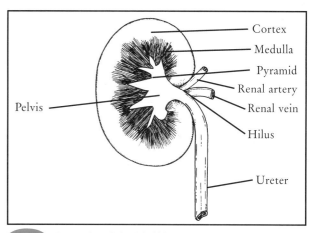

7.6 *Section through the right kidney.*

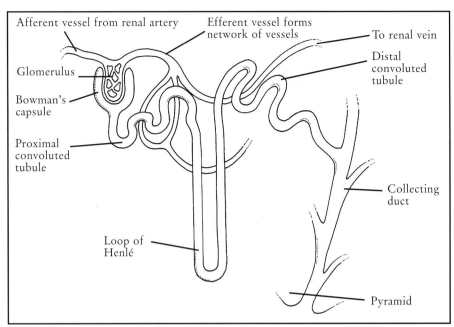

Afferent vessel from renal artery

Efferent vessel forms network of vessels

To renal vein

Distal convoluted tubule

Glomerulus

Bowman's capsule

Proximal convoluted tubule

Collecting duct

Loop of Henlé

Pyramid

The Bowman's capsule leads to a proximal convoluted tubule, a loop of Henlé, a distal convoluted tubule and a collecting duct. Several nephrons drain into one collecting duct, many of which drain into the pelvis of the kidney.

Formation of urine

Blood is at high pressure when it enters each glomerulus and most of the water and small dissolved substances are squeezed into the Bowman's capsule. Blood cells and most proteins in the plasma (the liquid part of the blood) are too large to be squeezed through; they remain in the blood. The liquid, called *glomerular filtrate*, drains along the renal tubule, where its composition is modified and most of the water is reabsorbed.

The formation of glomerular filtrate is a non-specific process and occurs due to blood pressure in the glomerulus, whereas the reabsorption of useful substances can be adjusted, depending the homeostatic balance.

The precise composition of urine depends on many factors:

- The amount of liquid/water recently taken in by the animal
- Types of food eaten
- Exercise status
- The acidity of the blood.

Filtrate is termed urine once it drains into the pelvis of the kidney.

The actual volume of urine that drains into the bladder is a fraction of the original filtrate. A large dog could produce 100 litres of filtrate per 24 hours, but urine volume is about 1–2 litres. This indicates how much water reabsorption occurs along every nephron tubule.

Reabsorption and secretion in the nephron

Useful substances are reabsorbed into blood capillaries surrounding nephrons. Other substances are secreted (pumped) into the filtrate from the surrounding capillaries to balance the composition and *pH* (acid/alkali balance) of the blood.

Hormones play an important role in regulating the final composition of urine on a daily basis. Without hormone regulation the animal could lose water and salts so quickly that death would occur.

- Antidiuretic hormone (*ADH*) regulates the amount of water in urine. When an animal needs to conserve water, more ADH is released, which acts on the distal convoluted tubule and collecting duct to increase water reabsorption into the blood
- The hormone *aldosterone* regulates the sodium and potassium balance. These electrolytes are essential to effective functioning of many systems, especially nerve and muscle action. The level of sodium in the blood also influences water retention and blood pressure.

The amount of acids or alkalis (bases) which are released into urine will depend on the acidity of the blood, which is kept as near to pH 7.4 as possible, otherwise homeostasis is upset.

- If the pH of blood drops below 7.4, then more acids will be excreted in the urine
- If the pH of blood becomes more alkaline (above 7.4), then more alkalis (bases) will be excreted.

The pH of urine of a cat or dog on a normal meat-based diet is between 5 and 7, as metabolic processes generally result in more acids being produced.

Figure 7.8 lists some of the main substances present in a filtrate sample below the Bowman's capsule, compared with those present in urine.

Fluid balance

Water losses over a 24-hour period for a healthy dog or cat are shown in Figure 7.9.

Some of the losses can be reduced by homeostatic mechanisms by the animal when water is in short supply. However, a loss of approximately 10 ml of urine/kg body weight per day is termed *obligate urine loss* and will be produced even during times of water deprivation. Respiratory water loss is also obligate or inevitable loss and cannot be reduced by homeostatic mechanisms. A healthy dog or cat therefore requires at least 50 ml of water/kg body weight per day to replace these losses.

Urine may be concentrated, dark and have a strong odour when the animal has consumed little fluid during the preceding 12 to 24 hours. If a lot of fluid is taken in, a large volume of paler urine will be produced.

Main substances present in filtrate and urine

Substance	Present in glomerular filtrate	Present in urine	Notes[1]
Water	+	+	Most of the water is reabsorbed. The hormone ADH regulates water reabsorption
Urea	+	+	Most urea remains in the urine
Amino acids	+	–	All reabsorbed
Glucose	+	–	All reabsorbed
Protein	+ (trace)	–	Reabsorbed
Salts: Sodium chloride Potassium	+ +	+ +	Most of these salts are reabsorbed. The levels of sodium and potassium are regulated by the hormone aldosterone (electrolyte balance)
Bicarbonate[2] (HCO_3^-)	+	+	Most reabsorbed
Hydrogen ions (H^+) and other acids[2]	+	+	Some hydrogen secreted into urine to regulate blood pH

1   Substances reabsorbed from filtrate are returned to the blood circulation
2   The balance of reabsorbed acids or alkalis present in urine is adjusted to maintain blood pH at 7.4; salts such as bicarbonate and acids such as hydrogen ions help to regulate blood pH between 7.35 and 7.45.

7.9   **Approximate fluid loss over 24 hours (ml/kg body weight per day)[1]**

Losses	Dog	Cat
Respiratory[2]/skin	20	20
Faecal	10–20	10–20
Urine[3]	20–60	10–20
Total	50–100	40–60

1   Approximate rate of urine production is 1–2 cm³/kg body weight/hour
2   Respiratory loss is obligate loss
3   10 ml/kg body weight/day is obligate urine loss

Some abnormalities of urine composition

Animals who develop *diabetes mellitus* (inability to regulate blood glucose) produce large volumes of dilute urine containing glucose. High glucose levels in blood interferes with normal reabsorption of water and some of the excess glucose is excreted in the urine. The urine of diabetic animals often has a characteristic sweet smell (like peardrop sweets).

Some animals produce *crystals* in urine. These may irritate the bladder, resulting in symptoms of cystitis (increased frequency of urination, bacterial infections, blood in urine). The animal can receive a special diet to minimize the formation of crystals.

Immunity and defence against disease

Immunity is the ability to resist disease. This section will consider how animals resist infections and overcome diseases caused by pathogens.

Infective microorganisms

Organisms that are too small to be seen with the naked eye are termed microorganisms or *microbes*.

Microbes that enter the body and cause diseases are called *pathogens*. Pathogens include bacteria, viruses, protozoa and fungi. (Some fungi produce large fruiting bodies, so not all fungi are microbes.)

If a pathogen gains entry to the body and overcomes defence mechanisms, then infection occurs and signs and symptoms of disease may develop. Disease due to infection causes stress while the animal overcomes the pathogen and restores homeostasis. It may take some time for recovery.

If ill health is due to infection caused by pathogens, care must be taken when handling and examining the animal as the disease may be transmissable (the pathogens could be transferred to another animal or human and cause disease in them). Until the cause of illness is diagnosed, procedures must be followed to minimize the risk of cross-infection between animals and between animals and humans:

- Isolate the sick animal
- Observe strict hygiene with handling and feeding routines
- Keep young children and pregnant women away from sick animals until veterinary diagnosis shows animals to be safe
- If disease is due to pathogenic infection, continue isolation and hygiene routines during treatment.

Non-specific defence mechanisms

Animals have a number of non-specific defence mechanisms that help to minimize invasion by any microorganisms, including pathogens (Figure 7.10).

Certain white cells are *phagocytes*; that is they are able to ingest some invading microbes and also debris from dead or infected cells. Phagocytosis is illustrated in Figure 7.11.

These mechanisms minimize the entry or multiplication of foreign particles, which may contain microbes, some of which may be pathogenic (disease-causing) in certain animals and harmless in other animal

7.10 Non-specific defence mechanisms

Structure/feature	Role in preventing entry of microorganisms
Skin	Forms a barrier
Skin secretions: sebum and sweat	Help to prevent growth of microbes
Blood clotting at wounds	Prevents blood loss and entry of microbes
Mucus secretion in respiratory system	Traps microbes during breathing. Mucus is then wafted to the throat and swallowed
Secretions on surface of eyes	Traps microbes. The enzyme lysozyme destroys some microbes
Wax in ear canal	Traps microbes
Stomach acids	Destroy many microbes on food before they multiply to infective levels
Phagocytes in blood (monocytes and neutrophils)	Ingest some microbes and cell debris
Macrophages in tissues	Ingest some microbes and cell debris

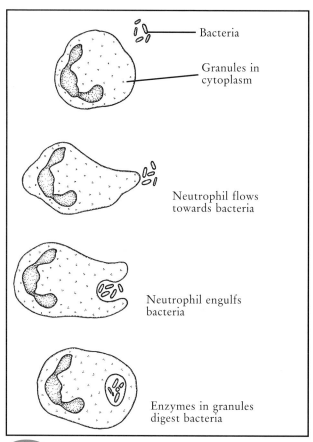

7.11 *Phagocytosis by a neutrophil.*

species. The absence of susceptibility in some animal species is called *innate immunity*. If the non-specific defence mechanisms fail, then the pathogen may multiply rapidly and cause disease.

Specific defence mechanisms

Animals have a number of specific defence mechanisms that help to minimize infections and disease and prevent reinfection with pathogens.

Specific defence mechanisms, which are activated when pathogens gain entry and start to multiply, are a function of the *immune system*. The blood and the lymphatic system contain specialized cells that mount a combined response to eliminate the disease-causing organism and resist future infections by that organism.

Specific mechanisms are less effective in certain situations:

- Young animals, which have a poorly developed immune system
- Aged animals, which are more susceptible to disease
- Sick animals.

Blood and lymph

The blood and the lymphatic system (described earlier) are both important for immunity. There are a number of different types of blood cell (Figure 7.12) but not all of them are directly involved in the defence against disease. Blood consists of:

- *Erythrocytes* (red blood cells): the most numerous cells in blood; they carry oxygen to all parts of the body
- *Leucocytes* (white blood cells): involved in the protection and defence of the body against diseases
- *Platelets* or *thrombocytes*: derived from larger cells (megakaryocytets) and are involved in blood clotting
- *Plasma*: the liquid part of blood.

Blood cells are suspended in a watery liquid (plasma) containing many substances – including antibodies, which can inactivate some pathogens.

Lymph contains antibodies, lymphocytes and other white cells which assist with the immune response.

Leucocytes (white blood cells)

Leucocytes are larger than erythrocytes but fewer in number. There are about 700 red blood cells for each white blood cell.

White cells form two groups:

- *Granulocytes*, occuring as neutrophils, basophils and eosinophils. Their cytoplasm, when stained, shows many granules and the nucleus is lobed
- Non-granular leucocytes (*agranulocytes*) are lymphocytes and monocytes. They have clear cytoplasm and a large unlobed nucleus.

The role of white blood cells is described in Figure 7.13.

Antigens and antibodies

An *antigen* is a protein or particle that causes a specific immune response by lymphocytes. *Antibodies* are complex proteins that are present in the blood plasma and lymph.

Microbes, tumour cells and cells invaded by viruses have proteins on their surfaces that are different from normal body cells. These are recognized as antigens (foreign to the body). The *B cells* (B-lymphocytes, Figure 7.13) produce specific antibodies that can destroy or inactivate the foreign particle or specific antigen. B cells are effective against many bacteria that invade the body.

Some *T cells* (T-lymphocytes, Figure 7.13) are able to destroy virus-infected cells and tumour cells without producing antibodies. Other T cells assist B cell immune responses.

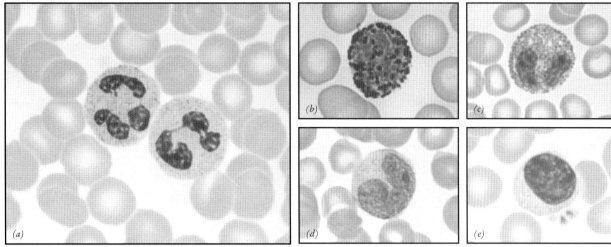

7.12 Blood cell types: (a) two neutrophils surrounded by erythrocytes; (b) basophil; (c) eosinophil; (d) monocyte; (e) lymphocyte.

7.13 White blood cell (leucocyte) types present in blood and lymph and their role in immunity

Type	Role
Granulocytes	
Neutrophils	Become phagocytic – they ingest bacteria and dead cells Release the enzyme lysozyme, which destroys certain bacteria
Basophils	Secrete histamine and accumulate at sites of inflammation Enable other white cells to assist with healing Generally thought to be involved with allergic responses Form *mast cells* when in tissues
Eosinophils	Increase when parasitic infections and allergies occur Help to reduce the effects of inflammation and allergic reactions Destroy antigen/antibody complexes
Agranulocytes (non-granular white blood cells)	
Monocytes	Become phagocytic – they ingest cell debris and bacteria in infected areas Assist B cells and T cells in specific immune responses Can move into tissues, where they are called *macrophages*, so play an important role in healing
Lymphocytes	Two types: B-lymphocytes or B cells, and T-lymphocytes or T cells
B cells	Produced and mature in the red bone marrow Produce specific proteins – *antibodies*, which inactivate *antigens* B cells produce long-lived memory cells for long-term protection
T cells	Mature in the thymus and spleen Inactivate antigens present on bacteria, viruses and tumour cells, through specific *cell-mediated* responses, without producing free antibodies Produce long-lived memory cells for long-term protection

The animal may be unwell while B cells and T cells increase in number to eliminate the antigen, but a small population of *memory cells* (Figure 7.13) remains to destroy the antigen more quickly next time. Because memory cells survive for long periods, they are activated rapidly when the same antigen challenges the immune system at a future date. B cells and T cells increase quickly and are able to eliminate the antigen before the full-blown disease develops. This explains why certain diseases are only contracted once in a lifetime.

- Immunity due to the activity of B cells and their antibodies is termed *humoral immunity*
- Immunity due to the activity of T cells is termed *cell-mediated immunity*
- B and T cells both produce long-lived memory cells which result in a rapid response to future invasions by a specific pathogen. This rapid response often prevents the disease from developing a second time.

Vaccination

Animals are vaccinated or inoculated against certain diseases and protection usually lasts for approximately one year. This procedure stimulates the animal's own B and T cells to increase in numbers when specially treated non-infective viruses and bacteria are used (a vaccine). Antibody levels are boosted by vaccination and the animal is able to resist the disease-causing organisms present in the normal population of animals. Regular and timely booster vaccination is important to maintain the correct level of resistance in the animal.

Figure 7.14 describes different types of immunity.

- *Active immunity* comes about through stimulation of the immune response (B and T cells) in the animal
- *Passive immunity* confers short-lived specific immunity, without stimulating the animal's own immune system.

Tumours

When cells multiply more quickly than they should, they may form a tumour. Some tumours are benign and slow growing but cause problems when the tumour presses on a nerve or blood vessel, for example. Other tumours are more aggressive, or malignant: the tumour may damage the organ where it develops and may form secondary tumours in

Type of immunity	Definition and explanation
Active	An active response by the immune system following exposure to specific antigens. Immunity may last up to a year or longer. May be naturally or artificially acquired
Naturally acquired	Active response following a natural exposure to antigens (an *infection*)
Artificially acquired	Active response following an artificial exposure to antigens (a *vaccination*)
Passive (artificial)	Readymade antibodies received from an external source (e.g. tetanus antibodies raised in horses and given to dogs following serious puncture wounds). Passive immunity declines and no specific B or T cells or memory cells are activated in the recipient
Passive (natural)	Antibodies that cross the placenta and are present in milk confer some ready-made immunity to a young animal while its own immune system matures
Innate	Certain species are immune to some diseases to which other animals are susceptible (e.g. canine distemper does not infect cats)

other systems by a process called *metastasis*. Malignant tumours are sometimes called cancer.

Normally cells that change and multiply at an abnormal rate are constantly eliminated by T cells (and other helping leucocytes) before they form tumours. As animals age they are less able to fight off infections and many other diseases, including developing tumours. The weakened defence system means that tumour cells may multiply more quickly than the body's defence system can cope with.

Further reading

Lane DR and Cooper B (eds) (1995) *Veterinary Nursing*, Chapters 14, 15, 22, 24. Butterworth-Heinemann, Oxford

Tortora GJ (1994) *Introduction to the Human Body: The Essentials of Anatomy and Physiology* 3rd edn. Harper Collins, London

Wilson KJW and Waugh A (1996) *Anatomy and Physiology in Health and Illness*, 8th edn. Churchill Livingstone, Edinburgh

8 Use of medicines

Sally Anne Argyle

This chapter is designed to give information on:

- The definition of the term 'veterinary medicine'
- The main categories of veterinary medicine
- The main routes used for the administration of drugs
- The advantages and disadvantages of each route of administration
- The equipment used in the administration of medicines
- Practical information regarding the administration of drugs
- The legislation and practicalities regarding the safe handling, storage and dispensing of veterinary medicines

Veterinary medicines

The definition of a veterinary medicine is 'any medicinal product intended for animals' (Bishop, 1998) and applies to veterinary medicinal products offered for sale *inter alia* (among others) in the form of proprietary medicinal products and readymade veterinary medicinal products.

The main categories of veterinary medicines are listed in Figure 8.1.

Routes of administration

The most frequently used routes of administration of drugs are summarized in Figure 8.2.

Oral administration

This is a frequently used route of administration.

- Drugs to be administered orally are most often in a solid form as a tablet or a capsule, or in a liquid form as a suspension or a solution
  - In a suspension the drug is dispersed in the fluid in the form of fine liquid or solid particles; the drug particles have a tendency to settle at the bottom of the container when the vessel in which the drug is contained is left standing
  - In a solution the drug is dissolved in the liquid, giving a homogeneous mixture
- Common sense should be exercised when handling any drugs. Special care should be taken by individuals with known sensitivities to particular drugs. For example, penicillin sensitivity is widespread in the general population and owners expected to administer drugs

should be informed. Ideally, gloves should be worn at all times
- It should be determined whether or not the drug should be given with food. For example, the absorption of the antifungal drug griseofulvin is enhanced by the presence of fatty food, whereas the antibacterial ampicillin is best given on an empty stomach
- Figure 8.3 illustrates how an animal may be restrained for the administration of a tablet or capsule:
  - The mouth is held open and the medicine is dropped or placed at the back of the tongue
  - The mouth should then be allowed to close but the head held slightly tipped back
  - Once the mouth is closed, the animal will swallow as a reflex action to the tablet or capsule on the back of the tongue
- Capsules should not be split
- Some tablets (for example, many of the cytotoxic drugs used to treat neoplasia) should not be divided
- Liquid suspensions should be well shaken to resuspend drug particles that will have settled to the bottom of the container
- Administration of liquid medication is best performed with a syringe; with certain preparations a plastic dropper is provided
- Liquids are best administered into the side of the mouth, at a slow rate, allowing the animal to swallow frequently
- A crop tube may be used for the oral administration of drugs to birds (see Chapter 4)
- Some drugs may be administered in the drinking water. This can be useful for the medication of large numbers of animals but is unreliable due to the variability in water intake.

8.1 Examples of some of the main categories of veterinary medicines

Category	Definition and role	Examples
Analgesics	Drugs designed to relieve pain	Opioids such as pethidine and morphine NSAIDs* such as ketoprofen and carprofen Local anaesthetics such as lignocaine
Anaesthetics	Drugs used to produce unconsciousness, immobility and a loss of sensation such as pain	Injectable agents such as propofol and thiopentone sodium Inhalational agents such as halothane and isoflurane
Antibacterials	Drugs that kill (bacteriocidal) or inhibit the growth (bacteriostatic) of bacteria	Sulphonamides and tetracyclines are bacteriostatic; ampicillin, amoxycillin and streptomycin are bacteriocidal
Antidiarrhoeals	Used in the treatment of diarrhoea	Loperamide, kaolin
Antidysrhythmics	Drugs used to abolish or control abnormal heart rhythms	Lignocaine, procainamide, tocainamide and mexiletine
Antiepileptics	Drugs used to prevent or abolish seizures	Phenobarbitone, primidone and phenytoin
Antifungals	Drugs that kill (fungicidal) or inhibit the growth (fungistatic) of fungi	Orally administered preparations such as griseofulvin Topically administered preparations such as ketoconazole
Antineoplastics/ Cytotoxic drugs	Drugs used to treat neoplasia	Cisplatin, cyclophosphamide, vincristine
Antitussives	Drugs that suppress coughing	Butorphanol and dextrometorphan
Anti-emetics	Drugs that prevent vomiting	Metoclopramide and acepromazine
Anti-inflammatories	Used to reduce inflammation	NSAIDs* such as ketoprofen and carprofen Corticosteroids such as prednisolone
Anti-ulcer drugs	For treatment and prevention of gastric ulcers	Cimetidine, sucralfate, omeprazole, misoprostil
Bronchodilators	Drugs that dilate the bronchial smooth muscle	Etamiphylline camsylate, clembuterol, theophylline
Cardiac drugs	Drugs that exert their effect on the cardiovascular system	Digoxin, enalapril, hydralazine
Diuretics	Drugs that enhance water loss through the kidneys	Frusemide, spironolactone, hydrochlorothiazide
Ectoparasiticides	Drugs used in the treatment and prevention of external parasite infestation (e.g. flea control)	Imidacloprid, fipronil, permethrin
Emetics	Drugs that induce vomiting	Xylazine
Endoparasiticides	Drugs used in the treatment and prevention of internal parasitic infections (e.g. tapeworm and round worm)	Piperazine, fenbendazole, praziquantal
Hormones	Substances produced endogenously (within the body) by endocrine glands. Naturally occurring or synthetic hormones may be administered exogenously	Oestradiol benzoate, proligesterone, methyltestosterone
Laxatives	Substances that aid the passage of faecal material	Liquid paraffin, lactulose, bran
Sedatives	Drugs used to calm an animal, often prior to anaesthetic induction or for minor procedures such as radiography	Acepromazine, xylazine
Vaccines	Substances that stimulate active immunity in the animal to an organism such as a bacterium, virus or parasite	Canine parvovirus vaccine, leptospirosis vaccine, parainfluenza virus vaccine

* NSAIDs = non-steroidal anti-inflammatory drugs

A summary of the main routes used for drug administration

Route	Detail	Advantages	Disadvantages
Oral	Tablets, capsules or liquid	No pain for the animal (versus injection) Owner may administer the drug	Some drugs cannot be given orally, e.g. may be broken down by the gastric acid such as penicillin G Animal may not be compliant, making dosing difficult, especially if the drug cannot be administered with food Gastrointestinal disease may intefere with drug absorption
By injection (parenteral)	Solutions or suspensions Examples of routes include: • Intradermal (i.d.) • Subcutaneous (s.c.) • Intramuscular (i.m.) • Intravenous (i.v.) • Intraperitoneal (i.p.)	Rapid systemic drug levels achieved, especially with i.v. route No reliance on gastrointestinal function	Pain of injection Local reaction to injection may occur Risk of self-injection Generally not suitable for owner administration Risk of damage to internal organs, e.g. i.p. injection
Intraosseus	Useful for administration of fluids and drugs to neonates or where it is not possible to access a peripheral vessel	Rapid access Useful in neonates and reptiles	More technically difficult than above
Intranasal	Limited to certain vaccines	Can provoke local immunity	Many animals resent this route
Rectal	Infrequently used Mainly confined to laxatives		
Transdermal	Mainly used for drugs that are metabolized by the liver so rapidly that oral administration of the drug is prevented	Ease of application	Risk of absorption by the administrator
Topical	Examples include drugs formulated as lotions, ointments, gels and shampoos	Ease of administration Direct delivery to required site Owner can administer	Absorption of drug through the skin of the administrator Animal can lick the drug Limited to sites that can be accessed, e.g. skin, ears, eyes
Inhalational	Limited to inhalational anaesthetics such as halothane, and some drugs administered by nebulization (e.g. gentamicin)	Nebulized drugs used to treat respiratory disease are delivered directly to required site of action, minimizing systemic side effects Non-invasive	Limited application Specialized equipment required

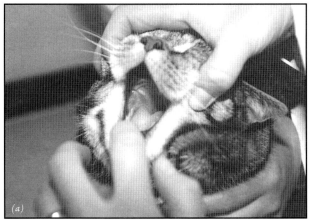
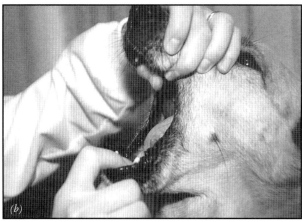

8.3 *Tablet administration. (a) Method used for restraint of a cat in order to administer a tablet or a capsule. (b) Similar method used to restrain a dog for the same purpose. In both cases the tablet or capsule may then be placed at the back of the tongue and the mouth allowed to close. The head should be kept tilted upwards until swallowing has occurred.*

Parenteral administration

This is a common method of drug administration.

Equipment

Hypodermic needles and syringes are the main pieces of equipment used to administer drugs parenterally. Figure 8.4 illustrates examples of hypodermic needles and syringes.

- Needles are sized according to their gauge (G). The gauge determines the bore of the needle. Commonly used sizes are 23 G, 21 G, 20 G, 18 G, 16 G and 14 G. The bore of the needle decreases with increasing gauge size. The needles have a bevelled end, which facilitates entry through the skin
- Each gauge can also come in a variety of lengths, commonly used ones being $^1/_2$ inch (12 mm), 1 inch (25 mm), $1^1/_2$ inch (40 mm).

For intravenous administration of drugs, a catheter may be used (Figure 8.5).

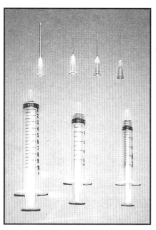

8.4 *Some examples of hypodermic needles and syringes frequently used for the parenteral administration of veterinary medicines. Needles (from left to right): 18 G, $1^1/_2$ inch (1.2 x 40 mm); 20 G, 1 inch (0.9 x 25 mm); 21 G, 1 inch (0.8 x 25 mm); 23 G, $1^1/_4$ inch (0.6 x 30 mm). Syringes (from left to right): 10 ml; 5 ml; 2.5 ml.*

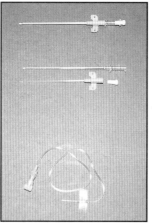

8.5 *Examples of catheters. Top: a fully assembled over-the-needle catheter with the stylet lying within the Teflon cannula. Centre: components of an over-the-needle cannula, with the stylet lying at the top; beneath it is shown the Teflon cannula, which is placed within the blood vessel and is secured in place by taping or stitching to the skin; to the right of the cannula lies the plug that seals it when it is not in use. Bottom: a butterfly cannula, which consists of the needle with two plastic flaps (hence butterfly), attached to a length of plastic tubing. The needle can be taped to the limb by the butterfly flaps. Also known as a scalp vein set.*

Practical points on parenteral administration

- Drugs for injection may come as solutions, emulsions or suspensions. Suspensions should be well shaken to resuspend the drug
- All equipment used for parenteral administration should be sterile and should not be reused
- Bottles containing drugs for parenteral administration are usually equipped with a rubber bung (Figure 8.6). To draw up the drug:
  - The bottle should be inverted

- The needle on the end of the syringe should be inserted into the bottle
- The plunger of the syringe should then be drawn out of the barrel of the syringe, drawing the drug into the syringe
- Drugs for parenteral administration may also come in individual glass vials
- Excess air should be removed from the syringe by inverting the syringe (needle uppermost) and gently tapping the barrel to bring the air to the top. The air can then be gently expelled without spraying the drug. The use of a sterile gauze pad to absorb any drug leakage from the needle is useful
- Care should be taken to avoid accidental self-injection and skin contact with the drugs being used (gloves should be worn)
- After use, all needles should be disposed of in a sharps bin (Figure 8.7).

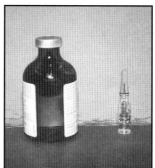

8.6 *Drug bottles. Left: a typical multidose bottle containing a drug in liquid form for parenteral administration. The bottle is equipped with a rubber bung through which the needle is placed, allowing the drug to be drawn up into a syringe. Right: a glass vial, designed for single use. The top of the vial is snapped off, the drug is used and then the empty vial is disposed of in a sharps disposal container.*

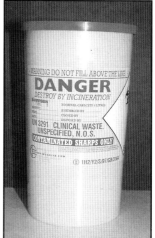

8.7 *Example of a yellow container used for the disposal of sharps such as used hypodermic needles, catheters and glass vials. Once full, these containers are sealed and incinerated.*

Sites for injection

 Follow the manufacturer's directions with regard to the route of administration. For example, some drugs are highly irritant and can only be given intravenously, or drugs recommended for intramuscular administration may be too poorly absorbed to achieve adequate levels in the blood if they are given subcutaneously.

Intradermal injection

This route is used primarily for allergy testing.

- Figure 8.8 demonstrates the site of the dermis in relation to the other skin layers
- Only very small volumes can be injected into the dermis.

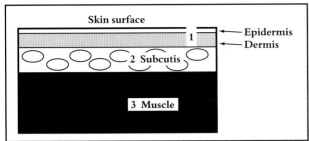

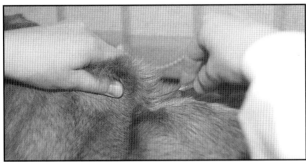

8.8 *The layers of the skin and underlying tissues, illustrating the site of (1) intradermal injection, (2) subcutaneous injection and (3) intramuscular injection.*

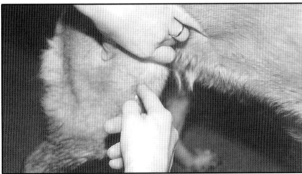

8.9 *For subcutaneous administration, the skin is pulled up and the needle is inserted into the skin tent. As in this example, a common site for subcutaneous injection is under the loose skin overlying the shoulders. The dog's head is to the left and tail to the right.*

Subcutaneous injection

This is often performed at the scruff of the neck, but may be performed at any site where there is sufficient loose skin.

- Figure 8.8 shows the location of the subcutis in relation to the other skin layers
- The skin is raised with one hand and the needle is inserted under the skin. Negative pressure should be applied to the syringe to ensure that the needle has not been placed in a blood vessel. The plunger should then be depressed slowly to discharge the drug from the syringe
- Absorption of the drug is quite slow from this site
- Subcutaneous injections tend to elicit lees pain than other parentetal routes
- Figure 8.9 illustrates the technique for subcutaneous injection.

Intramuscular injection

This is the injection of the drug into a muscle mass.
The best sites are those with a large muscle bulk.

- A commonly used site in the dog and cat is the muscle mass at the front of the thigh. The muscles here are the quadriceps (Figure 8.10)
- In birds, the pectoral muscles (those overlying the breast) are preferred
- Intramuscular injection is quite painful and only small volumes can be injected at a given time. For example, approximately 1.5 ml would be the maximum desirable volume for intramuscular injection into the hindlimb of a medium-sized dog
- Care should be taken to avoid blood vessels (apply negative pressure on the syringe prior to injection). The inadvertent insertion of the needle into a blood vessel is much more likely using this route than the subcutaneous route.

Intravenous injection

This involves injection directly into a vein.

- The most commonly used vessels in dogs and cats are the cephalic vein, the jugular vein and the lateral saphenous vein (Figures 8.11, 8.12 and 8.13). The marginal ear vein is commonly used in rabbits (Figure 8.14)

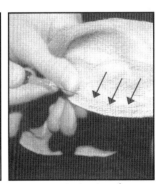

8.10 *Site for intramuscular injection in the hindlimb of a dog.*

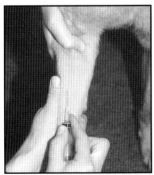

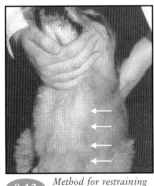

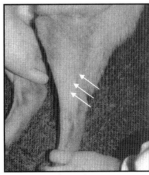

8.11 *The cephalic vein, which runs down the anterior aspect of the front limb, is commonly used for drug administration. Note how the person restraining the animal raises the vein with their thumb. The person administering the injection then uses their thumb alongside the vessel to stabilize it while the tip of the needle is placed into the vein.*

8.12 *Method for restraining an animal to allow injection into a jugular vein. The animal could also be restrained in lateral recumbency. The thumb of the hand at the bottom of the picture is applying pressure to raise the vein. Normally the hair overlying the vessel would be clipped allowing better visualization and a cleaner site. The white arrows indicate the approximate location of the vein.*

8.13 *The saphenous vein runs down the lateral (outer) aspect of the hindlimb. Usually the animal is held in lateral recumbency and the vein is raised by applying pressure behind the stifle joint. The white arrows indicate the position of the vein.*

8.14 *Injection into the marginal ear vein on the inner aspect of a rabbit's ear. The vessel is raised by the application of pressure at the ear base. The black arrows indicate the location of the vein.*

- This route of administration bypasses the need for drug absorption and so rapid systemic drug levels are achieved
- This route is much more suitable for the administration of large volumes of drug
- A catheter should be used at all times for the administration of drugs into the jugular vein, since due to the mobility of the vessel the risk of perivascular leakage is too great when using a needle
- The vessel is raised by an assistant. It may be necessary to clip or shave the hair overlying the vessel for better visualization. The skin is swabbed with 70% ethanol and the tip of the needle or catheter is placed in the vein. At this point, if a needle attached to a syringe is being used, then once it is confirmed that the needle tip is in the vessel (negative pressure on the syringe draws blood back into the hub of the needle), the assistant removes the pressure from the vessel so that the drug may be injected into the vein
- Injection of the drug should be performed slowly unless it is specified otherwise.

 Some drugs are extremely irritant. This includes many of the cytotoxic drugs such as vincristine and doxorubicin. These should be administered using intravenous catheters to avoid the risk of perivascular leakage of the drug. It is best to flush these catheters with non-heparinized 0.9% sterile saline as some of the drugs (e.g. doxorubicin) precipitate in the presence of heparin.

Intraperitoneal injection
This is administration of the drug into the peritoneal cavity.

- It is mainly used for the intraperitoneal administration of fluids in small patients and neonates and the administration of injectable anaesthetics in small mammals
- There is a risk of penetration of abdominal viscera
- This route provides a large surface area for drug absorption
- The best position is with the animal's forelimbs raised off the ground; the needle is inserted just caudal to the umbilicus angling the needle cranially.

Intraosseus injection
The drug is delivered directly into the bone marrow cavity.

- This is a useful route when it is not possible to access a peripheral vein such as the cephalic or the saphenous (a common situation in neonates)
- Sites used include the trochanteric fossa of the femur, the proximal tibia and the greater tubercle of the humerus.

Intranasal administration
This route is used for the administration of certain vaccines, such as the *Bordetella bronchiseptica* vaccine in dogs.

- A special delivery nozzle is supplied with the vaccine for delivery into the nasal cavity
- The nozzle is attached to the syringe containing the vaccine
- With the animal's head tipped upwards, the tip of the nozzle is inserted gently into one of its nostrils
- The vaccine is then delivered into the nasal cavity.

Rectal administration
This route of drug administration is less frequently used in animals than in humans.

- The lining of the large intestine provides a large surface area for the absorption of drugs delivered by this route
- Enema solutions are delivered per rectum
- Gloves should be worn
- Urinary catheters or rubber tubing, in conjunction with syringes, may be used for the administration of solutions that are not already supplied in long-nozzled delivery tubes designed for the purpose.

Transdermal administration
This route, in which the drug is applied on the skin to be absorbed through the skin and act systemically, is not commonly used in veterinary medicine.

- Examples of drugs administered in this way are glyceryl trinitrate (a drug used in heart failure to dilate the veins) and ivermectin (a drug used against worms)
- Care should be exercised to protect the administrator from absorbing the drug
- The drug is usually applied to a site that is inaccessible to the animal (for example, the inner aspect of the ear flap – the pinna) and that has minimal hair cover (clipping may be required).

Topical administration
This commonly used route encompasses the administration of drugs to the ear, the eye and the skin.

- Topical application is commonly used in the treatment and prevention of skin conditions
- Care should be taken to avoid contact with the skin of the person administering the treatment
- Gloves should be worn
- Excess hair may need to be clipped from the site to allow access to the skin
- There is a wide variety of formulations for topical administration, including the following:
  - Creams – water-miscible, non-greasy and easily removed by washing and licking
  - Ointments – greasy, insoluble in water and generally anhydrous; more difficult to remove than creams
  - Dusting powders – finely divided powders
  - Lotions – aqueous solutions or suspension, evaporating to leave a thin film of drug at the site
  - Gels – semi-solid aqueous solutions, easy to apply and remove
  - Sprays
  - Shampoos.

Ophthalmic administration (application to the eye)
Figure 8.15 demonstrates the administration of an eye preparation.

 Care should be taken to avoid contact between the dispenser / container and the surface of the eye, as this would contaminate the container and may also traumatize the eye.

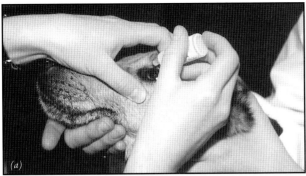

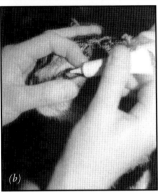

 Administration of (a) eye drops to a dog and (b) eye ointment to a cat.

- The eyelids are held apart with the thumb and the index finger
- Liquid solutions (eye drops) are dropped on to the surface of the eye; generally one or two drops is sufficient
- Eye ointment is semi-solid and more greasy in consistency. A length of ointment can be squeezed on to the lower palpebral surface (lower eyelid border); when the animal blinks, the ointment is distributed over the eye surface.

Aural administration (application to the ear)

Ear disease is extremely common in small animals and this is a frequently used route of administration.

> ⚠ Do not poke anything like a cotton bud into the ear.

- Any loose dirt or debris should be removed from the ear using a tissue or a piece of cotton wool
- The pinna of the ear is grasped gently and pulled upwards while the animal is well restrained

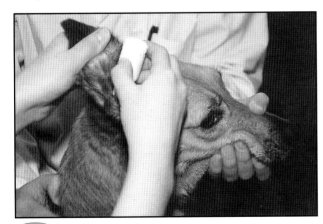

8.16 Administration of ear ointment.

- The tip of the dispenser is then placed into the vertical canal of the ear and the drug is administered to the ear (Figure 8.16)
- The base of the ear is gently massaged to distribute the medication within the ear canal.

Inhalation

Administration of drugs by inhalation is mainly confined to gaseous and volatile anaesthetics such as halothane, isoflurane and nitrous oxide. The equipment required for the administration of these is covered in Chapter 8 of *BSAVA Manual of Veterinary Nursing*.

Nebulization

A nebulizer (Figure 8.17) produces small droplets forming a mist in which the drug is contained. The mist can then be inhaled by the animal.

- Nebulization is useful in the treatment of respiratory disease as an adjunct to systemic treatment
- This route is useful for the administration of drugs that are very toxic when administered systemically. A good example of this would be the antibacterial gentamicin, which can be associated with nephrotoxicity (toxicity to the kidneys) when administered systemically.
- Care must be taken to prevent exposure of personnel.

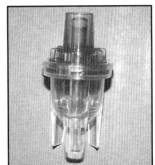

8.17 A nebulizer. The nebulizer unscrews so that the drug solution can be placed in the central chamber. One end is then connected to an oxygen supply and the other to a face mask. The oxygen flowing through the nebulizer creates a mist containing the drug, which is then inhaled by the animal.

Legislation

The legislation regarding the handling, usage, storage, dispensing, disposal and prescribing of veterinary medicines is covered in some detail in Chapter 2 of *BSAVA Manual of Veterinary Nursing*. Due to the importance of this topic, pertinent points are also outlined here.

Relevant legislation includes:

- Medicines Act 1968
- Medicines (Restrictions on the Administration of Veterinary Medicinal Products) Regulations 1994
- Misuse of Drugs Act 1971
- Health and Safety at Work Act 1974
- Control of Substances Hazardous to Health Regulations 1988.

Figure 8.18 lists the legal categories of veterinary medicines.

Handling of veterinary medicines

Control of Substances Hazardous to Health Regulations 1988

COSHH regulations relate to work involving substances that are deemed to be hazardous to health. These include

8.18 Legal categories of veterinary medicines

Category	Definition	Examples
General Sales List (GSL)	Sale of these is unrestricted. May be sold by a veterinary surgeon to anyone, whether they are a client or not	Nitroscanate, a wormer used in dogs Piperazine citrate, a wormer used in dogs and cats Some shampoos and ear cleaning preparations
Pharmacy only (P)	Only supplied by veterinary surgeons to animals under their care. May also be supplied over the counter by pharmacists	Few veterinary drugs fall into this category
Pharmacy and Merchant's List (PML)	Supplied by veterinary surgeons to animals under their care. May also be supplied by pharmacists or registered merchants. A small range of anthelmintics may also be sold by registered merchants and saddlers to owners of dogs, cats and horses	Many of the worming drugs and ectoparasiticides
Prescription only (POM)	Supplied by veterinary surgeons to animals under their care. May also be supplied by pharmacists but only on a veterinary prescription	Antibacterial drugs, animal vaccines
Controlled drugs (CD)	Drugs capable of being abused. Under the control of the Misuse of Drugs Act. Divided into five Schedules:	
	• **Schedule 1** Veterinary surgeons have no authority to possess these	Cannabis, LSD
	• **Schedule 2** A requisition in writing required to obtain these and need to be recorded in a register and kept in a locked receptacle	Morphine, pethidine
	• **Schedule 3** As for Schedule 2 but transactions do not need to be recorded in a register	Pentobarbitone, buprenorphine
	• **Schedule 4** Exempt from most restrictions of controlled drugs	Benzodiazepines
	• **Schedule 5** Exempt from all controlled drug requirements except the need to keep invoices for 2 years	Preparations containing cocaine, codeine and morphine at less than a specified amount

certain veterinary medicines and animal products. It is the employer's responsibility to perform a risk assessment of each of these substances used. Manufacturers of veterinary products provide a product safety data sheet to aid this risk assessment. *The employer must aim to prevent or control exposure of employees to these substances by information, instruction and training.* A responsibility also extends to the client and the client should therefore be clearly informed with regard to the safe handling and disposal of the medicine.

 Anyone involved in the handling or dispensing of veterinary medicines should be trained. Qualified veterinary nurses may supply POM products provided they do so under the authority of a veterinary surgeon.

Practical points for handling and dispensing of medicines

- Direct contact between the skin of the person dispensing the drug and the drug itself should be avoided. This can be achieved through wearing protective clothing such as disposable gloves, or by using pill counters
- The veterinary surgeon should be notified of skin abrasions and the dispensing of drugs should be avoided under these circumstances

- Particular care should be taken with drugs marked teratogenic (capable of causing a malformation in the developing embryo) or carcinogenic (capable of causing cancer)
- The data sheet should always be consulted, especially if the individual dispensing the drug is not familiar with the particular drug in question
- Drugs should be appropriately labelled and dispensed in an appropriate container (see separate section)
- The client should be given clear instructions with regard to the safe handling, storage and disposal of the medicine (for example, some products should be kept refrigerated). It may be necessary to give the client disposable gloves for the application of certain products for external application.

Cytotoxic drugs

Cytotoxic drugs, such as cyclophosphamide, require extreme care in handling and administration as many are highly toxic and irritant.

- Appropriate protective clothing should be worn
- The drugs should be prepared in a designated area
- Tablets must never be divided or crushed
- These drugs should not be handled by pregnant women.

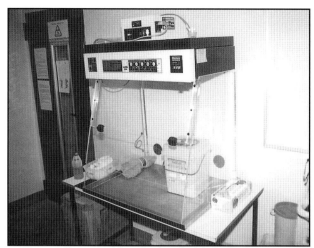

 Self-contained fume hood used solely for the dispensing of cytotoxic drugs. The hood contains a sharps bin and a filter is attached to the top of the hood. The stainless steel base allows for easy cleaning.

Figure 8.19 illustrates a self-contained fume hood which may be used to dispense cytotoxic drugs. All procedures are carried out within the hood, which is provided with a filter, thereby protecting the individual from inhalation of the drug. It also clearly allows the designation of an area in which cytotoxic drugs are to be handled.

Labelling

Details covering prescription writing and labelling are given in Chapter 2 of *BSAVA Manual of Veterinary Nursing*, which also gives the requirements for the labelling of veterinary medicines. Figure 8.20 gives an example of a label for a veterinary drug. Abbreviations commonly used in prescription writing are shown in Figure 8.21.

```
For Animal Treatment Only
Mr Ebb's dog Flo
21 Seaside Lane
Beach Town
1/1/2000


20 Ampicillin tablets 250mg
1 tablet twice daily without food

Keep all medicines out of
the reach of children

S.A. Argyle, MRCVS
Veterinary Surgeon
1 Seaside Lane
Beach Town
```

8.20 *Example of the correct labelling of a veterinary medicine.*

8.21 Abbreviations commonly used in prescription writing

Abbreviation	Latin phrase	Meaning
bid	*bis in die*	Twice daily
od	*omne die*	Every day
qid	*quater in die*	Four times daily
sid	*semel in die*	Once daily
tid	*ter in die*	Three times daily

Essential information which *must be legally provided* on the label includes:

- The statement 'For animal treatment only'
- The name and address of the owner and the identity of the animal (i.e. the animal's name)
- The date
- The statement 'Keep all medicines out of the reach of children'
- The name and address of the veterinary surgeon.

Information that it is *recommended* should appear on the label includes:

- Details of the drug (name, strength and amount)
- Instructions for administration
- Instructions for storage.

Containers

Many of the veterinary medicines may be dispensed from bulk containers and should therefore be packaged in suitable containers when dispensed to the public.

- Reclosable child-resistant containers made of light-resistant glass, rigid plastic or aluminium should be used. Elderly or infirm clients may require more easily opened containers and discretion may be operated in these circumstances
- Blister-packed medicines may be dispensed in paperboard cartons or wallets
- Paper envelopes and plastic bags are not acceptable as sole containers of products
- Creams, dusting powders, ointments, powders and pessaries should be supplied in wide-mouthed jars made of glass or plastic
- Light-sensitive medicines should be dispensed in opaque or dark-coloured containers
- Certain liquids for external use, as specified under the Medicines (Fluted Bottles) Regulations 1978, should be dispensed in fluted bottles (with vertical ridges), so that they are discernible by touch. These bottles are no longer in production and so may be difficult to obtain at present. If possible, these liquids should therefore be dispensed in the manufacturer's container.

Calculation of drug dosages

The ultimate responsibility for the calculation of the correct drug dosage for an animal rests with the veterinary surgeon. Nurses performing this task should always check with the veterinary surgeon responsible for the case.

The calculation of a dose for a particular animal is usually worked out in terms of the weight of the drug per kilogram body weight of the animal.

Example

A puppy weighing 5 kg requires worming with piperazine citrate. The dose rate is 125 mg/kg. The tablets give 500 mg each. How many tablets are required to worm this puppy?

The dose will be the dose rate multiplied by the weight of the puppy:

Dose = 125 x 5 = 625 mg.

The number of tablets will be the dose divided by the tablet weight:

Number of tablets = 625/500 = 1¼ tablets.

Calculation of drug dosages is covered in more detail in Chapter 2 of *BSAVA Manual of Veterinary Nursing*.

Storage of veterinary medicines

- Drugs should be stored correctly for several important reasons:
  - To ensure the optimum shelf life of the drug and to protect it from damage due to inappropriate storage
  - To protect the public from access to potentially dangerous drugs and to protect the employer and employees on the premises
  - To allow effective monitoring of drug stocks, which is essential for stock control and the monitoring of expiry dates
- Store in accordance with the manufacturer's instructions
- Refrigeration must be available and maintained between 2°C and 8°C. Refrigerators should be fitted with a maximum/minimum thermometer to allow monitoring of the temperature. Insulin and vaccines are examples of products that must be kept refrigerated
- The designated storage area must be inaccessible to the public
- Storage areas should be kept clean and should be well ventilated. Eating or drinking should be forbidden in this area
- Flammable products should be stored in appropriate cabinets
- Dates of delivery should be logged and marked on products. For multi-use products, date of first use should be marked on the product
- Products returned by clients should not be reused as they may have been inappropriately stored

- An effective stock control system should be implemented that allows routine checking and detection of products requiring reordering or approaching their expiry date
- Controlled drugs (see Figure 8.18) in Schedule 2 and some in Schedule 3 must be stored in a locked cabinet that is fixed in position, e.g. attached to a wall. Keys for this cabinet should only be available to the veterinary surgeon or an authorized person designated by the veterinary surgeon. It is recommended that other drugs such as ketamine, which are liable to abuse although not classed as controlled drugs, should also be stored in a locked cabinet
- Drugs in consulting rooms and in vehicles should be kept to a minimum and should not include controlled drugs
- P, PML and GSL drugs may be displayed to the public but only 'dummy' packs may be used
- POM drugs may not be displayed to the public, but posters advertising them may be displayed within the veterinary practice since this is only advertising to clients and not the public.

Further reading

Bishop Y (1998) *The Veterinary Formulary*, 4th edn. The Pharmaceutical Press, Wallingford

Bishop Y (1998) *British Veterinary Association Code of Practice on Medicines.* BVA, London

McCurnin DM (1998) (ed.) *Clinical Textbook for Veterinary Technicians,* 4th edn. WB Saunders, Philadelphia

NOAH (1995) *Animal Medicines: A User's Guide*

Gorman NT (1998) (ed.) *Canine Medicine and Therapeutics,* 4th edn. Blackwell Science, Oxford

9 Animal first aid

Sue Dallas

This chapter is designed to give information on:

- Definition of the term first aid and its limitations
- Reasons for patient evaluation
- The need for obtaining a good case history, and what should be included
- Allowed emergency procedures to maintain life until the veterinary surgeon arrives
- Basic resuscitation techniques
- Emergency procedures for common first aid situations

Introduction

First aid is defined as the immediate treatment of injured animals or those suffering from sudden illness.

Although veterinary nurses do not have greater legal powers than lay people, in situations requiring first aid they will have far greater knowledge of anatomy and physiology, and of the specific emergency first aid techniques required until the arrival of a veterinary surgeon.

In practice, nurses may be faced with emergency situations requiring evaluation and stabilization until the arrival of the veterinary surgeon. Due to the nature of these emergencies it is important that:

- A part of the practice is set up with the required equipment and drugs
- A triage of treatment is formulated (the process of examination and rapid classification of emergency cases by the urgency with which treatment is required)
- A plan for initial evaluation of a severely injured animal is established and followed.

When evaluating the patient, it must be borne in mind that some situations will allow plenty of time to attend to the injuries or problems, whereas other situations are so severe that the animal will die if urgent and emergency care is not initiated immediately (Figure 9.1).

If possible, always have a detailed case history ready for the veterinary surgeon's arrival. This should include:

- Name and address of owner
- Telephone numbers (home, work, mobile phone)
- Species, breed, age and sex of injured animal
- Idea of the extent of injury
- Time of admission.

9.1 Evaluation and urgency

Life-threatening:

- Cardiopulmonary arrest (heart and breathing have stopped)
- Airway obstruction
- Respiratory arrest
- Haemorrhage from a major artery or vein
- Anaphylaxis (acute allergic reaction).

Immediate action:

- Multiple deep lacerations, haemorrhage, with hypovolaemia (low blood volume circulating in the blood vessels)
- Profound shock
- Penetrating wounds of the thorax or abdomen
- Head injuries
- Respiratory distress
- Spinal injury.

Urgent:

- Extensive muscular or skeletal injuries
- Acute to overwhelming infection
- Compound fractures
- Dystocia (difficulty during parturition)
- Spinal cord injury with paralysis
- Shock (early stages)
- Collapse due to accident or illness.

Less urgent:

- Fractures and dislocations
- Severe diarrhoea and vomiting
- Deep puncture wounds
- Foreign body in ear or eye.

Objectives and limitations of first aid

The aims of first aid are:

- To preserve life
- To prevent further suffering
- To promote recovery.

In order to manage a first aid situation, the nurse should always try to:

- Be calm and confident
- Be in command of the situation
- Use initiative
- Show sympathy.

Previous knowledge that is useful includes:

- A good understanding of the anatomy and physiology of the body
- Knowledge of one's own limitations in situations requiring first aid
- Knowledge of how much a nurse can do legally
- Safe handling procedures to ensure that no one else is injured.

Difficulties with first aid situations include people as well as animal patients – for example, a person reporting or arriving with the animal not being the owner, or the owner being upset and requiring sensitive handling and support.

Handling and transport of injured animals

Initially it is important that an injured animal is not moved until it has been examined. There are exceptions to this rule but only if the animal's life would be in further danger if it was not moved.

Injured animals are usually in pain, shocked and frightened. This means that they may attack anyone who tries to approach or handle them.

- Slow deliberate movements are essential
- When approaching, use a calm soothing voice
- The animal should be handled as little as possible. If the animal is not already at the clinic, the owner should be instructed to transport it with consideration to obvious injuries at all times (Figures 9.2 and 9.3)
- If the owner can check the airway, breathing and heart before transport, then initial help can be given at an early stage. This assists nursing staff to prepare for their arrival.

Transport

- Small dogs, cats and smaller pets are safely transported in a basket or pet carrier. If a container is not available, the animal should be picked up in a manner that provides support around its chest and hindquarters. It should be supported by the handler's body
- Medium-sized dogs with minor injury may be able to walk. If this is not possible, then they should be lifted

 9.2 Basic rules of transportation

- Do not obstruct breathing or airway by bending the animal's neck
- Support the animal's back and body
- Retain its body temperature
- Keep the weight off any obviously fractured limb
- Muzzle a dog if necessary to prevent injury from biting.

> ⚠ Muzzling is contraindicated in cases of dyspnoea (difficulty in breathing) or epistaxis (bleeding from the nostrils) and for brachycephalic (short-nosed) breeds.

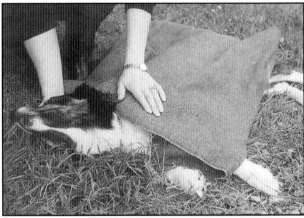

9.3 *Maintain body temperature to prevent shock from becoming established.*

into the handler's own body with an arm around the front of the forelegs and an arm around the hindlegs (provided this is not contraindicated by the injuries) (Figure 9.4)

- Large and giant dogs that are unable to walk should be lifted by at least two people using a stretcher or blanket:
  - The blanket should be spread beside the animal
  - The animal should be slid on to the blanket (taking care not to lift the body up), still in the position in which it was lying
  - The corners of the blanket can now be lifted by two to four people, depending on the size of the animal.

> ⚠ Always lift in a correct manner, so that the handler's own back is not at risk (Figure 9.5).

General procedure on arrival at the clinic

Recovery position
Unless it is contraindicated, always start by placing the animal into the recovery position (Figure 9.6):

1. Lie the animal on its right side
2. Ensure that its head and neck are straightened
3. Draw the tongue forward so that it hangs out of the side of the animal's mouth
4. Remove any collar or harness.

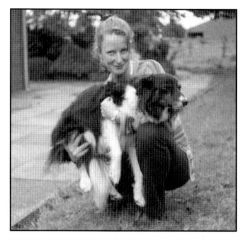

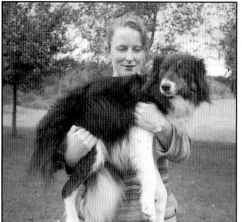

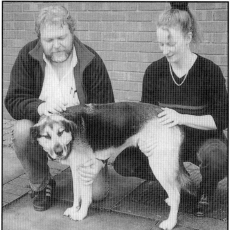

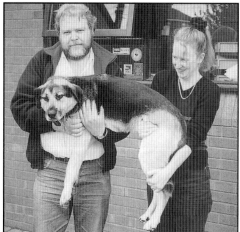

9.5 Lifting a large dog requires two people. Each handler keeps their back straight for safety during lifting.

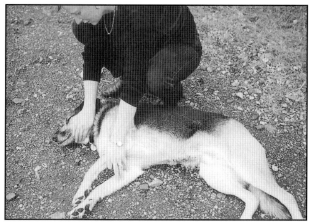

9.6 Place the animal in the recovery position. The tongue should now be drawn forward and the collar removed.

Evaluation

The initial positioning should be followed by evaluation of all areas of the animal (Figure 9.7). All findings should be recorded:

- External haemorrhage (bleeding)
- Colour of mucous membranes (Figures 9.8 and 9.9)
- Capillary refill time (when the gum over the top canine tooth is pressed, the time it takes to go pink again, i.e. for the blood vessels to refill)
- Rate and quality of pulse
- Breathing – note whether it is normal speed, slow or fast, and whether there is evidence of dyspnoea
- Body temperature – take the rectal temperature
- Level of consciousness
- Unusual odours (on the body or coming from the mouth).

9.7 A CRASH PLAN

A	=	Airway
C	=	Cardiovascular (check the apex beat of the heart)
R	=	Respiratory (presence/absence of breathing)
A	=	Abdomen (look, but do not palpate)
S	=	Spine (look for any deformity, but do not palpate)
H	=	Head (look for deformity, and level of consciousness)
P	=	Pelvic and anal areas (look for sign of injury)
L	=	Limbs (check for deformity)
A	=	Arteries and veins (check for signs of dehydration and shock)
N	=	Nerves that are peripheral (check for ability to move limbs and tail)

9.8 Colour of mucous membranes

- *Pale* – indicates shock, haemorrhage or anaemia
- *Cyanotic* – with a blue tinge, due to lack of oxygen at tissue level
- *Jaundiced* – seen as a yellow tinge, due to excess bile pigment in the circulation
- *Injected/red* – bright red, seen after overexercise, hyperthermia (heat stroke) or pyrexia (fever)
- *Congested* – dark red, seen with cardiovascular insufficiency.

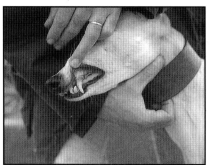

9.9 *Checking the colour of mucous membranes and capillary refill time.*

Cardiopulmonary resuscitation (CPR)

Cardiopulmonary resuscitation (Figures 9.10–9.13) should be attempted in all cardiac arrests, unless otherwise directed by the veterinary surgeon. Cardiopulmonary arrest is when the heart and breathing have stopped. The object is to restore heart and lung action and to prevent irreversible brain damage. Following cardiac arrest, this damage would usually occur within 3–4 minutes; therefore being adequately prepared is the most important step in managing a cardiac emergency.

9.10 ABC – the basic cardiopulmonary technique

A = **A**irway – clear it of any obstruction, such as saliva, vomit, the patient's own tongue or any other material that could block the trachea or throat

B = **B**reathing – start artificial respiration (Figure 9.11) and assist with oxygen, if available

C = **C**irculation – if the heart has stopped start cardiac compression (Figures 9.12 and 9.13).

9.11 Artificial respiration

1. Place in recovery position (on its right side, head and neck extended and tongue drawn forward) (Figure 9.6)
2. Clear airway
3. Place hand over ribs, behind shoulder bone, and compress chest with a sharp downward movement (Figure 9.12)
4. Allow chest to expand and then repeat the downward movement at intervals of 3–5 seconds, until breathing restarts.

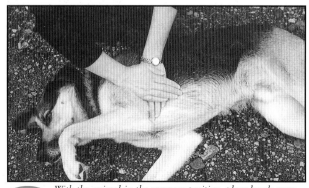

9.12 *With the animal in the recovery position, place hands over ribs, behind shoulder bone, and compress the chest.*

9.13 Cardiac compression techniques

Small dogs and cats

1. Place in recovery position (Figure 9.6)
2. Take hold of chest (thorax) between thumb and fingers of one hand, just behind elbows. Support animal's body with other hand on spine to prevent it moving away
3. Squeeze thumb and fingers of first hand together, over heart, to compress chest and heart
4. Repeat this action at rate of approximately 120 times per minute.

Medium-sized dogs

1. Place animal in recovery position (Figure 9.6)
2. Put heel of one hand on its chest, just behind elbow, and place other hand on top of first hand
3. Press down on chest with firm sharp movements
4. Repeat this action at rate of about 80–100 times per minute.

Large dogs and fat dogs

1. Put dog on its back, with head lowered
2. Place heel of one hand on abdomen end of chest and put other hand on top of that hand
3. Press firmly on chest, pushing hands forwards (towards head of animal). This method requires some strength
4. Repeat chest pressure at rate of 80–100 times per minute.

Whatever the size of the animal

- Apply compressions for about 15 seconds at a time
- Then stop and check for a pulse
- Continue until pulse returns
- Seek veterinary attention as soon as possible.

Asphyxia (suffocation)

Interference with respiration or breathing can occur in the upper respiratory tract (nose, mouth and throat) or lower respiratory tract (trachea, bronchi and lungs). It can involve a simple physical blockage of air conduction to the lungs or interference with the transference of air through the alveoli (air sacs), preventing gaseous exchange.

Signs and causes

Signs of asphyxia (which is suffocation, resulting from failure to oxygenate the blood) are:

- Cyanosis (blue mucous membranes)
- Dyspnoea (difficulty in breathing)
- Tachypnoea (increased rate of inspiration, which is also shallow).

The respiratory and cardiovascular systems are closely linked, and so a change in one is usually reflected in the other. Change in breathing ability can be mirrored in the pulse rate (speed) and character (strong, weak or thready), and in the colour of the mucous membranes, as the blood gas levels become abnormal.

Causes of asphyxia include:

- Obstruction of the air passage to the lungs
- Pressure on the chest or neck region, possibly due to a road traffic accident (RTA), causing collapse of air passage
- Medical conditions that may cause fluid build-up in the thorax
- Paralysis of the respiratory muscles caused by electrocution, spinal injury or poisons
- Direct thoracic injury, such as diaphragmatic hernia (the diaphragm, which separates the thorax and abdomen, is torn) or pneumothorax (air free in the thorax) due to trauma to lung tissues
- Drowning
- Inhaling of poisonous gases such as carbon monoxide, which will interfere with the uptake of oxygen by the haemoglobin (red pigment) in red blood cells
- Disease of the central nervous system (CNS).

Dyspnoea (difficulty in breathing)

Structures associated with the respiratory tract, such as the pleura (membrane covering the lungs) or ribs, can affect breathing. Damage or disease in either of these parts of the system makes breathing difficult and painful.

Diseases not associated with the respiratory tract, such as heart disease, anaemia (lack of red cells or haemoglobin in the blood) or gastric dilation and torsion (when the stomach fills with gas and twists), can have an effect on the breathing.

Action

Whatever the cause of breathing difficulty, it should be taken very seriously and viewed as an emergency. If the breathing has stopped then it must urgently be restarted.

Resuscitation methods include the use of drugs that stimulate the heart and the breathing, but these must be administered only by a veterinary surgeon. For first aid, therefore, manual techniques such as Airway/Breathing/Circulation (ABC) apply (see Figure 9.10).

Haemorrhage

Haemorrhage is bleeding from a damaged blood vessel in any part of the body due to injury or a disease condition.

Even slight bleeding, over a long period, could result in eventual death, and certainly sudden severe blood loss will cause death.

Signs

General signs of life-threatening haemorrhage are:

- Pale mucous membranes
- Rapid weak pulse and altered breathing pattern
- Subnormal temperature
- Slow capillary refill time
- Inability to rise.

Evaluation

Record information on the following:

- Type of blood vessel damaged (whether an artery, vein or capillary)

- When the bleeding started (for example: immediately; within the past 24–48 hours; several days before)
- In relation to the body, is the bleeding visible (external) or possibly hidden and into a body cavity (internal)?

Different types of haemorrhage are described in Figure 9.14.

9.14 Types of haemorrhage

- *Arterial* – bright red blood, in spurts synchronized with heart beat
- *Venous* – dark red blood, with definite bleeding point and steady flow
- *Capillary* – bright red blood, oozing slowly with no definite bleeding point.

- *Primary* – haemorrhage as direct result of a blood vessel having been damaged
- *Secondary* – haemorrhage that restarts several days after injury, due to infection
- *Reactionary* – haemorrhage that restarts within 24 hours of the initial injury, due to rise in blood pressure that displaces clot formation

- *External* – haemorrhage seen on surface of body or coming from body opening (mouth, nose, urethra, anus)
- *Internal* – haemorrhage into a body cavity, therefore unseen during examination.

Action

Methods of haemorrhage control include applying digital pressure, the use of pressure bandages, using pressure points or (rarely) applying a tourniquet.

Digital pressure

Fingers are used to control the bleeding (Figure 9.15), but care is required to ensure that there is no foreign body embedded in the wound, as this pressure would push it deeper into the tissues.

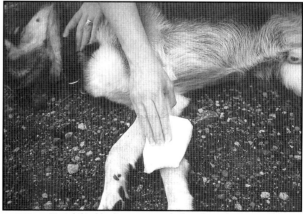

9.15 *To inhibit bleeding: use a pad of swabs and press on the affected area.*

Pressure bandages

These are applied to extremities such as limbs, and are used to constrict the surface circulation temporarily, helping to limit the loss of blood. A pressure bandage is applied over plenty of padding material backing the wound dressing, tightly bandaged in place until a veterinary surgeon arrives (see Chapter 1 in *BSAVA Manual of Veterinary Nursing* for details).

Pressure points

Pressure is applied on an artery (where it passes over a bone) to the body extremities. The supply of blood to forelimbs, hindlimbs or tail can then be temporarily constricted to reduce blood loss. The pressure required must be sufficient to prevent the flow of blood through the artery.

Pressure points are:

- The brachial artery – distal third of humerus, medial to the shaft
- The femoral artery – proximal third of the femur, medial aspect of the thigh
- The coccygeal artery – underside of the tail, at the root or base.

Tourniquet

A tourniquet is used to cut off the circulation supply to the tissues below its application site. However, this technique should *not* be employed, except in extreme circumstances.

Poisons

A poison or toxin is a substance that, on entry to the body in sufficient amounts, has a harmful effect on the individual. An antidote is a substance that counteracts a poison.

Animals can be poisoned by any of a multitude of potentially toxic substances. Sources might include poisonous plants, or toxic chemicals used on or stored near the animal (kitchen or utility room cupboards). These chemicals might be pesticides for the garden, paint, cleaning solutions for brushes, or many other household products.

Signs

Very few poisons produce distinctive signs. Most cause non-specific signs, such as:

- Becoming excited or depressed
- Becoming weak and ataxic (unsteady on the feet)
- Salivating, development of vomiting or having diarrhoea
- Abdominal pain and convulsions
- Evidence of shock (pale, loss of body temperature, slow capillary refill time)
- Convulsions.

Evaluation

Find out from the owner:

- Whether there have been any changes in routine at home or in the walk route
- Whether any medication has been given
- Full details about the animal concerned – age, sex, breed and species
- Details of symptoms and any actions taken by the owner
- A full case history – this is very important to the veterinary surgeon's diagnosis, unless the chemical is already known and named.

Always save any material passed by the animal (vomit, urine or faeces) for forensic testing if required.

Action

If the owner is able to tell staff what the poison was, then treatment should be started sooner rather than later:

- Place the animal in the recovery position (see Figure 9.6)
- Keep it warm to reduce shock (see Figure 9.3)
- Provide comfort companionship – never leave the patient unattended (in case its condition suddenly worsens).

 The animal should not be made to vomit, except on instructions from a veterinary surgeon.

Burns

Burns cause destruction of tissue by extreme localized *dry* heat. The severity of a burn is measured by the depth of tissue and the proportion of surface area affected. The full extent of the injury is often not apparent until several days after the accident.

Signs

- Loss of coat or fur; skin change
- Swelling
- Redness and heat
- Local infection
- Pain and signs of shock.

Evaluation

The depth of the injury may be described as:

- Superficial – penetrating no deeper than the skin surface
- Deep – penetrating through the skin, subcutaneous tissues, fat, muscle and even to bone.

The physical extent of the injury is also important, as the extensive pain and fluid loss (in the form of plasma from the damaged blood vessels) can lead to serious dehydration and shock.

Action

While waiting for the arrival of a veterinary surgeon:

- Cool and flush the area with cold water for 10 minutes if immediately post injury. This will reduce the swelling and plasma loss, and also provide some pain control
- Cover with moist sterile dressing or clingfilm to prevent any contamination
- Prevent self-mutilation
- To prevent shock, keep the animal warm (but do not use direct heat)
- Restrict the animal's movement to lessen the pain
- Do not leave unattended
- Comfort the patient
- Prepare fluid therapy equipment if burns are extensive or shock is severe.

Scalds

Scalds are caused by *moist* heat, such as steam or hot liquids. The signs for scalds can be similar to those for burns, but with scalding the coat is not singed.

It is important with both types of injury that the area affected is covered with a dressing to prevent contamination.

Insect stings

Most insect stings are painful but harmless. However, it is possible that an animal may have an allergic reaction to insect venom; therefore any stings near the airway in particular must be considered serious. Appropriate action for anaphylaxis (life-threatening allergic reaction) should be initiated (ABC – see Figure 9.10).

 Never squeeze the venom sack if it is embedded in the animal's skin. Such action may inject more venom into the animal.

- *Wasp stings* are alkaline, therefore treat with an acid solution (e.g. a vinegar compress)
- *Bee stings* are acid, therefore treat with an alkali (e.g. bicarbonate of soda compress).

If it is unclear what the biting insect was, then a cold compress should be applied to reduce the pain and swelling to the affected area.

Fractures and dislocations

Signs

- Pain
- Shortening or lengthening of limb
- Deformity
- Abnormal position of bone or joint
- Loss of use of the part
- Crepitus (crackling sound).

Causes of fracture
A fracture is a crack or break in a bone. Causes include:

- *Direct violence* (such as in an RTA) – the bone breaks at the place to which violence is applied
- *Indirect violence* – the fracture occurs some distance from the area where force was applied (for example, an animal landing on a hard surface with the break occurring to bones further up the limb)
- *Muscular action* or *fatigue fracture* – seen after muscular contraction during a race, particularly in the Greyhound and Whippet
- *Pathological* or *spontaneous fracture* – may be due to an existing bone disease or a condition that weakens the structure of the bone. These fractures often occur during a normal limb movement.

Causes of dislocation
Dislocation refers to the displacement of one or more bones forming a joint. Causes of dislocation include:

- Direct violence (e.g. RTA)
- Indirect violence (e.g. falling)
- Pathological displacement (e.g. hip dysplasia, an inherited factor – the joint and bone that should be in contact are so deformed that they cannot stay in contact)
- Congenital displacement (e.g. luxating patella – the patella, i.e. kneecap, is dislocated from the groove in the femur, often due to poor alignment in the stifle joint).

Action
Emergency treatment for fractures and dislocations is as follows:

- Arrest any haemorrhage
- Clean any wounds to the area and cover with sterile dressing to prevent contamination
- Confine the animal, to prevent movement
- Monitor and observe until arrival of a veterinary surgeon.

Sprains and strains

Sprains always involve a joint, with damage to ligaments and other tissues that are stretched and torn during the injury. Recovery and repair to some of these tissues are slow, due to continued use of the area and because some of the tissues (ligaments) are naturally slow to heal. Sprains occur most commonly in the lower limbs to the carpus (wrist) area and the tarsus (hock) area.
Strains involve tearing and stretching damage to muscles, often close to joints. They can occur anywhere in the body.

Signs

- Pain
- Swelling
- Lameness.

Action

- Initial care involves the application of a cold compress to the area, to reduce the swelling and pain
- Prevent use of the affected limb
- Confine to a kennel with plenty of bedding
- Comfort the patient
- Treat for any shock.

Wounds

A wound is a break in the continuity of a tissue anywhere in the body, internal or external. In a first aid situation this will usually mean a break in the skin or mucous membrane, but the term also applies to damage to other tissues or organs in the body.
Wounds may be:

- *Open* – damage to the skin and underlying tissues
- *Closed* – they do not penetrate the whole thickness of the skin.

Action

- Arrest any haemorrhage
- Check for foreign bodies
- Flush the wound, preferably using 0.9% sodium chloride (normal saline)
- Cover with a sterile dressing
- Keep the animal warm
- Comfort and monitor the patient.

Eye injuries

Signs

Both eyes should be examined and compared, and any differences noted:

- Obvious loss of vision
- Tissue swelling (oedema) (Figure 9.16)
- Bleeding around the eye
- Abnormal size and position of the eyeball within the orbit.

Causes

- Direct violence
- Indirect violence
- Chemical exposure
- Foreign body in eye.

Evaluation

Take a history from the owner, concerning:

- The type of trauma
- When it occurred
- Whether there has been any exposure to chemicals
- Whether there are any pre-existing eye problems.

The animal should be approached slowly – and warned of any approach. Most eye injuries are quite painful, and if the animal has considerable sight impairment it will also be frightened and could injure any handler.

Action

For emergency treatment:

- Keep the eye moist with sterile fluid
- Prevent self-mutilation
- Do not leave unattended
- Keep warm and quiet.

 Prolapse: do not attempt to force the eye into the socket. Pull eyelids over gently, to cover the eye.

Penetrating wounds to the thorax and abdomen

Thorax

Signs

- Breathing painful and will be seen as rapid and shallow
- Affected animals often reluctant to move
- May adopt a sitting position.

Action

- Cover the wound
- Keep the animal quiet and calm
- Allow it to choose its own resting position
- Keep it warm.

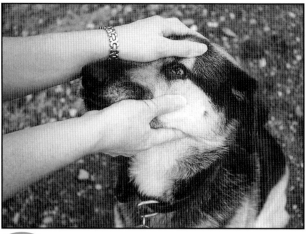

9.16 *Examining the eye for signs of tissue swelling.*

Abdomen

Signs and causes

An open wound to the abdomen is seen, allowing abdominal tissues and organs to protrude.

Causes of abdominal rupture include:

- Road traffic accident
- Bite wounds
- Stab or staking injuries
- Breakdown of surgical site.

Complications include:

- Drying
- Swelling of exposed tissues
- Contamination or infection
- Self-inflicted damage.

Action

- Clean the wound
- Cover exposed tissue with swabs soaked in saline warmed to body temperature, or boiled water
- Do not leave unattended
- Treat for shock
- Seek veterinary help urgently
- Prevent self-mutilation.

Unconsciousness

Unconsciousness may render the brain:

- Depressed, as seen in central nervous system injury (head injury, or resulting from asphyxia as in drowning)
- Active, seen in convulsions or epileptic type fits and in electrocution.

Causes of unconsciousness include:

- Epilepsy
- Lack of oxygen
- Poisoning
- Electrocution.

Action

- Place in recovery position (see Figure 9.6)
- ABC (see Figure 9.10)
- Examine for signs of injury
- Keep warm
- Do not leave unattended.

Asphyxiation by drowning

Asphyxiation occurs when the lungs fill with water, preventing exchange of oxygen and carbon dioxide. Although most animals can swim for short distances, exhaustion will overtake them if they are unable to climb out of the water, followed by panic and the inability to float.

Action

As soon as the unconscious animal is removed from the water:

- Place in recovery position (see Figure 9.6)
- Draw the tongue forward
- Gravity-drain water from the lungs by holding the animal upside down, or proceed with artificial respiration (see Figure 9.11)

- Treat for shock, dry the animal and keep it warm
- Seek veterinary attention urgently.

Fits or seizures (epileptic-type fit)

Action

- Do not restrain
- Subdue light and reduce noise
- Clear a space by moving furniture back
- Observe but do not handle
- If the animal's breathing becomes obstructed, clear the airway
- Handle only when the animal responds to its name and or attempts to stand.

Further reading

Bell C (1993) *First Aid and Health Care for Dogs*. Lutterworth Press, Cambridge

Kirk B and Bistner S (1985) *Handbook of Veterinary Procedures and Emergency Treatment*. WB Saunders, Philadelphia

Lane DR and Cooper B (eds) (1999) *Veterinary Nursing*, 2nd edn. Butterworth–Heinemann, Oxford

The law relating to working with small animals

George Malynicz

This chapter is designed to give information on:

- What law is and how laws are made
- The law and small animals
- The law and working with animals

Introduction

Laws are changing all the time. Even lawyers have trouble keeping up and so this chapter, which is written by a veterinary surgeon, should be treated as no more than a rough guide. More information can be found in any law library or the library of the Royal College of Veterinary Surgeons.

What is the law and how are laws made?

Common law

This is a system of laws that has evolved over hundreds of years by the decisions of judges in court. It is based on decisions from previous cases where similar issues arose. Most civil law, where one person sues another, is dealt with under common law.

Statute law

The United Kingdom does not have a written constitution. The members we elect to Parliament can make, change or repeal any laws, known as Acts, and it is up to the courts to carry them out. Acts are supported by Regulations which spell out in detail what the Act is about. Regulations do not have to be passed by Parliament but can be decided on by a Government Minister. The law in England and Wales is sometimes slightly different from that in Scotland and Northern Ireland but the principles remain the same.

European Union law

This is a system of law that applies to all members of the European Union and takes precedence over laws made by those countries. There are many areas, in particular relating to employment, where EU law has been incorporated into the laws of the United Kingdom.

The law and small animals

The law relating to small animals can be grouped into four main areas:

- Protection of the public from disease and danger
- Protection of the public from damages and nuisance
- Animal welfare and cruelty
- Statutory bodies working with animals.

Protection of the public from disease and danger

Animal Health Act 1981

This is the main piece of legislation concerned with preventing disease from entering the country as well as controlling specified diseases within England and Wales. The Minister for Agriculture has very wide powers under the Act to prevent such diseases from spreading. These powers include destruction and disposal of the animals and disinfection of areas that might be contaminated. The Minister may issue legally binding Orders under these powers.

As far as pets are concerned, rabies has always been considered the main threat. The Act provides for the control of rabies and its impact on animal quarantine. It gives the Minister power to prescribe and regulate: the muzzling of dogs and keeping them under control; the seizure, detention and disposal of stray dogs; and the wearing of dog collars with name tags. Local authorities and the police, acting on behalf of the Minister, are empowered to enforce the Act.

It should be noted that the whole policy on rabies quarantine is currently under consideration.

Dangerous Dogs Act 1991, and Dangerous Dogs (Amendment) Act 1997

These two Acts:

- Prohibit people from owning or keeping dogs of a breed or type intended for fighting. The types of dog that

come under the Act include pit bull terrier, Japanese Tosa, Dogo Argentino and Fila Braziliero. Dogs of these types or breeds have to be neutered, identified and insured, and kept muzzled and on a lead in public places
- Enable restrictions to be made for other types of dogs that are dangerous to the public
- Make it an offence to have *any* dog that is dangerously out of control in a public place.

Dangerous Wild Animals Act 1976

This Act regulates the keeping of certain kinds of dangerous wild animals. A schedule is in force which lists a large number of mainly imported wild animals that are considered dangerous. The local authority can issue a license to keep such animals if it believes that they do not pose a threat to the public and can be well cared for.

Guard Dogs Act 1975

This Act is designed to ensure that the public is not endangered by guard dogs. Guard dogs are not allowed to be set loose on premises unless there is someone there capable of controlling them. If guard dogs are used on premises a notice must be displayed to the public.

Protection of the public from damages and nuisance

Animals Act 1971

This Act covers the whole area of civil liability for damage caused by animals. Damage includes death or injury (including mental) to people or to livestock (including farm animals in general but not pets) and property damage. Under the Act, the term 'animals' includes dangerous species that are not normally domesticated (such as foxes) as well as animals that belong to a normally harmless species (such as dogs) but which are known by the keeper to be dangerous. Owners of dangerous animals have a duty of care to inform people who may come into contact with such an animal that it is dangerous.

Thousands of farm animals are killed by dogs every year. Farmers are entitled to protect their stock against dangerous animals, and even to kill such animals in certain defined circumstances. However, if they have to kill an animal they must report the matter to the police.

It cannot be assumed that those who work with animals have voluntarily accepted that their work carries a risk. Employers are required to protect their staff from damage through proper training on how to handle dangerous animals and through the provision of physical and chemical restraints.

Dogs (Fouling of Land) Act 1996

This Act prevents fouling by dogs of land to which there is public access. Guide dogs are exempt. Local authorities are charged with implementing the Act.

Animal welfare and cruelty

Keeping animals commercially

The following legislation provides a framework of standards for keeping domestic or captive animals as a business.

Animal Boarding Establishments Act 1963

This regulates the keeping of boarding establishments for animals. It applies only to cats and dogs. Boarding kennels and catteries have to be licensed by the local authority, which is required to inspect the premises. The rules also apply to animals boarded at veterinary surgeries, or at boarding establishments managed or owned by veterinary surgeons.

Breeding of Dogs Act 1973, and Breeding of Dogs Act 1991

These regulate the commercial breeding of dogs and provide for inspection of premises at which dogs are bred and for control over the transport of puppies. A breeding establishment is defined as any place, including a private home, where three or more bitches are kept for breeding. The local authority is required to inspect and license breeding establishments.

Pet Animals Act 1951, and Pet Animals (Amendment) Act 1983

These regulate the sale of pet animals in pet shops and prohibit the sale of pets in public places. Pet shops have to be licensed. The local authority has been delegated the power to administer these Acts.

Cruelty

The main legislation controlling cruelty to animals is the Protection of Animals Act 1911. Related statutes are:

- Protection of Animals (Amendment) Act 1927
- Protection of Animals (Cruelty to Dogs) Act 1933
- Protection of Animals Act 1934
- Protection of Animals Act 1954
- Protection of Animals (Anaesthetics) Act 1954
- Animals (Cruel Poisons) Act 1962
- Protection of Animals (Anaesthetics) Act 1964
- Protection of Animals (Penalties) Act 1987
- Protection of Animals Act 1988.

There have been a number of supplementary Acts and amendments which have clarified and extended the original 1911 Act. The object of legislation is to prevent cruelty to animals and to reduce suffering. Animals suffering from the effects of cruelty may be destroyed or otherwise disposed of by a veterinary surgeon following a request by the police. Under the Acts it is a crime to abuse animals physically or mentally. Specific legislation has included:

- Prohibition of the use of animals for fighting or baiting, or the holding of rodeo-style events, or advertising such meetings
- The performance of operations on animals without due care and humanity (the Protection of Animals (Anaesthetics) Act 1954 does allow for some minor surgery to be carried out without anaesthetics but castration of dogs and cats must always be carried out by veterinary surgeons using anaesthesia)
- A ban on killing of mammals, including vermin, by cruel or caustic poisons such as phosphorus.

Research using animals

Some of the scientific research carried out on animals has the potential to cause suffering. This research includes that done to develop medicines for the treatment of diseases in humans and animals. The research is licensed and monitored by the Home Office and is subject to specific legislation.

Animals Scientific Procedures Act 1986

This makes provisions for the protection of animals used for experimental purposes. It applies to all vertebrates – not just mammals – and covers not only experiments and genetic studies but also the use of animals for the production of medicines. Because this Act recognizes that animal suffering may take place it is very strictly controlled and laboratories can be banned from research. Each research project and procedure must be licensed by the Home Office and so must the premises and the individual research workers. Research will not be allowed on animals unless every alternative method of getting the information has been considered. Animals must be obtained from designated sources; the use of strays in experiments is strictly forbidden. Any animal in severe pain or distress must be euthanased and most are euthanased at the end of use.

Statutory bodies working with animals

People's Dispensary for Sick Animals Act 1949

This Act incorporates and confers powers upon the People's Dispensary for Sick Animals (PDSA). This is the largest charity providing free veterinary attention for people unable to afford the fees of private veterinary surgeons.

Royal Society for the Prevention of Cruelty to Animals Act 1932

This Act incorporates and confers powers upon the Royal Society for Prevention of Cruelty to Animals. The RSPCA has a very wide mandate, ranging from prosecution of cruelty cases under the cruelty legislation listed above to political lobbying on animal welfare issues, including promoting the sale of meat that has been produced under sound welfare conditions (the 'Freedom meats' campaign).

Veterinary Surgeons Acts

These include:

- Veterinary Surgeons Act 1881
- Veterinary Surgeons (Amendments) Act 1920
- Veterinary Surgeons Act 1948
- Veterinary Surgeons Act 1966
- Veterinary Surgeons Act 1981.

They established the Royal College of Veterinary Surgeons and its Council. The College was given the power to teach and examine people and register and charge them for membership of the College, while restricting the practice of veterinary surgery by unqualified people. The College was also empowered to discipline its members.

Health and safety

Employers are responsible for the safety of their employees. The duties that employers owe to those that work for them are established in common and statute law. The duty to provide employees with a safe place of work is implied under common law. If an employer fails to do so and an employee is injured, the employer can be sued for damages by the employee. The main statute covering this area is the Health and Safety at Work Act 1974 (HSAWA) and its Regulations.

Common law duties for health and safety

Employers have a duty to take all reasonably practicable steps to protect the health and safety of their employees. What is 'reasonable' must take into account any hazards and the cost of eliminating them. Employers must formally consider the amount of risk and the likelihood of harm to those in their employment, and take reasonable steps to minimize or eliminate those risks. Employers are not required to, and could not, provide an absolute guarantee of their employees' health and safety. Furthermore, employers cannot be held liable for a risk that could not have been foreseen. For example, if a chemical used at work had been considered safe and was later found to cause cancer, employers could not be held liable unless they had continued to use the chemical. The common law duty is a personal one between the employer and each employee and is not escaped by making someone else (the manager, for example) responsible for health and safety.

The requirement to provide a safe place in which to work can be considered under three headings:

Safe premises and equipment

Employers must provide a reasonably safe workplace for their workers and others who come on to the premises. Equipment or plant used at work must be safe and properly maintained. Employers must take out insurance against personal injury to their employees, as laid down in the Employers Liability (Compulsory Insurance) Act 1966.

Safe working systems

This involves a wide range of activities, including working instructions, training, supervision and the provision of protective clothing.

Competent fellow workers

Employees have a right to expect that their fellow workers are not so incompetent that they are dangerous; or, if they are not fully competent, that they are supervised.

Health and Safety at Work Act 1974

The HSAWA reinforces the common law duty of the employer on health and safety but it has one important distinction: it creates a partnership between employer and employee regarding safety. Both parties are required to cooperate in developing safety at work. Employers have a statutory duty of care for the health and safety of their employees, who in turn have a statutory responsibility to cooperate with the employer in meeting these obligations. This is achieved by the joint development of a written safety policy for a workplace.

The difference between the common law and HSAWA duties is that failure to adopt the latter is a crime punishable by up to two years in prison.

Duties

Employers have certain duties to their workers and those coming on to their premises:

- To develop a health and safety policy together with employees or their union representatives
- To provide safe premises, equipment and substances
- To have safe working procedures
- To provide a safe environment
- To advise of any hazards that cannot be avoided
- To prevent the emission of noxious substances, such as clinical wastes.

For their part, employees must:

- Take reasonable care of themselves, their fellow workers and the public
- Help the employer by following laid-down health and safety procedures.

Regulations under Health and Safety at Work Act

There are regulations under the HSAWA that affect those who work with animals. Each regulation is supported by an approved Code of Practice. Some of the more important are discussed below.

Health and safety arrangements

This is concerned with the management (plans, controls and reviews) of health and safety at the workplace.

- Individuals must be appointed with responsibility for health and safety
- Emergency procedures must be set up and all staff provided with information about any potential hazards and how to prevent them
- A formal record must be made of all accidents and this must be analysed from time to time
- Staff are required to warn employers of any health and safety problems
- The employer must make sure that staff are sufficiently trained in their work not to put themselves or others at risk
- Employees are expected to follow any health and safety instructions.

Risk assessment

Employers are required to carry out formal risk assessments on every aspect of their work. This means that they have to identify all the potential hazards in the workplace. Each hazard must be analysed for how severe its effects would be if it were to take place and how likely it is to happen.

Health surveillance

Where hazards have been identified in the risk assessment, employers should arrange medical check-ups for their employees. Staff should notify their manager if they react to any drugs or chemicals.

Provision and use of work equipment

This concerns ensuring that equipment used at the workplace is safe. It covers such things as annual testing of electrical equipment, autoclaves and protective devices and the setting up of proper procedures and training in using equipment. Arrangements must be in place for the safe disposal of used equipment such as glassware and needles.

Manual handling

Mishandling of heavy or awkward loads leads to a large number of injuries. Examples include lifting heavy animals or oxygen cylinders. Employers are required to set up systems that minimize the risks of injury. Employees are required to use any equipment, such as trolleys or stretchers, provided by the employer to reduce the risks of manual handling.

Workplace

This covers three main subjects: the working environment, safety and facilities.

The working environment

This has to meet certain standards of ventilation, temperature, lighting, size and hygiene. Eating and drinking are not allowed where animals are kept.

Safety

This is to protect employees from injuries resulting from slipping, falling and bumping into things, and also to protect them from things falling on them.

Facilities

There must be enough toilets, wash basins, drinking water, changing rooms and rest rooms. If the workforce numbers more than five people, separate toilets have to be provided for men and women.

Personal protective equipment at work

Employers must provide their staff with approved personal protective equipment to protect them from risks such as infection from animal secretions which can carry zoonotic diseases and other hazardous substances. Equipment includes uniforms, disposable gloves, masks used while scaling and polishing teeth, and goggles for use when handling liquid nitrogen sprays.

Display screen equipment

This is designed to protect people who work for long periods at computer screens. The employer must provide comfortable working conditions, good lighting, prescribed breaks and free eye tests.

Control of Substances Hazardous to Health 1994 (COSHH)

COSHH regulations are designed to protect employees from the risks of working with hazardous substances. The risk is the likelihood that the substance will harm people by causing problems such as allergy, asthma, poisoning, cancer or infection. Substances hazardous to health are those that can cause harm. The most hazardous substances have been identified under Schedule 1 in the Chemicals (Hazard Information Packing for Supply) Regulations (CHIP), available from the Health and Safety Executive, and carry a warning label showing them to be 'Very Toxic', 'Toxic', 'Harmful', 'Irritant' or 'Corrosive'.

There are also some other hazardous substances, such as dusts and biological agents, which, because they are not used in trade, do not carry any warnings. For many substances there are Approved Codes of Practice, which provide detailed instructions on how to handle the substance safely.

The duties of employer and employee under COSHH are quite similar to those under the broader HSAWA 1974 and include:

- The need to carry out a full risk assessment of all substances hazardous to health. Where a hazardous substance has been bought it will come with a data sheet, or the manufacturer must provide one
- Defining what precautions need to be in place to protect employees. These might include such things as protective clothing or additional ventilation
- Making sure that all precautions laid down are actually used by the employees. Failure to do so is a disciplinary matter

- Monitoring exposure of employees to hazardous substances and carrying out health surveillance of staff as appropriate
- Training all staff so that they understand the risks to which they are exposed and the precautions in place to minimize that risk. They should study the risk assessments and the relevant data sheets and be involved in developing the safety procedures and precautions.

Ionizing Radiations Regulations 1985

Radiography is widely used in veterinary practice for diagnosis of diseases. Because X-rays are dangerous and cannot be seen, heard, felt or smelt there are statutory Regulations and an Approved Code of Practice (ACP) to protect people working with them. The Regulations are administered by the Health and Safety Executive (HSE) and the National Radiological Protection Board. It is the employer's responsibility to make sure they are followed.

The Regulations have three objectives:

- To discourage the use of X-rays except where there are good clinical reasons
- To reduce the exposure of people to X-rays
- To make sure that exposure *never* gets above certain safe limits.

The ways in which the Ionizing Radiations Regulations protect people working with X-rays from radiation fall into two main classes: organizational and physical.

Organizational arrangements and working practices

The Regulations and ACP lay down strict procedures which have to be followed when setting up and using X-rays in a practice. These are designed to make sure that:

- The HSE knows that X-rays are used at certain premises
- An expert in radiology – the *Radiation Protection Advisor* (RPA) – is involved in all stages of planning and designing the X-ray facility, developing a set of safe working practices known officially as the *Local Rules*, monitoring exposure and dealing with incidents when things have gone wrong
- One person – the *Radiation Protection Supervisor* – is responsible for the day-to-day management of the radiography at the premises according to the Local Rules
- Everyone working with X-rays is properly trained and understands the Local Rules
- Anyone working on a regular basis with X-rays wears a *personal dosemeter* to measure exposure and that these are checked monthly or quarterly
- Plans are available in case of emergency, such as breakdown of the equipment
- Suppliers of X-ray equipment provide a critical report showing that the machine has passed various safety tests.

Physical protection against radiation

The Ionizing Radiations Regulations deal with the premises where X-ray equipment is used, warnings and signs to protect people from accidental exposure, the X-ray equipment itself and other equipment used in the X-ray process. The RPA should be involved in advising on appropriate standards on these matters (National Radiological Protection Board, 1988).

- *Premises*: the Regulations lay down how thick the protective barriers (brick, concrete flooring, lead, etc.) should be to contain the X-rays emitted
- *Signage*: signs must be fixed to all doors leading to the X-ray room. Automatic warning lights or lit signs must come on whenever the X-ray machine is actually emitting X-rays
- *Maintenance of X-ray equipment* must be to the standards set down by the RPA
- *Ancillary equipment* such as the X-ray table and cassettes must be suitable for the purpose
- *Processing equipment* should be of a high standard and used correctly to provide diagnostic X-rays without having to repeat them
- *Fast film* should be used with screens to cut down the time of exposure
- *Special clothing* (such as aprons) to protect the wearer from X-rays should be worn during radiography.

Employment

This section gives some insight into the legal aspects of work. Because the employment relationship is based on contract, the basic source of employment law in the United Kingdom is the common law. A contract is a freely entered agreement between two equal parties. In employment situations this often is not the case and the employer brings to the contract of employment more power than the employee. In order to secure definite minimum rights for employees statutes were introduced for their protection which override any common law rules. These include the Employment Relations Act 1996 (ERA) and the Industrial Tribunals Act 1996. The European Union is very active in making laws about employment.

The contract of employment

All employees are employed under a contract which must meet the requirement of the ERA. It is usually a formal contract in writing setting out the duties and obligations that have been agreed to by both parties – the *express* terms of the contract. Other conditions, known as the *implied* terms of the contract, exist even though they are not actually written down in the contract. These are conditions that apply to both parties. See also *BSAVA Manual of Advanced Veterinary Nursing*.

Express terms

Express terms vary quite a lot but usually state: the names and addresses of the parties; the date when employment began; details of wages, salaries, commissions, hours of work, duties, holidays and overtime; and overtime pay, sick pay, pensions and other entitlements such as membership of health insurance schemes. Some of these would have appeared in the advertisement for the job; some should have been discussed and agreed to during the job interview. Other details may consist of terms and conditions, notices and circulars.

Implied terms

Apart from what is written into the employment contract, there are duties implied by statute and common law on both employers and employees. Employers must pay their employees their wages, and provide them with suitable safe working conditions. The employees must obey reasonable and lawful instructions, exercise reasonable care and attention at work, and not accept gifts or secret commissions or disclose confidential information to competitors.

Statutory terms

These are implied terms of employment that have the force of statutory law behind them. Employment rights increase with length of service up to a maximum of 2 years, after which the full rights shown below apply.

- When applying for work, employees cannot be discriminated against on the grounds of sex, race or disability
- On being appointed to a new job, employees have a right to:
    - an itemized payslip
    - time off for certain public duties such as jury service
    - belong to and participate in a trade union.
- After 4 weeks of employment, employees have the right to 1 week's notice of termination
- Within 2 months from the start of employment, employers must provide a written contract showing the employee's terms and conditions of employment. The disciplinary rules may be simplified for businesses with fewer than 20 employees (which would include many veterinary practices)
- The recent Working Time Regulations (1998) placed a limit on working time of 48 hours a week and made special provisions for night workers
- After 2 years with the same employer, unless they commit a gross misconduct, employees are protected from unfair dismissal or being made redundant without compensation. This applies to part-time and full-time employees. If dismissed, an employee is entitled to 2 weeks' notice plus 1 week for every year worked thereafter, up to a maximum of 12 weeks.

Termination of contract of employment

Either party may terminate the contract of employment by giving notice as required under the contract. Failure to give adequate notice or money in lieu of notice (except in the case of gross misconduct) would leave the employer open to action for wrongful dismissal. If the employer terminates the contract, the employee is dismissed. Dismissal exists when:

- The employer serves notice on the employee that the contract of employment is being terminated
- The employer fails to renew a fixed-term contract that has expired
- A redundancy situation has developed
- The employee resigns because of things the employer has done to make it difficult to continue working (this is known as constructive dismissal)
- The employer fails to allow a woman to return to work after maternity leave.

Wrongful dismissal

Dismissal without notice or money in lieu of notice can only be justified in law where the employee has been guilty of gross misconduct. Employees who feel they have been wrongfully dismissed have up to 6 years to sue their employer for breach of contract.

Unfair dismissal

Unfair dismissal takes place when an employer dismisses a worker without good reason. There are a number of grounds for dismissal that may be considered fair under the Act, including the following:

- The employee lacked the capability or qualifications for the work
- The conduct of the employee was unsatisfactory
- The employee was redundant
- The employment contravened legal obligations
- Other valid reasons.

Employees who think they have been dismissed unfairly can bring an action against their employer to an *Industrial Tribunal*. In deciding whether or not the dismissal was unfair the Tribunal will consider the truth and fairness of the reasons given by the employer as well as the disciplinary procedures that led up to the dismissal.

The *Advisory Conciliation and Arbitration Service* (ACAS) has produced guidelines on disciplinary procedures which are fair to both parties. Employees must be made aware of these procedures. They include giving warning to the employee that there is a problem. These warnings must be both verbal and in writing. Employees may be accompanied by a trade union official or friend at disciplinary hearings.

Discrimination

Discrimination exists when an employer treats one employee or group of employees differently because of their sex, race or physical attributes rather than their ability to do the job. There is considerable statutory protection against discrimination (Sex Discrimination Act 1975, Race Relations Act 1976 and Disability Discrimination Act 1995) but there is no provision against discrimination on the grounds of age. Detailed advice on discrimination matters is available from the National Disability Council, the Equal Opportunities Commission and the Council for Racial Equality.

Protection against discrimination starts at the selection process and lasts as long as the employee is with the same employer. Employees who think they have suffered from discrimination can bring an action against an employer to an Industrial Tribunal.

There are three kinds of discrimination:

- Direct discrimination occurs when one employee is treated differently from another because of race or gender
- Indirect discrimination occurs where a condition of employment applies to all employees but people of one race or gender are less able to fulfil the condition
- Victimization takes place where employees are treated less favourably because they have in the past complained of discrimination.

Equal pay

Historically, women have been paid less for doing the same work as men. The Equal Pay Act 1970 and various European Directives require that where a woman does the same job as a man, or another job that has been rated as equivalent under a job evaluation scheme, she should be paid the same as a man. If a woman feels that she is doing a job that is equivalent to a man's but her employer refuses to submit to independent evaluation of the post, she can make a claim for equal value to an Industrial Tribunal.

Disability discrimination

The Disability Protection Act 1995 protects people with disabilities against discrimination. A disabled person is one whose normal activities are permanently reduced by their physical or mental handicaps. Difficulties with mobility, manual dexterity, coordination, talking, seeing, hearing and learning all count as disabilities. If a disabled person applies for a job and is rejected, or is dismissed, on the grounds that making the necessary changes to the buildings and working procedures would be unreasonably costly, the applicant can complain to an Industrial Tribunal. Businesses with fewer than 20 employees are exempt from the provisions of the Act.

Further reading

National Radiological Protection Board (1988) *Guidance Notes for the Protection of Persons Against Ionising Radiations arising from Veterinary Use.* HMSO, London

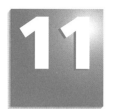

11 Veterinary terminology

Paula Hotston Moore

This chapter is designed to give information on:

- Word roots
- Prefixes and suffixes
- How to understand and recognize common veterinary words
- Common abbreviations.

Introduction

Veterinary terminology is a completely new language. This chapter will explore how medical terms are constructed. Once an understanding of some basic body parts and their terms are learned, words can begin to be built up. A long, confusing medical term can be broken down into sections to obtain its meaning.

The main section of the word is the *word root* and it is this which gives the word its meaning. A prefix or suffix is added to the word root at the beginning or end to change its meaning.

- A *prefix* is added in front of the main word root to form the first part of the word. Many words used in everyday language are formed as a word root with a prefix in front (e.g. *tri*cycle; *anti*social; *dis*advantage; *un*acceptable)
- A *suffix* is added to the end of the word root to form the last part of the word (e.g. mov*able*; charm*ing*; happ*iness*; baro*meter*).

Example
Word root:	NATAL ('birth')
Prefix:	ANTE ('before')
New word:	ANTENATAL ('before birth')

Some words have both a prefix and a suffix which combine to alter the meaning of the word root.

Example
Word root:	STRESS
Prefix:	UN ('not')
Suffix:	FUL ('complete')
New word:	UNSTRESSFUL

Many word roots change their spelling slightly to accommodate the addition of a prefix or suffix, to allow ease of pronunciation. This is called the *combining form*.

Example
Word root:	NATURE
Combining form:	NATUR
New word:	NATURALLY (not 'natureally')

The following sections relating to terminology for body systems give:

- The word root
- The Greek or Latin origins
- The meaning.

This is followed by examples of words that combine the root with various prefixes and suffixes to form new words. The prefix (e.g. 'peri~') or suffix (e.g. '~itis') and its meaning are given in the first two columns; the combined word and its meaning are given in the last two columns.

Body systems

The heart

Word root: **cardia** From: **Greek *kardiakos*** Meaning: **heart**			
brady~	slow	BRADYCARDIA	slow heart rate
tachy~	fast	TACHYCARDIA	fast/increased heart rate
myo~	pertaining to muscle	MYOCARDIUM	heart muscle
~itis	inflammation of	CARDITIS	inflammation of the heart
~logy	study of	CARDIOLOGY	study of the heart
~pathy	disease of	CARDIOPATHY	disease of the heart
~megaly	enlargement of	CARDIOMEGALY	enlargement of the heart
~graph	instrument that records	CARDIOGRAPH	instrument that records the heart
~gram	record of	CARDIOGRAM	record or radiograph of the heart
~dynia	pain	CARDIODYNIA	heart pain
~al	belonging to	CARDIAL	belonging to the heart
endo~/ ~itis	inner, within/ inflammation of	ENDOCARDITIS	inflammation of inner lining of heart wall
peri~/ ~al	near, around/ belonging to	PERICARDIAL	around the heart
myo~/ ~itis	pertaining to muscle/ inflammation of	MYOCARDITIS	inflammation of the heart muscle
electro-/ ~graph	having electricity/ instrument that records	ELECTROCARDIOGRAPH	instrument that records electrical activity of the heart
electro~/ ~gram	having electricity/ record of	ELECTROCARDIOGRAM	a recording of the electrical activity of the heart

Word root: **angio** From: **Greek *angeion*** Meaning: **vessel**			
~oma	tumour	ANGIOMA	tumour of a blood vessel
~gram	record of	ANGIOGRAM	record or radiograph of a blood vessel
~graphy	description of	ANGIOGRAPHY	process of taking a description, recording or radiography of blood vessels
~plasty	reconstructive surgery	ANGIOPLASTY	reconstructive surgery of blood vessels

Word root: **vascul** From: **Latin *vasculum*** Meaning: **blood vessel**			
		VASCULAR	relating to blood vessels
cardio~	pertaining to the heart	CARDIOVASCULAR	pertaining to the heart and blood vessels
~itis	inflammation of	VASCULITIS	inflammation of a blood vessel

Word root: **ven** From: **Latin *vena*** Meaning: **vein**			
intra~	into	INTRAVENOUS	into a vein

Word root: **phleb** From: **Greek _phleps_** Meaning: **vein**			
~itis	inflammation of	PHLEBITIS	inflammation of a vein

Word root: **haem** From: **Greek _haima_** Meaning: **blood**			
~logy	study of	HAEMATOLOGY	study of blood
~thorax	chest, pleural cavity	HAEMOTHORAX	blood in the chest
~rrhage	excessive flow	HAEMORRHAGE	excessive flow of blood, process of bleeding
~uria	pertaining to urine	HAEMATURIA	presence of blood in urine
~oma	tumour, growth	HAEMATOMA	accumulation of blood in tissues, forming solid swelling
~lysis	breakdown of	HAEMOLYSIS	breakdown of blood

The respiratory system

Word root: **pneumo** From: **Greek _pneumon_** Meaning: **lung**			
		PNEUMONIA	inflammation of the lungs
~itis	inflammation of	PNEUMONITIS	inflammation of the lungs
~thorax	chest, pleural cavity	PNEUMOTHORAX	presence of air or gas in the pleural cavity

Word root: **pnoea** From: **Greek _pnoe_** Meaning: **breathing**			
a~	without	APNOEA	absence of breathing
dys~	difficulty	DYSPNOEA	diffuculty in breathing
tachy~	fast	TACHYPNOEA	fast breathing rate
brady~	slow	BRADYPNOEA	slow breathing rate

Word root: **thorac** From: **Greek _thorax_** Meaning: **chest**			
~otomy	surgical incision into	THORACOTOMY	surgical incision into thorax

Word root: **rhin** From: **Greek _rhis_** Meaning: **nose**			
~scope	instrument for examining	RHINOSCOPE	instrument used for internal examination of nose
~itis	inflammation of	RHINITIS	inflammation of the nose

Word root: laryng
From: Greek *laryngos*
Meaning: larynx

~itis	inflammation of	LARYNGITIS	inflammation of the larynx
~scope	instrument for examining	LARYNGOSCOPE	instrument used for internal examination of larynx

Word root: trache
From: Greek *tracheia*
Meaning: trachea

~otomy	surgical incision into	TRACHEOTOMY	surgical incision into trachea
~itis	inflammation of	TRACHEITIS	inflammation of the trachea
laryngo~/ ~itis	pertaining to the larynx/ inflammation of	LARYNGOTRACHEITIS	inflammation of the larynx and trachea

Word root: bronch
From: Greek *bronchos*
Meaning: bronchi

~itis	inflammation of	BRONCHITIS	inflammation of the bronchi
~scope	instrument for examining	BRONCHOSCOPE	instrument used for internal examination of bronchi

The digestive system

Word root: oesophag
From: Greek *oisophagos*
Meaning: oesophagus

~itis	inflammation of	OESOPHAGITIS	inflammation of the oesophagus
~otomy	surgical incision into	OESOPHAGOTOMY	surgical incision into oesophagus

Word root: gastr
From: Greek *gaster*
Meaning: stomach

~itis	inflammation of	GASTRITIS	inflammation of the stomach
~pathy	disease of	GASTROPATHY	disease of stomach
~scope	instrument for examining	GASTROSCOPE	instrument used for internal examination of the stomach
~ectasia	dilation of	GASTRECTASIA	dilation of stomach
~ostomy	surgical creation of opening into part of body	GASTROSTOMY	surgical creation of an opening into the stomach
~pexy	surgical fixation of	GASTROPEXY	surgical fixation of the stomach

Word root: enter
From: Greek *enteron*
Meaning: intestine

~itis	inflammation of	ENTERITIS	inflammation of the intestine
~tomy	surgical incision into	ENTEROTOMY	surgical incision into intestine
~ectomy	removal of	ENTERECTOMY	removal of part of intestine
gastr~/ ~itis	pertaining to the stomach/ inflammation of	GASTROENTERITIS	inflammation of the stomach and intestine
gastr~/ ~logy	pertaining to the stomach/ study of	GASTROENTEROLOGY	study of the stomach and intestines
gastr~/ ~pathy	pertaining to the stomach/ disease of	GASTROENTEROPATHY	disease of the stomach and intestine

Word root: hepat
From: Greek *hepar*
Meaning: liver

~itis	inflammation of	HEPATITIS	inflammation of the liver
~cyte	cell	HEPATOCYTE	liver cell

Word root: pancrea
From: Greek *pankreas* ('all flesh')
Meaning: pancreas

~itis	inflammation of	PANCREATITIS	inflammation of the pancreas

Word root: lapar
From: Greek *lapara*
Meaning: flank

~otomy	surgical incision into	LAPAROTOMY	surgical incision into the abdomen
~scope	instrument for examining	LAPAROSCOPE	instrument used for internal examination of the abdomen

Word root: periton
From: Greek *peritonaion* ('stretched around')
Meaning: peritoneum

~itis	inflammation of	PERITONITIS	inflammation of the peritoneum

The urinary system

Word root: nephr
From: Greek *nephros*
Meaning: kidney

~itis	inflammation of	NEPHRITIS	inflammation of the kidney
~logy	study of	NEPHROLOGY	study of the kidney
~ectomy	removal of	NEPHRECTOMY	removal of the kidney
~lithiasis	formation of calculus (urolith, stone)	NEPHROLITHIASIS	formation of a calculus in the kidney

The reproductive system

Word root: ovar
From: **Latin *ovum* ('egg')**
Meaning: **ovary**

~iectomy	surgical removal of	OVARIECTOMY	surgical removal of ovary
~itis	inflammation of	OVARITIS	inflammation of the ovary
~ian	relating to	OVARIAN	relating to the ovary

Word root: oo
From: **Greek *oion***
Meaning: **egg**

| ~genesis | development of | OOGENESIS | development process of eggs in ovary |
| ~cyte | cell | OOCYTE | egg cell |

Word root: uter
From: **Latin *uterus***
Meaning: **womb**

| intra~ | within | INTRAUTERINE | within the uterus |

Word root: hyster
From: **Greek *hystera***
Meaning: **uterus**

~ectomy	surgical removal of	HYSTERECTOMY	surgical removal of the uterus
~otomy	surgical incision into	HYSTEROTOMY	surgical incision into the uterus
ovario~/	relating to the ovary/	OVARIOHYSTERECTOMY	surgical removal of ovaries and uterus
~ectomy	surgical removal of		

Word root: metr
From: **Greek *metra***
Meaning: **uterus**

py~	denoting pus	PYOMETRA	accumulation of pus in the uterus
~itis	inflammation of	METRITIS	inflammation of the uterus
endo~/	inner, within/	ENDOMETRITIS	inflammation of inner lining of the uterus
~itis	inflammation of		

Word root: oestrus
From: **Latin *oestrus*, Greek *oistros***
Meaning: **female sexual impulse**

		OESTRUS	stage of oestrous cycle when female is receptive to male ('on heat')
poly~	many	POLYOESTROUS	having several consecutive oestrous cycles per annum
mono~	one, single	MONOESTROUS	having a single oestrous cycle occurring two or three times per annum
an~	without	ANOESTRUS	absence of oestrus, reduced ovarian activity
pro~	before	PRO-OESTRUS	stage of oestrous cycle when development of ovarian follicles begins, prior to oestrus

Word root: **vagina**
From: **Latin** *vagina*
Meaning: **sheath**

per	through	PER VAGINA	through the vagina
~itis	inflammation of	VAGINITIS	inflammation of the vagina

Word root: **mamma**
From: **Latin** *mamma*
Meaning: **milk gland**

~graphy	description of	MAMMOGRAPHY	process of taking a recording of the mammary gland

Word root: **mastos**
From: **Greek** *mastos*
Meaning: **breast**

~itis	inflammation of	MASTITIS	inflammation of the mammary gland
~ectomy	surgical removal of	MASTECTOMY	surgical removal of a mammary gland

Word root: **natal**
From: **Latin** *natalis*
Meaning: **birth**

ante~	before	ANTENATAL	before birth
neo~	new, recent	NEONATAL	newborn

The skeletal system

Word root: **oste**
From: **Greek** *osteon*
Meaning: **bone**

peri~	around	PERIOSTEUM	layer of connective tissue covering bone
~malacia	softening of	OSTEOMALACIA	softening of bone
~cyte	cell	OSTEOCYTE	bone cell
~itis	inflammation of	OSTEITIS	inflammation of bone
~blast	formative cell	OSTEOBLAST	cell responsible for formation of bone
~lysis	breakdown of	OSTEOLYSIS	breakdown of bone
~oma	tumour of	OSTEOMA	benign bone tumour
~dys/ ~trophy	difficulty/ development	OSTEODYSTROPHY	abnormal bone development
~sarcoma	malignant tumour of connective tissue	OSTEOSARCOMA	malignant tumour of bone

Word root: **myel**
From: **Greek** *myelos*
Meaning: **marrow**

~malacia	softening	MYELOMALACIA	abnormal softening of bone marrow
osteo~/ ~itis	relating to bone/ inflammation of	OSTEOMYELITIS	inflammation of bone marrow

Word root: **chondr** From: **Greek *chondros*** Meaning: **cartilage**			
~cyte	cell	CHONDROCYTE	cartilage cell
~genesis	formation of	CHONDROGENESIS	formation of cartilage
~itis	inflammation of	CHONDRITIS	inflammation of cartilage
osteo~/ ~itis	relating to bone/ inflammation of	OSTEOCHONDRITIS (OCD)	inflammation of bone around a joint

Word root: **spondyl** From: **Greek *sp(h)ondylos*** Meaning: **vertebra**			
~itis	inflammation of	SPONDYLITIS	inflammation of the synovial joints in the vertebral column
~lysis	breakdown of	SPONDYLOSIS	degeneration of intervertebral discs

Word root: **arthr** From: **Greek *arthron*** Meaning: **joint**			
~itis	inflammation of	ARTHRITIS	inflammation of a joint
~desis	surgical fusion of bones	ARTHRODESIS	surgical fusion of bones across a joint space
~pathy	disease of	ARTHROPATHY	disease of a joint
~plasty	plastic surgery	ARTHROPLASTY	surgical construction of new joint; remodelling of diseased joint
~otomy	surgical incision into	ARTHROTOMY	surgical incision into a joint

The endocrine system

Word root: **thyroid** From: **Greek *thyreoeides*** Meaning: **shield-shaped**			
hyper~	excessive, abnormally high	HYPERTHYROID	with excessive amounts of thyroid hormone in the bloodstream
hypo~	abnormally low	HYPOTHYROID	with abnormally low amounts of thyroid hormone in the bloodstream
para~	adjacent to	PARATHYROID	next to thyroid glands
~ectomy	surgical removal of	THYROIDECTOMY	surgical removal of thyroid gland
~itis	inflammation of	THYROIDITIS	inflammation of the thyroid gland

Word root: **pituita** From: **Latin *pituita*** Meaning: **phlegm**			
hypo~	abnormally low	HYPOPITUITARISM	condition caused by subnormal activity of pituitary gland
hyper~	excessive, abnormally high	HYPERPITUITARISM	condition caused by overactive pituitary gland

The nervous system

Word root: **neur** From: **Greek *neuron*** Meaning: **nerve**			
		NEURON(E)	nerve cell
~algia	pain	NEURALGIA	nerve pain
~logy	study of	NEUROLOGY	study of nerves
~oma	tumour	NEUROMA	benign tumour of nerves
~osis	denoting a condition	NEUROSIS	functional disorder of nervous system
~itis	inflammation of	NEURITIS	inflammation of a nerve
~pathy	disease of	NEUROPATHY	disease of the nervous system

Word root: **cephal** From: **Greek *kephale*** Meaning: **head**			
hydro~	denoting water or watery fluid	HYDROCEPHALUS	abnormal increase in cerebrospinal fluid present in brain
brachy~	short	BRACHYCEPHALIC	with short wide skull or head (e.g. in Pekingese dogs)
dolicho~	long	DOLICHOCEPHALIC	with long narrow skull (e.g. Irish Wolfhound)
mesati~	middle	MESATICEPHALIC	with skull intermediate between brachy- and dolichocephalic (e.g. Beagle)
~itis	inflammation of	CEPHALITIS	inflammation of the brain

Word root: **encephal** From: **Greek *enkephalon* ('in the head')** Meaning: **brain**			
~itis	inflammation of	ENCEPHALITIS	inflammation of the brain
~malacia	softening of	ENCEPHALOMALACIA	degeneration or softening of the brain
~oma	tumour	ENCEPHALOMA	benign brain tumour

Word root: **mening** From: **Greek *meninx*** Meaning: **membrane**			
~oma	tumour	MENINGIOMA	benign tumour of the meninges
~encephal/ ~itis	pertaining to/ inflammation of	MENINGOENCEPHALITIS	inflammation of the meninges and brain

Word root: **plegia** From: **Greek *plege* ('a blow')** Meaning: **paralysis**			
para~	beside, near	PARAPLEGIA	paralysis of both hindlimbs
tetra~	four	TETRAPLEGIA	paralysis of all four limbs
hemi~	half	HEMIPLEGIA	paralysis of one side of the body (left or right)

The ear

Word root: **aur** From: **Latin** *auris* Meaning: **ear**			
~al	relating to	AURAL	relating to the ear
~icle	diminutive	AURICLE	visible part of external ear
~scope	instrument for examining	AURISCOPE	instrument used for internal examination of ear

Word root: **oto** From: **Greek** *ous* Meaning: **ear**			
~scope	instrument for examining	OTOSCOPE	instrument used for internal examination of ear
~itis	inflammation of	OTITIS	inflammation of the ear

The eye

Word root: **ophthalm** From: **Greek** *ophthalmos* Meaning: **eye**			
~logy	study of	OPHTHALMOLOGY	study of the eye
~scope	instrument for examining	OPHTHALMOSCOPE	instrument used for internal examination of eye

Word root: **ocul** From: **Latin** *oculus* Meaning: **eye**			
~ar	relating to	OCULAR	relating to the eye
~motor	movement	OCULOMOTOR NERVE	nerve concerned with movement of eye muscles

Word root: **blephar** From: **Greek** *blepharon* Meaning: **eyelid**			
~itis	inflammation of	BLEPHARITIS	inflammation of the eyelid
~spasm	involuntary movement	BLEPHAROSPASM	involuntary spasm or twitching of the eye muscle around the eyelid

Word root: **conjunctiv** From: **Latin** *conjunctum* ('joined') Meaning: **conjunctiva**			
~itis	inflammation of	CONJUCTIVITIS	inflammation of the conjuctiva

The mouth

Word root: **gloss** From: **Greek *glossa*** Meaning: **tongue**			
~itis	inflammation of	GLOSSITIS	inflammation of the tongue
~pharyngeal	of the pharynx	GLOSSOPHARYNGEAL	relating to the tongue and pharynx

Word root: **gingiv** From: **Latin *gingiva*** Meaning: **gum**			
~itis	inflammation of	GINGIVITIS	inflammation of the gums

The skin

Word root: **derm** From: **Greek *derma*** Meaning: **skin**			
epi~	above	EPIDERMIS	outer layer of skin
~itis	inflammation of	DERMATITIS	inflammation of the skin
~logy	study of	DERMATOLOGY	study of the skin
~mycosis	fungal infection of	DERMATOMYCOSIS	fungal infection of the skin

Word root: **kerat** From: **Greek *keras*** Meaning: **horn**			
hyper~	excessive	HYPERKERATOSIS	overproduction of the horny layer of the skin

Word root: **seb** From: **Latin *sebum* ('suet')** Meaning: **sebum**			
		SEBACEOUS	containing or secreting fatty or oily matter
~rrhoea	excessive flow	SEBORRHOEA	excessive secretion of sebum

Tumours

A tumour is any abnormal swelling on or in the body.
Tumours are classed as malignant or benign.

Definitions

malignant tumour	A tumour that invades and destroys tissue in which it originates and then spreads to other sites in the body	**metastasis**	The spread of malignant tissue to other areas of the body
benign tumour	A tumour that does not destroy tissue or produce harmful effects	**prognosis**	An assessment of the outcome of a disease

Classification of tumours

adenocarcinoma	Malignant tumour of glandular tissue	malignant melanoma	Malignant skin tumour of melanocytes
adenoma	Benign tumour of glandular tissue	melanoma	Benign skin tumour of melanocytes
carcinoma	Malignant tumour of epithelial tissues	osteosarcoma	Malignant tumour of osteoblasts
fibroma	Benign tumour of fibrous tissue	papilloma	Benign tumour of epithelial cells, often wart-like in appearance
fibrosarcoma	Malignant tumour of fibrous tissue	sarcoma	Malignant tumour arising from connective tissue
lipoma	Benign tumour of adipose cells	squamous cell carcinoma	Malignant tumour of squamous epithelium commonly affecting skin, mouth and conjunctiva
lymphosarcoma	Malignant tumour of lymphatic tissue		

Abbreviations

a.c.	Before food
ACD	Acid citrate dextrose (an anticoagulant)
ad lib	*Ad libitum* — freely as wanted
b.d.s.	To be taken twice daily
bid	Twice daily
BIOP	Been in owner's possession
BSAVA	British Small Animal Veterinary Association
BVA	British Veterinary Association
BVNA	British Veterinary Nursing Association
CD	Controlled drugs
CNS	Central nervous system
COSHH	Control of Substances Hazardous to Health
CPD	Continual professional development
CPDA	Citrate phosphate dextrose adenine (an anticoagulant)
CPR	Cardiopulmonary resuscitation
CURTD	Canine upper respiratory tract disease
CVP	Central venous pressure
EDTA	Ethylenediamine tetraacetic acid (an anticoagulant)
e.o.d.	Every other day
FeLV	Feline leukaemia virus
FIA	Feline infectious anaemia
FIP	Feline infectious peritonitis
FIV	Feline immunodeficiency virus
FLUTD	Feline lower urinary tract disease
FURTD	Feline upper respiratory tract disease
g	Gram
GDV	Gastric dilation and volvulus
GI	Gastrointestinal
GSL	General sale list (medicines)
h	Hour
Hb	Haemoglobin
HSE	Health and Safety Executive
IC, i.c., i/c	Intracardiac
ICU	Intensive care unit
IM, i.m., i/m	Intramuscular
IP, i.p., i/p	Intraperitoneal
IPPV	Intermittent positive pressure ventilation
IU	International units
IV, i.v., i/v	Intravenous
KC	Kennel Club

kg	Kilogram
kV	Kilovolt
mA	Milliampere
mAs	Milliampere second
mcg	Microgram
MCV	Mean cell volume
m.d.u.	Use as directed
mg	Milligram
ml	Millilitre
mm	Millimetre
mm	Mucous membrane
NAD	No abnormalities detected
NPO	Nil per os (nil by mouth)
NSAID	Non-steroidal anti-inflammatory drug
NYD	Not yet diagnosed
o.d.	Every other day
P	Pharmacy only (medicines)
p.c.	After food
PCV	Packed cell volume
pd	Polydipsic
PML	Pharmacy merchant's list (medicines)
POM	Prescription-only medicine
pu	Polyuric
q.d.s.	To be taken four times daily
q.4 h.	Every 4 hours
qid	Four times a day
rbc	Red blood cell
RCVS	Royal College of Veterinary Surgeons
RPA	Radiation protection adviser
RPS	Radiation protection supervisor
RTA	Road traffic accident
SC, s.c., s/c	Subcutaneous
sid	Once a day
sol.	Solution
t.d.s.	To be taken three times daily
tid	Three times a day
TPR	Temperature, pulse and respiration
uid	Once daily
v	Volume
wbc	White blood cell
w/v	Weight/volume (percentage of weight of drug per volume of solution)

Terms of description, position and direction

abduct	Move a part of the body away from the midline	lateral	Relating to a part of the body furthest from the midline
acquired	Condition that develops due to external factors	medial	Relating to parts of the body nearest the median plane
acute	Condition of sudden onset	median	Situated in the plane that divides the body into a left and right half
adduct	Move a part of the body towards the midline	oral	Relating to the mouth
anterior	Relating to the front part of a limb or organ (not in common use)	palmar	Relating to the back of the front foot
axis	Imaginary line through a part of the body about which the part moves	plantar	Relating to the back of the hind foot
		posterior	Situated at the rear of the body or organ
bilateral	Relating to both sides of the body	primary	Condition that happens first, or that arises from changes within the body part affected and not elsewhere
caudal	Relating to the tail end of the body		
chronic	Condition present for some time and with a slow onset	proximal	Situated close to the midline of the body
congenital	Present at birth	rostral	Relating to the nose or front end of the head
cranial	Relating to the head or front end of the body	sternal	Relating to the sternum (the bone lying in the ventral midline of the thorax)
distal	Situated away from the midline of the body		
dorsal	Relating to, being near, or on the back	superficial	On or near the surface
		unilateral	Affecting one side only
inherited	Condition that arises from the genetic makeup of the individual	ventral	Relating to the undersurface of the body

Further reading

Lane D and Cooper B (1999) *Veterinary Nursing*, 2nd edn. Butterworth-Heinemann, Oxford

The Concise English Dictionary (1986) Omega Books, Ware

Index